Connective Tissue Diseases of the Skin

CLINICAL DERMATOLOGY

Series Editor

ALAN R. SHALITA, M.D.

Professor and Chairman
Department of Dermatology
State University of New York
Health Science Center at Brooklyn
Brooklyn, New York

1. Cutaneous Investigation in Health and Disease: Noninvasive Methods and Instrumentation, *edited by Jean-Luc Lévêque*
2. Irritant Contact Dermatitis, *edited by Edward M. Jackson and Ronald Goldner*
3. Fundamentals of Dermatology: A Study Guide, *Franklin S. Glickman and Alan R. Shalita*
4. Aging Skin: Properties and Functional Changes, *edited by Jean-Luc Lévêque and Pierre G. Agache*
5. Retinoids: Progress in Research and Clinical Applications, *edited by Maria A. Livrea and Lester Packer*
6. Clinical Photomedicine, *edited by Henry W. Lim and Nicholas A. Soter*
7. Cutaneous Antifungal Agents: Selected Compounds in Clinical Practice and Development, *edited by John W. Rippon and Robert A. Fromtling*
8. Oxidative Stress in Dermatology, *edited by Jürgen Fuchs and Lester Packer*
9. Connective Tissue Diseases of the Skin, *edited by Charles M. Lapière and Thomas Krieg*
10. Epidermal Growth Factors and Cytokines, *edited by Thomas A. Luger and Thomas Schwartz*

ADDITIONAL VOLUMES IN PREPARATION

Connective Tissue Diseases of the Skin

edited by

Charles M. Lapière

University of Liège
Sart Tilman, Belgium

Thomas Krieg

University of Cologne
Cologne, Germany

Marcel Dekker, Inc. New York • Basel • Hong Kong

Library of Congress Cataloging-in-Publication Data

Connective tissue diseases in the skin / edited by Charles M. Lapière,
Thomas Krieg.
p. cm.—(Clinical dermatology ; 9)
Includes bibliographical references and index.
ISBN 0-8247-9133-9 (alk. paper)
1. Skin—Pathophysiology. 2. Connective tissues—Diseases.
I. Lapière, Charles M. II. Krieg, T. III. Series.
[DNLM: 1. Connective Tissue Diseases. 2. Skin Diseases. 3. Skin—physiopathology. 4. Skin—anatomy & histology. W1 CL69L v.9 1993
/ WR 100 C752 1993]
RL96.C65 1993
616.7′7—dc20
DNLM/DLC
for Library of Congress 93-4532
CIP

The publisher offers discounts on this book when ordered in bulk quantities. For more information, write to Special Sales/Professional Marketing at the address below.

This book is printed on acid-free paper.

Marcel Dekker, Inc.
270 Madison Avenue, New York, New York 10016

Current printing (last digit):
10 9 8 7 6 5 4 3 2 1

PRINTED IN THE UNITED STATES OF AMERICA

Foreword

Although connective tissues comprise the predominant constituents in skin, it is only in the past 10 to 15 years that considerable knowledge about the morphology, biochemistry, molecular biology, and function of its various components has been elucidated. Much of this knowledge derives from the painstaking isolation of various collagen types, elastic fibers, and proteoglycans through biochemical and immunological techniques, their visualization by rotary shadowing electron-microscopic techniques and, most recently, through identification, cloning, and sequencing the many genes that code for these molecules. Much has also been learned about the posttranstational events that alter the collagen gene products. Through these types of studies the molecular basis for several connective tissue diseases, such as Ehlers-Danlos disease, Marfan's syndrome, and osteogenesis imperfecta, has been elucidated.

Many of these same leaps of knowledge have also recently been attained regarding the skin basement membrane zone. Although its major structural components were identified about 20 years ago, its chemical constituents have been biochemically and molecularly identified only in the past ten years. Here again, this knowledge has impacted in the clinic in helping to elucidate the molecular basis for various forms of inherited as well as acquired blistering diseases.

The pathophysiology of some major diseases of connective tissue, most notably scleroderma, awaits elucidation. Utilizing molecular biological and immunological techniques, an understanding of this disease as well as the critical events in wound healing and the entire concept of aging of skin will hopefully be forthcoming in the near future.

Charles M. Lapière and Thomas Krieg have contributed significantly to our understanding about skin connective tissue. It is because of their knowledge of and respect within this field that they have been able to assemble contributors who bring up-to-date information as well as a glimpse into the future.

Stephen I. Katz, M.D., Ph.D.
National Cancer Institute,
Bethesda, Maryland

Connective tissue has a complex structure and is composed of a large number of different constituents, such as collagens, elastic fibers, the basement membrane, and the interfibrillary ground substance. Many diseases, inherited or acquired, are known to be due to disturbances in the structure or biosynthesis of these connective tissue components.

I still remember very clearly when collagen fibers were considered to be nothing more than crystalloid structures without any metabolic activity. However, our view of these aspects has changed dramatically in the last few decades. Our knowledge of the different constituents of the dermal connective tissue and its physiological control mechanisms has grown enormously. Progress in this field has been strongly influenced by advances in laboratory techniques in the basic sciences (e.g., biochemistry, immunology, gene technology, and electron microscopy).

Among those who deserve great merit in promoting this field of dermatology through excellent scientific work, Charles M. Lapière and Thomas Krieg have to be mentioned both as researchers and clinicians. Their attempts in integrating our fast-growing knowledge regarding the biology of connective tissue and the fundamental pathological processes underlying diseases of the skin have been very successful. Personally, I am glad to have been able to work with Thomas Krieg for a long time in my department at the University of Munich and that we could host Charles Lapière as a guest professor several times. This friendly scientific interaction was possible due to a generous grant by the Alexander von Humboldt Foundation and turned out to be very stimulating and fruitful.

The editors have been successful in realizing a book that provides information not only on biology and pathophysiology of connective tissue, but also on diseases—including clinical morphology, pathogenesis and new therapeutic concepts. It is fascinating to see how much progress has been reached in the last years toward a better understanding of the biology and pathology of the extracellular matrix.

FOREWORD

This book represents an important step in the development of this field of dermatology. Many expert contributors of worldwide reputation have written excellent chapters. This book will be of great value to all physicians and scientists interested in physiology and pathophysiology of connective tissue of the skin. It may also stimulate interdisciplinary cooperation between different fields of medicine and basic research. Congratulations to the editors.

O. Braun-Falco, M.D.
University of Munich
Munich, Germany

Preface

The goal of this book is to introduce biochemistry, biology, and pathology of the extracellular matrix to all those who do not have close contact with this exciting and rapidly developing field. For a long time, the extracellular matrix in skin has been overlooked by many scientists and dermatologists. This is due to the fact that diseases involving the extracellular matrix were thought to be less common than others and that the different functions of the extracellular matrix were not understood. This changed after it became clear that the extracellular matrix has many unexpected biological functions and plays a key role in a large variety of diseases ranging from inborn disorders and the invasive growth and metastasis of tumors to the development of fibrosis.

This book was written by dermatologists for dermatologists and scientists interested in the skin. It should be used as a guide for solving clinical problems and as a tool to enter the field of clinical and more basic research. Most of the topics in this book are covered by investigators who have contributed greatly to the advances in their respective fields. Each chapter focuses on a defined topic and many include the authors' own views of forthcoming developments. The accompanying lists of references are purposely selective rather than complete and contain key review articles.

Some of the editorial work for this book was done in Munich during a sabbatical period when Charles M. Lapière was awarded a Research Prize from the Alexander von Humboldt Foundation.

We also would like to thank the authors for their participation and to acknowledge the help of H. Cuaz and the team of Marcel Dekker, Inc., for the editing of this work.

Charles M. Lapière
Thomas Krieg

Contents

Contributors

Adriana Albini, Ph.D. Instituto Nazionale per la Ricerca sul Cancro, Genoa, Italy

Eugene A. Bauer, M.D. Department of Dermatology, Stanford University School of Medicine, Stanford, California

Marie-Luce Bochaton-Piallat, Ph.D. Department of Pathology, University of Geneva, Geneva, Switzerland

Hans-Joachim Böhme, M.D. Institute of Biochemistry, University of Leipzig, Leipzig, Germany

Monika Borchert, Ph.D. Department of Dermatology, University of Munich, Munich, Germany

Leena Bruckner-Tuderman, M.D., Ph.D. Department of Dermatology, University Hospital Zürich, Zürich, Switzerland

Bernard Coulomb, Ph.D. Laboratory of Dermatology, INSERM 312, Hôpital Henri Mondor, Créteil, France

Frank DeLustro, Ph.D. Department of Scientific Affairs, Collagen Corporation, Palo Alto, California

Louis Dubertret, M.D. Department of Dermatology, Hôpital St. Louis, Paris, France

Christopher Edwards, Ph.D. Department of Dermatology, University of Wales College of Medicine, Cardiff, Wales

Michael Fazio, M.D. Department of Dermatology, Jefferson Institute of Molecular Medicine, Thomas Jefferson University, Philadelphia, Pennsylvania

Raul Fleischmajer, M.D. Department of Dermatology, Mount Sinai School of Medicine, New York, New York

Giulio Gabbiani, M.D., Ph.D. Department of Pathology, University of Geneva, Geneva, Switzerland

Rosalind A. Grymes, Ph.D.* Department of Dermatology, Stanford University School of Medicine, Stanford, California

Konrad Herrmann, M.D. Department of Dermatology, University of Leipzig, Leipzig, Germany

Stefania Jablonska, M.D. Department of Dermatology, Warsaw School of Medicine, Warsaw, Poland

Veli-Matti Kähäri, M.D., Ph.D. Department of Dermatology, Jefferson Institute of Molecular Medicine, Thomas Jefferson University, Philadelphia, Pennsylvania

Hynda K. Kleinman, Ph.D. Laboratory of Developmental Biology, National Institute of Dental Research, National Institutes of Health, Bethesda, Maryland

Thomas Krieg, M.D. Department of Dermatology, University of Cologne, Cologne, Germany

Annemarie Kronberger, Ph.D. Department of Dermatology, Stanford University School of Medicine, Stanford, California

Charles M. Lapière, M.D., Ph.D. Department of Dermatology, Centre Hospitalier Universitaire de Liège, University of Liège, Sart Tilman, Belgium

Ronald Marks, MBBS, FRCP, FRCPath Department of Dermatology, University of Wales College of Medicine, Cardiff, Wales

Cornelia Mauch, Ph.D. Department of Dermatology, University of Cologne, Cologne, Germany

Antonella Melchiori, Ph.D. Instituto Nazionale per la Ricerca sul Cancro, Genoa, Italy

Betty V. Nusgens, Ph.D. Department of Dermatology, Centre Hospitalier Universitaire de Liège, University of Liège, Sart Tilman, Belgium

Aarne Oikarinen, M.D., Ph.D. Department of Dermatology, University of Oulu, Oulu, Finland

Edward J. O'Keefe, M.D. Department of Dermatology, University of North Carolina, Chapel Hill, North Carolina

Silvio Parodi, M.D. Istituto Nazionale per la Ricerca sul Cancro, Genoa, Italy

F. Michael Pope, M.D., FRCP Dermatology Research Group, M.R.C. Clinical Research Centre, Harrow, England

Yves Sarret, M.D. Department of Dermatology, Hôpital Edouard-Herriot, Lyon, France

Hiroshi Shinkai, M.D., Ph.D. Department of Dermatology, Oita Medical University, Oita, Japan

**Present affiliation*: Life Sciences Division, NASA-Ames Research Center, Moffett Field, California

Samuel J. Stegman, M.D.† Department of Dermatology, University of California, San Francisco, California
Jouni Uitto, M.D., Ph.D. Department of Dermatology, Jefferson Institute of Molecular Medicine, Thomas Jefferson University, Philadelphia, Pennsylvania
Fenella Wojnarowska, M.D. Department of Dermatology, The Churchill Hospital, Oxford, England
David T. Woodley, M.D. Department of Dermatology, Northwestern University, Chicago, Illinois

† Deceased

1

Collagens: Their Structure and Metabolism

Cornelia Mauch and Thomas Krieg
University of Cologne, Cologne, Germany

Collagen is not a single entity but represents a family of genetically different proteins. [1]. Common to all is their unique triple helical structure, which requires the presence of glycine at every third position of the amino acid sequence and a high amount of proline and hydroxyproline. All collagens are built up by three α-chains, which form the triple helix. In some, however, this structure can be interrupted by globular domains or these domains of different size are located at the ends of the molecule. Following protein synthesis, individual collagen chains are posttranslationally modified. After secretion into the extracellular space, the molecules aggregate to a macromolecular structure.

All together at least 14 different collagen types have been identified and characterized. They differ in the amino acid sequence of the α-chains, in their tissue distribution, and also in their biological functions (Table 1.1). According to their structure and distribution, they can be classified into three groups: the fiber-forming collagens I, II, III, and V; the large nonfibrillar collagens, which include the basement membrane collagen IV as well as types VI and VIII; and the minor collagens, including types VII, XIII, and XIV and the cartilage collagens IX, X, XI, and XII.

Table 1.1 The Collagen Family

Type	Chains	Localization
I	α_1(I), α_2(I)	Skin, tendon, bone
II	α_1(II)	Cartilage
III	α_1(III)	Skin, internal organs, vessels
IV	α_1(IV), α_2(IV)	Basement membranes
V	α_1(V), α_2(V), α_3(V)	Skin, muscle, tendon, vessels, cornea
VI	α_1(VI), α_2(VI), α_3(VI)	Microfibrils, skin, cartilage
VII	α_1(VII)	Anchoring fibrils
VIII	α_1(VIII)	Endothelial cells
IX	α_1(IX), α_2(IX), α_3(IX)	Hyaline cartilage, type II associated
X	α_1(X)	Hypertrophic cartilage
XI	α_1(XI), α_2(XI), α_3(XI)	Hyaline cartilage, type II associated
XII	α_1(XII)	Tendons, skin, periosteum, ligaments perichondrium
XIII	α_1(XIII)	Fetal tissue, endothelial cells, type I associated
XIV	α_1(XIV)	Fetal skin, tendon, type I associated

STRUCTURE OF THE FIBER-FORMING COLLAGENS I, II, III, V, AND XI

The interstitial collagen types I, II, and III are most abundant in different connective tissues and have been studied in detail. Their gene and protein structures as well as their macromolecular organization are well known.

GENES OF THE INTERSTITIAL COLLAGENS

Collagen genes have been found to be unusually large and to vary from 35,000 base pairs (bp) to 18,000 bp. Their structure is highly complex, containing many exons and large introns. The coding sequence accounts only for 20–30% of the genes. Analysis of the aminoterminal sequences revealed the presence of several repeating units; the most important one is the 234 residue D unit, which is essential for the self-assembly of the molecules into higher molecular structures. Also the procollagen peptides show a good correlation between the structural elements on the protein level and the gene structures [1].

STRUCTURE OF INTERSTITIAL COLLAGENS

The interstitial collagens are all built up of three α-chains that are triple-helical. They have a length of 300 Å and a diameter of 14 Å. Type I collagen α-chains contain 1014 amino acids for the α_1 (I) chain, whereas the α_1 (III) chain accounts for 1023 residues. At both ends the molecules have short, nonhelical sequences that contain a hydroxylysine residue involved in cross-linking and also provide the molecule with a certain flexibility. In addition the cleavage site for the propeptidase is found in this domain [1–3].

The interstitial collagens are synthesized as a precursor form called procollagen, which contains at both ends large peptides attached to the flexible nonhelical terminal region of the molecules. These peptides have several functions: they prevent macromolecular organization intracellularly, control fibril formation in the extracellular space, and play a role in chain selection and triple helix formation. In addition, after cleavage they act as feedback inhibitors and can control collagen biosynthesis [4]. The structure of the N-terminal procollagen peptides of the α_1 (I) and the α_1 (III) chains is complex, bearing helical and nonhelical domains (Fig. 1.1). The triple-helical part contains 48 amino acid residues for the α_1 (I) and 39 for the α_1 (III) chain; the globular domain contains 66 and 68, respectively. In the α_2 (I) chain the globular part is missing, whereas type II collagen chains contain a globular domain and a triple-helical domain somewhat larger than the region of the α_1 (I) and α_1 (III) chains.

Most of the sequence information available for the carboxy-terminal procollagen peptides has been deduced from cDNA clones. The size of these peptides is very similar for all chains (246–247 amino acid residues). They contain eight cysteine residues; six form intrachain disulfide bonds whereas two build interchain bridges. These peptides were found to be biologically active and are thought to play an important role in controlling the formation of the triple helix. It has recently been established that the carboxyterminal peptides are involved

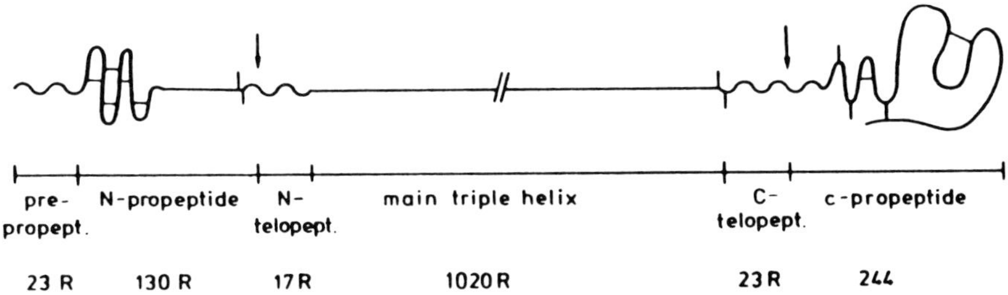

Figure 1.1 Schematic representation of the prepro α_1(III) chain of collagen. Because of the strong homology between all the fiber forming collagen types I, II, and III, α_1(III) is representative of all alpha-chains. It contains a large triple-helical part, bearing short non-triple-helical telopeptides at both ends. The N- and C-terminal propeptides are cleaved off during fibril formation and play a role in regulation of fibrillogenesis and collagen biosynthesis. R, amino acid residues.

in the physiological control of collagen synthesis as already demonstrated for the aminoterminal peptides.

The macromolecular assembly of the collagen molecules into fibrils is regulated by the amino acid sequences and the distribution of hydrophobic and polar charged residues. These amino acids are located in 4 regions of the molecule, which are each 234 residues long and designated as D 1,2,3, and 4 (Fig. 1.2). Therefore, the molecules aggregate in parallel, in a D-staggered way with an overlap region between the adjacent molecules; these overlapping terminal sequences are important for the cross-link formation, which occurs between the hydroxylysine residues 87 and 930 of the triple helix with the hydroxylysine aldehydes in the C-and N-terminal telopeptides. The molecules are then lightly bonded in the cross-link area. The close association of the molecules with an overlap in the fibrils is the molecular explanation for the cross-striation pattern observed on electron microscopic examination [3].

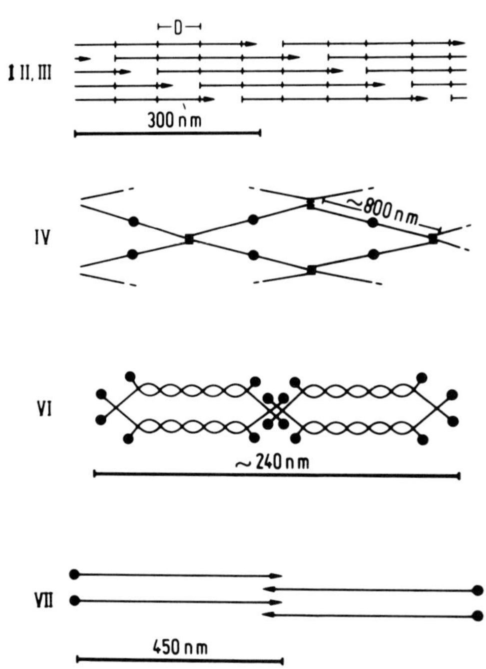

Figure 1.2 Macromolecular organization of fibrillar collagens I–III, the basement membrane collagen IV, microfibrils forming type VI collagen, and the type VII collagen-forming anchoring fibrils.

TISSUE DISTRIBUTION OF THE INTERSTITIAL COLLAGEN TYPES

Type I collagen is widely distributed through most connective tissues of an organism. It is the major collagen found in bone, tendon, ligaments, and skin, but it is also present in muscles, internal organs, and blood vessels [3]. Type I collagen is thought to guarantee the mechanical strength of the tissue. Although most of collagen I is composed of two identical α_1-and one α_2-chains, α_1 (I)$_3$ trimers exist, which have been isolated in small quantities from different tissues including dermis and were found to be synthesized also by several cell strains. With regard to posttranslational modifications of type I collagen molecules, differences have been observed between various organs. The physiological function of these differences is not yet known, but they could account to a certain extent for the difference in fibril formation observed in different tissues.

Type III collagen was first isolated from fetal tissues but is also present in most organs of adults. Type III is always found as homotrimers α_1 (III)$_3$. The three α-chains are covalently linked to each other by one disulfide bridge. Type III is extracted in high amounts from muscles, internal organs, and the vessel wall. It is also present in skin and accounts for 20–30%. Type III procollagen has also been found to be synthesized by several cells in culture. In contrast, no type III collagen has been found in bone, dentin, ligaments, and cartilage. Type III collagen is thought to form fibrils with a smaller diameter than type I fibrils. Recently it became evident that both collagen types can contribute to the same fibrils and it was assumed that the content of type III might regulate the size of the fibrils [5,6]. It has been concluded indirectly that type III collagen is responsible for the flexibility of the tissue since it is found in higher amounts in tissues that need a certain extensibility to fullfil their biological functions.

Type II is always found as a homotrimer α_1 (II)$_3$ and represents the predominant collagen type in the cartilage. It is highly hydroxylated, contains many hydroxylysine residues, which are glycosylated and galactosylated. It forms thin fibrils with a weak cross-striation pattern and aggregates with proteoglycans. Type II collagen is found in the elastic and fibrous cartilage, in the intervertebral disk, but also in the vitreous body of the eye [2,8].

Two other fibrillar collagen types were described and have been found to be associated with type I and type II collagen fibrils. Type V collagen contains several molecules with genetically different chains, which have not been studied in detail. Six chains are known, from which α_1 (V), α_2 (V), and α_3 (V) have been characterized. All different chains can assemble into the same or different molecules. Although homotrimers and different heterotrimers have been found, α_1 (V)$_2$ α_2 (V) seems to be the most common composition. Recent studies on in vitro fibrillogenesis of type I collagen indicated that type V also can interact with type I collagen and might be involved in controlling the diameter of type I collagen fibrils [6]. Type V collagen has been isolated from several tissues, including skin, and is found to be present in higher amounts in muscle and amniotic membranes. It is thought to be cell-associated; its detailed function, however, is not known. Type V may represent a component of the extracellular cytoskeleton or be integrated in the fine reticular network of connective tissue [9].

Type XI collagen is composed of three different chains. The α_1- and α_2-chains were found to be closely related to the α_1-and α_2-chains of type V collagen, whereas α_3 (XI) is an overglycosylated form of the α_1 (II) chain. Type XI collagen contributes 5–10% of the total collagen in chicken hyaline cartilage and it was speculated that it is involved in controlling the diameter of type II collagen fibrils. The cDNA sequence of α_1 (XI) and α_2 (XI) has recently been established and localized on the chromosomes 1 and 6 [10].

THE BASEMENT MEMBRANE COLLAGEN

Type IV collagen differs in its molecular and macromolecular structure from the other collagens. The molecule is 400 nm long and carries at its C-terminal end a noncollagenous globule, the NC1 domain. The triple-helical domain is interrupted by several nonhelical segments that allow a higher structural flexibility of type IV collagen [11].

Type IV collagen contains two different chains, two α_1-and one α_2-chain, which are both 1700 amino acids long. The primary structure has been established by protein and DNA sequencing for most of both chains. Besides the NC1 domain mentioned above, the molecule contains the 7S region, which represents the cross-linking area and the major triple helical part with several nonhelical interruptions. These interruptions are mainly located near the N-terminus and are strictly conserved between different species, which indicates that this region is involved in cross-linking, whereas the adjacent nonhelical area appears to be responsible for the flexibility of the molecule. The arrangement of these structures results in an overlap between 2 adjacent molecules of about 10 amino acid residues with disulfide bridges between the cysteine residues 12 and 98, which is then followed by a kink of 40 degrees. The NC1 domain is 229 residues long and contains a high proportion of cysteine and hydrophobic amino acids (Fig. 1.3).

The macromolecular organization of type IV collagen is still not completely understood and different models have been emphasized. Type IV collagen probably aggregates end-to-end: four molecules are then cross-linked via the 7S region, whereas two molecules join at the NC1 region. This results in formation of a network that fits into the lamina densa of the basement membrane (Fig. 1.2). Alternatively, dimers of type IV collagen associate side-by-side with a stagger

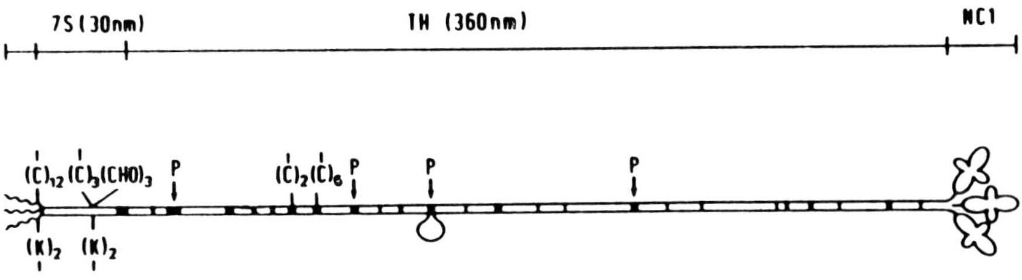

Figure 1.3 Schematic model of a collagen IV molecule. Black bars along the triple helix (TH) indicate imperfections in the Gly—Y repeat. Cross-linking can occur via cysteine (C) or lysine/hydroxylysine (K) residues. CHO, N-linked carbohydrate. P, pepsin-sensitive bonds. Reproduced from [25] with permission.

of 170 nm. When the carboxyl globular regions are associated with flexible regions of the molecules, vertices of a hexagonal lattice can be formed [10,11].

THE MINOR COLLAGENS

The intima collagen, type VI, was first isolated from aortic intima but then found in many other tissues, including the skin. Although type VI collagen is not fully characterized, it seems to represent a unique collagen that differs in principle from all other collagen types. The triple helix is considerably shorter and has a length of approximately 103 nm. The molecular weight of the molecule was determined to be 36 kDa; the individual α-chains account for 110–140 kDa. Smaller fragments (30–40 kDa) result from treatment with pepsin or collagenase. Of all collagens type VI contains by far the highest noncollagenous portion [12].

The formation of a macromolecular organization of type VI collagen molecules is highly complex. Dimers can be formed by an antiparallel and lateral aggregation of two molecules, which are staggered against each other by 30 nm. Tetramers are formed by a parallel aggregation of dimers with their ends in register. Further aggregation of tetramers to linear fibrillar strands occurs by an end-to-end alignment (Fig. 1.2).

Immunofluorescence and immune electron microscopic studies indicate that type VI collagen is widely distributed in connective tissue and is arranged in a microfibrillar structures. In skin and other connective tissues fibrous forms with a periodicity of 100 nm have often been observed. These cross-striated structures agree well with the model of type VI collagen; further proof has been obtained by immune electron microscopy, which showed that type VI collagen antibodies reacted with these structures.

Type VII collagen was first isolated from human placenta. It turned out to have the largest triple-helical length of all collagens. The triple-helical domain is 450 nm and contains three α-chains with a molecular weight (MW) of 170 kDa, which are connected by disulfide bonds [13,14]. Type VII collagen probably also has globular domains at both ends that seem to carry antigenic determinants. Recently type VII collagen was identified as the epidermolysis bullosa acquisita (EBA) antigen (for details see Chap. 4.)

Type VII collagen was then found to be restricted to the basement membrane zone of stratifying epithelia. The segment-long spacing crystallites of type VII collagen molecules exhibit a very similar pattern on electron microscopic studies to anchoring fibrils. In addition, antibodies against type VII collagen were found to bind to anchoring fibrils on immune electron microscopic examination. The molecules probably interact end-to-end with an antiparallel orientation and overlap by about 60 nm. This arrangement is then stabilized by intermolecular disulfide bonds. By further lateral aggregation, the molecules are connected to each other in a complex network anchoring the basement membrane in the anchoring plaques in the papillary dermis [13] (Fig. 1.2).

Type VIII collagen is synthesized by endothelial cells and contains globular and triple-helical domains. Three triple-helical regions each with a MW of 40 kDa are separated by small globular parts of about 10 kDa. Recent studies on the sequence of the cDNA indicate a strong homology with the α_1 (X) gene, which indicates that both collagen types belong to the same subclass within the collagen gene family [15].

Type X collagen was originally described as 1α-, 2α-, 3α-chain collagen, short chain, or G collagen. Type X collagen is synthesized in large quantities in chondrocytes from hypertrophic cartilage. It has a triple helix of 139 nm and a globular domain at one end. The helix is composed of 3 identical α-chains with a MW of 53 kDa. The macromolecular organization of type X is not known, but the molecules tend to aggregate with their globular domains. Type X might have important functions in the calcification of cartilage. The molecule is much shorter than the interstitial collagens; however, there are indications that it can interact with type II collagen fibrils and prevent their calcification [16].

Type XIII collagen is a new short-chain collagen and was detected from cDNA sequencing. The α_1 (XIII) gene has some features found in genes for fibrillar collagens but also features that are distinctly different. It consists of three identical α-chains and the deduced polypeptide has three collagenous domains and four noncollagenous domains. It is transcribed in several mRNAs probably generated by alternative splicing. Very little is known about the biological function of type XIII collagen; however, transcripts of this gene have been localized in fetal tissues in bone, cartilage, skin (epidermis and hair follicles), and striated muscle [17].

THE FACIT COLLAGENS IX, XII, AND XIV

The FACIT collagens include different nonfibrillar collagens found to be associated with the fibrillar collagens I and II. The structure of these molecules can be classified into three functional regions. One region contains the triple-helical domains interacting with the collagen fibrils. A second triple-helical domain projects out of the fibril and a third nontriple-helical region mediates the interaction with other matrix components or with cells. The triple-helical domains are separated by short nonhelical sequences. In addition to the similarities in their structures, they share a strong homology at the DNA level within different domains of the molecules. Therefore, the term fibril-associated collagens with interrupted triple helices (FACIT) has been proposed for this group [8,10].

Type IX was previously named HMW, LMW, M, J, or K collagen and has been isolated as pepsin fragments from cartilage. Based on biosynthetic labeling and cDNA sequencing it then became clear that these fragments belong to one molecule, which is composed of three genetically distinct α-chains. The intact type IX collagen molecule is composed of three triple-helical domains interspersed with four noncollagenous domains. It has recently been shown that the α_2(IX) chain contains chondroitin sulfate and dermatan sulfate residues, which are covalently bound. It is also now clear that type IX collagen is located at the surface of type II collagen fibrils. Both collagen types are oriented in the same direction and are covalently linked to each other (Fig 1.4). Type IX collagen also can bind other matrix proteins (e.g., proteoglycans via the N-terminal noncollagenous domain). These interactions play an important role in the organization of connective tissue in cartilage, where a close interaction of collagen and proteoglycans is required [8,18].

Type XII collagen has been discovered as a new collagen by cDNA cloning

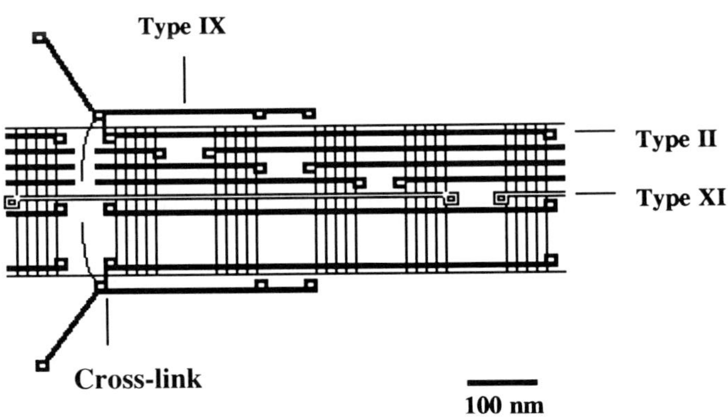

Figure 1.4 Model for the macromolecular organization of a thin collagen fibril in hyaline cartilage. The location of type XI collagen in the fibril is not known, and it may be either within the fibril, as shown, or on the surface of the fibril. The scale applies to the length of the molecules. Their diameters are exaggerated for clarity. The fibril is represented with the overlap region *shaded* and the gap region *clear* (from [8] and [18]).

from chick embryonic tendon mRNA. The deduced sequences displayed striking similarities to chick type IX collagen. Lateron type XII collagen was isolated from tendons and was localized by immunofluorescene studies in type I collagen-containing connective tissues such as tendons, ligaments, perichondrium, and periosteum. Type XII collagen is composed of three identical α-chains. Rotary shadowing and electron microscopy demonstrated that the molecule has the structure of a cross, consisting of a short triple-helical central part and three non-triple-helical arms. These large nonhelical domains are thought to interact with other matrix proteins or with cells. Similar to the interaction of type IX and II collagen, type XII was found to be localized on the surface of type I collagen fibrils. However, the chondroitin sulfate attachment site of a cross linking to the banded cartilage fibril does not exist in type XII collagen and therefore does not become cross-linked to type I fibrils. The biological function of this collagen is not yet understood; however, it may be involved in the interaction of cells with the fibrils [10, 19, 20].

Type XIV collagen was recently described as a novel collagen shown to be similar to but distinct from type XII collagen. Like type XI collagen, it is a homotrimeric molecule with the chain composition $\alpha_1(XIV)_3$ and represents a small percentage of the total collagen extractable from fetal skin or tendon [10, 21].

COLLAGENS IN SKIN

The macromolecular organization of the connective tissue in the dermis varies considerably (Fig. 1.5). The papillary layer, adjacent to the epidermal basement membrane, appears as a loose connective tissue network, containing thin collagen fibrils. In contrast, the reticular layer shows a dense connective tissue matrix with thick, regularly oriented bundles of fibrils. Below the reticular layer, in the subcutaneous fat tissue, the collagen molecules are found in fibrous trabeculae as well as in fine woven matrix surrounding the adipocytes. To a certain degree their varying macromolecular organization is reflected by a specific distribution of collagen types [3]. Human skin contains at least nine different collagen types. Type I accounts for about 80% and type III collagen for 15% which is found, however, to accumulate in the papillary dermis. Types V, VI, XII, and XIV are found in the dermis as minor collagens; type VII is restricted to the dermoepidermal basement membrane zone of blood vessels and epidermal cells. Type VIII is synthesized by endothelial cells in the vessels.

BIOSYNTHESIS OF COLLAGENS

After transcription, a complex splicing process converts pre-mRNA into mature mRNA, which is transported out of the nuclei and translated into the procollagen

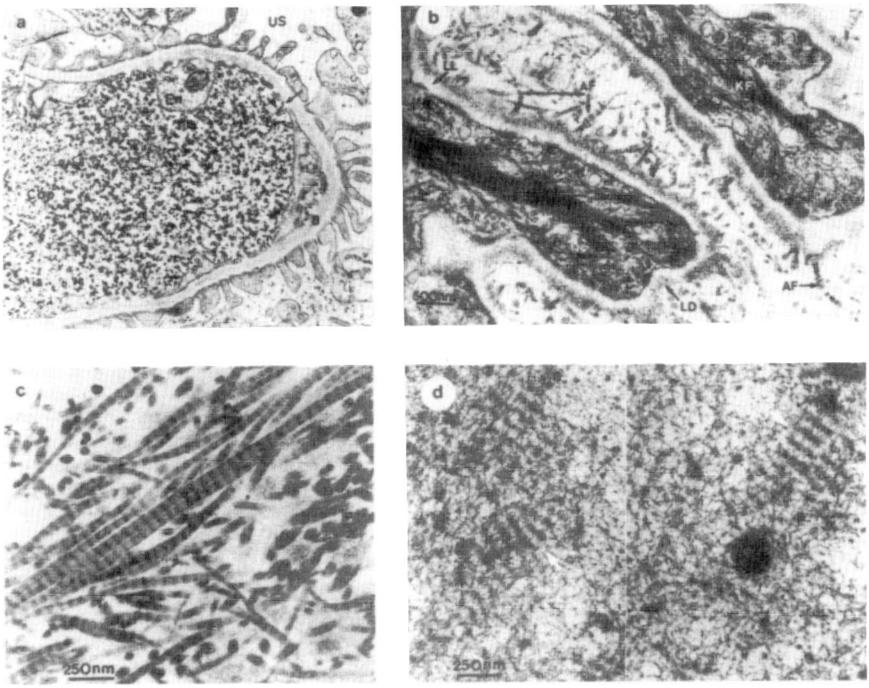

Figure 1.5 Electron microscopic appearance of the diversity of connective tissues. a. Basement membranes serve as barrier in the kidney. b. A basement membrane separating epidermis and dermis in the skin. LD, lamina densa; AF, anchoring fibrils. c. Interstitial collagen displays the characteristic cross-striation pattern. d. Type VI collagen microfibrils.

chains at the polysomes of the rough endoplasmic reticulum. During growth of the nascent polypeptide chains, several posttranslational modifications take place. These are enzymatically controlled and include the hydroxylation of proline residues, lysine residues, and also their glycosylation and galactosylation. All these processes are terminated by the triple helix formation. Then the molecules are secreted out of the cell. In the extracellular space further modifications take place before the molecules can aggregate into their characteristic macromolecular organization (Table 1.2) [4, 9, 22].

Hydroxylation of Proline and Lysine Residues

Hydroxylation of proline and lysine involves several enzymes, which are already well characterized. The prolyl-4-hydroxylase is a tetramere (240 kDa) composed of 4 subunits (64 and 60 kDa). Prolyl-3-hydroxylase has a MW of 160 kDa and

Table 1.2 Biosynthesis of Collagens

Intracellular steps	
	DNA
	|
	Pre-mRNA
	|
	mRNA
	|
	Alpha-chains
	|
	1. Hydroxylation of proline and lysine 2. Glycosylation of hydroxylysine
	|
	Chain selection and triple helix formation
	|
	Secretion of procollagen molecules
Extracellular steps	
	Cleavage of N- and C-terminal propeptides
	|
	Fibril formation by lateral and end-to-end aggregation
	|
	Oxidation of Lys- and Hyl-residues
	|
	Cross-linking
	|
	Stable fibrils

the lysylhydroxylase composed of 2 identical subunits has a MW of 190 kDa. Probably several isoenzymes exist, which are specific for different connective tissues.

The prolyl-4-hydroxylase is specific for hydroxylating peptide-linked prolyl residues located before a glycine residue; in contrast, the prolyl-3-hydroxylase is limited to those prolyl residues found in X-position when the Y-position is occupied by 4-hyp. The lysylhydroxylase has a similar specificity to prolyl-4-hydroxylase and recognizes X-Lys-Gly peptides. All three enzymes need molecular oxygen, α-ketoglutarate, and ascorbic acid as cofactors. α-Ketoglutarate is stoichimetrically decarboxylated and oxidized during hydroxylation.

Glycosylation of Hydroxylysine Residues

Several of the hydroxylysine residues are glycosylated and galactosylated. This reaction is catalyzed by two different enzymes. Galactose is transferred to hydroxylysine residues by hydroxylysyl-galactosyltransferase and then galactosylhydroxy-lysyl glucosyltransferase mediates glycosylation of some galactosylhydroxylysine residues. Not very much information is available concerning galactosyl transferase. Glucosyltransferase, however, is known to consist of one polypeptide chain with a MW of 70,000. The enzymes use the free ε-amino group of the hydroxylysine residue and UDP-glucosides as carbohydrate donors. Zn^{2+} is required as a cofactor but other metal ions can also be used. Activity of the transferase is terminated by formation of the triple helix.

Chain Selection, Helix Formation, and Secretion of Procollagen

C-Terminal procollagen peptides are thought to play an important role in chain selection and in initating helix formation, which then does not need any further enzymatic control. The molecular details of selecting the right α-chains, however, are not yet understood.

After protein synthesis and completion of the intracelllular posttranslational modifications, procollagen molecules are secreted out of the cell via the Golgi apparatus.

Cleavage of the Propeptides

In the extracellular space N- and C-terminal procollagen peptides have to be removed before fibril formation can take place. This process involves two specific enzymes, the procollagen N-proteinase and the procollagen C-proteinase, which are to a certain degree specific for the different collagens. The type III N-proteinase and the type I procollagen C-proteinase have already been purified and were found to have a molecular mass of 70 and 80 kDa, respectively. A procollagen N-proteinase has been isolated from chick embryo tendons and was characterized as a 500 kDa protein with a 90 kDa chain as the major active recognize polypeptide. All these enzymes are endopeptidases that require Ca^{2+} and recognize specifically a cleavage site located in the terminal nonhelical regions of the molecules. For the N-proteinases the triple helical conformation of the substrate is required.

For type I procollagen the N-terminal procollagen peptides are cleaved first. The N-terminal procollagen peptides for type III collagen can sometimes remain attached to the molecules in the tissue and are only slowly removed [4, 23]. It has been suggested that removal of N- and C-terminal propeptides has an important influence on the control of fibril formation.

Cross-Link Formation

After cleavage of the procollagen peptides, the collagen molecules arrange themselves into macromolecular structures. This process is exclusively regulated by the distribution of charged amino acid residues on the molecules. The aggregates then serve as substrate for enzymes introducing cross links to stabilize the collagen fibrils. The initial event during this process is the oxidative deamination of the ϵ-amino group in certain lysine and hydroxylysine residues to the corresponding aldehyde. These aldehydes then react with another lysine or hydroxylysine residue to form a Schiff's base, which then undergoes an Amadori rearrangement. In addition several other cross-link components have been isolated, which can originate from the aldehydes. The oxidative deamination is catalyzed by the lysyl oxidase, which contains copper and requires molecular oxygen. It can be present in different forms revealing a MW of 30–60 kDa.

COLLAGEN DEGRADATION

Degradation of collagen can occur intracellularly. This mechanism has been observed also for other proteins. However, its biological role is not yet understood.

Degradation of mature collagen fibrils in the extracellular space requires the mammalian collagenase, which cleaves the interstitial collagens at a defined position releasing two fragments of one and three-quarter lengths that are available to other proteases (see Chap. 6).

REGULATION OF COLLAGEN SYNTHESIS

The complex metabolism of collagen requires several control elements that can operate on different levels. Investigation of the transcriptional and translational control mechanisms became feasible due to the development of molecular biological techniques. Several collagen genes have been isolated and the promoter regions have been cloned. It is already well known that distinct sequences in the promoter are involved in the expression of type I collagen; also enhancer regions have been defined and several nuclear proteins that control gene expression were partially characterized. Determination of protein synthesis and mRNA levels in different cellular systems revealed a close correlation, indicating that the transcriptional control determines the quantity of collagen synthesized. There is, however, also evidence that in some systems other factors are operating at posttranscriptional levels. This has been shown for chondrocytes switching from synthesis of type II collagen to type I and also for tendon fibroblasts [4, 10, 24].

It has been mentioned above that during biosynthesis of the collagen molecule several posttranslational modifications occur, which influence the quantity and quality of the synthesized collagen. Of particular importance is the hydroxylation of proline residues by the prolylhydroxylase, since formation of hydroxyproline determines the stability of the helix. Unstable molecules can be rapidly degraded either directly in the cell or in the extracellular space. An essential cofactor is therefore ascorbate, which has a major effect on collagen synthesis. Fe^{2+} and Cu^{2+} serve as cofactors for prolylhydroxylase and lysylhydroxylase, respectively. A lack of Cu^{2+} results in reduced cross linking and a rapid turnover of collagen.

REFERENCES

1. Kühn K. The collagen family—variations in the molecular and supramolecular structure. In: Kühn K, and Krieg T, eds. Connective tissue: biological and clinical aspects. Rheumatology. An Annual Review 1986; 10: 29–69.
2. Kühn K. The classical collagens: types I, II and III. In: Mayne R, Burgeson RE, eds. Structure and function of collagen types. Orlando, FL: Academic Press, 1987: 1–42.
3. Miller EJ. Chemistry of the collagens and their distribution. In: Piez KA, Reddi AH, eds. Extracellular Matrix Biochemistry 1983; 41–81.
4. Nehrlich AG, Pöschl E, Voss T, Müller PK. Biosynthesis of collagen and its control. In: Kühn K, and Krieg, T, eds. Connective tissue: biological and clinical aspects. Rheumatology. An Annual Review 1986; 10: 70–90.
5. Fleischmajer R, Perlish JS, Faraggiana T. Rotary shadowing of collagen monomers, oligomers, and fibrils during tendon fibrillogensis. J Histochem Cytochem 1990; 39: 51–58.
6. Birk DE, Fitch JM, Babiarz JP, Doane KJ, Linsenmayer TF. Collagen fibrillogenesis in vitro: interaction of types I and V collagen regulates fibril diameter. J Cell Sci 1990; 95: 649–57.
7. Rest van der M, Mayne R. Type IX collagen. In: Mayne R, Burgeson RE, eds. Structure and function of collagen types. Orlando, FL: Academic Press, 1987: 195–221.
8. Mayne R. Cartilage collagens. Arthritis Rheum 1989; 32:241–6.
9. Burgeson RE, Morris NP. The collagen family of proteins. In: Uitto J, Perejda AJ, eds. Connective tissue disease. Molecular pathology of the extracellular matrix, vol 12. The biochemistry of disease. New York: Marcel Dekker, 1986: 3–28.
10. Vuorio E, de Crombrugghe. B Annu Rev Biochem 1990; 59: 837–72
11. Timpl R, Dziadek M. Structure, development and macromolecular pathology of basement membranes. Int Rev Exp Pathol 1985; 29: 1–34.
12. Timpl R, Engel J. Type VI collagen In: Mayne R, Burgeson, RE, eds. Structure and function of collagen types. Orlando, FL: Academic Press, 1987: 105–43.
13. Burgeson RE. Type VII collagen. In: Mayne R, Burgeson RE, eds., Structure and Function of collagen types. Orlando Fl:, Academic Press, 1987 105–44.
14. Sakai LY, Leen DR, Morris NP, Burgeson RE. Type VII collagen is a major structural component of anchoring fibrils. J Cell Biol 1986; 103: 1577–86.

15. Yamaguchi N, Mayne R, Ninomiya Y. The α1 (VIII) collagen gene is homologous to the α1(X) collagen gene and contains a large exon encoding the entire triple helical and carboxy-terminal non-triple helical domains of the α1 (VIII) polypeptide. J Biol Chem 1991; 266: 4508–13.
16. Schmid TM, Linsenmayer TF. Type X collagen. In: Mayne R, Burgeson RE, eds. Structure and function of collagen types. Orlando, FL: Academic Press, 1987.
17. Tikka L, Pihjajaniemi T, Henttu P, Prockop DJ, Tryggvason K. Gene structure for the α1 chain of a short-chain collagen (type XIII) with alternatively spliced transcripts and translation termination codon at the 5 end of the last exon. Biochemistry 1988; 85: 7491–5.
18. Rest van der M, Mayne R. Type IX collagen proteoglycan from cartilage is covalently cross-linked to type II collagen. J Biol Chem 1988; 263: 1615–8.
19. Gordon MK, Gerecke DR, Olsen BR. Type XII collagen: distinct extracellular matrix component discovered by cDNA cloning. Proc Natl Acad Sci USA 1987; 84: 6040–4.
20. Lunstrum GP, Morris NP, McDonough AM, Keen DR, Burgeson RE. Identification and partial characterization of two type XII-like collagen molecules. J Cell Biol 1991; 113: 963–9.
21. Dublet B, van der Rest M. Type XIV collagen, a new homotrimeric molecule extracted from fetal bovine skin and tendon, with a triple helical disulfide-bonded domain homologous to type IX and type XII collagens. J Biol Chem 1991; 266: 6853–8.
22. Kivirikko KI, Myllylä R. Biosynthesis of the collagens. in: Piez A, Reddi AH, eds. Extracellular matrix biochemistry 1983; 83–118.
23. Hojima Y, Mckenzie J, vau der Rest M, Prockop D. Type I procollagen N-proteinase from chick embryo tendons. J Biol Chem 1989; 264: 11336–45.
24. Wu Ch, Donovan CB, Wu GY. Evidence for pretranslational regulation of collagen synthesis by procollagen peptides. J Biol Chem 1986; 261: 10482–4.
25. Martin G. R., Timpe R., Kühn K. Basement membrane proteins: molecular structure and functions. Adv Prot Chem 1988; 39: 1–50.

2

Proteoglycans: Structure, Biosynthesis, and Degradation

Hiroshi Shinkai
Oita Medical University, Oita, Japan

The term *mucopolysaccharide* has been used to describe polysaccharides with a mucinous or viscous nature. The term *glycosaminoglycan* was introduced to differentiate the large polysaccharides containing repeating disaccharide units as their most characteristic feature from polysaccharide chains of other mammalian glycoconjugates. Most glycosaminoglycans are bound to protein and therefore known as proteoglycans. They are produced by various types of cells and represent macromolecules involved in the structure of the pericellular and extracellular matrix. Proteoglycans are specified by the nature of the polypeptide and the number and chemical form of the bound glycosaminoglycans [1]. The covalently bound sugar chain may be chondroitin sulfate, dermatan sulfate, keratan sulfate, heparan sulfate, or heparin. Several types of proteoglycans carry two or more different side chains. The most abundant glycosaminoglycan in skin is hyaluronic acid devoid of significant polypeptide core. Each proteoglycan has received a given name (Table 2.1).

The proteoglycans play multiple roles as structural components of the polymers, ensuring their architectural organization [2], acting as an integral component of the cell membrane involved in adhesion and control of the cellular phenotype [3], as anticoagulant, and as binding molecules for growth factors [4]. The main function of hyaluronic acid is related to its osmotic properties, which confer on the tissue turgidity and resistance to pressure.

Table 2.1 Proteoglycans Related to Skin

Name	GAG	Location	Function
Decorin	CS/DS	Fibroblasts, fibers	Adhesion, structure
Biglycan	CS/DS	Fibroblast, fibers	Adhesion, structure
Versican	CS	Fibroblast	Adhesion
Fibromodulin	KS	Fibroblast, fibers	Adhesion, structure
Fibroglycan	HS	Fibers	Adhesion
Syndecan	CS/HS	Fibroblast	Adhesion
Betaglycan	CS/HS	Fibroblast	Receptors TGF-b
Glypican	HS	Fibroblast	Membrane-bound
Basement membrane proteoglycan	HS	Basement membrane	Structure

These various proteoglycans are specified by a unique protein core and GAGs of defined composition. CS, chondroitin sulfate; DS, dermatan sulfate; KS, keratan sulfate; HS, heparan sulfate (see Fig. 2.1).

STRUCTURE AND COMPOSITION OF THE GLYCOSAMINOGLYCANS

Glycosaminoglycans are composed of uronic acid (D-glucuronic acid, L-iduronic acid, or both) and hexosamine (D-glucosamine or D-galactosamine). The hexosamine residues are commonly N-acetylated, although most of the anion groups in heparin and heparan sulfate are N-sulfated. Sulfate is also found as *o*-sulfate ester in all members of the group, except in hyaluronic acid, and generally located on carbon 4 or 6 of the hexosamine moiety and on carbon 2 of the iduronic acid moiety (Fig. 2.1). There are several distinct glycosaminoglycans in the connective tissues (Table 2.2). Glycosaminoglycans in the dermis are composed mainly of hyaluronic acid and dermatan sulfate, with smaller amounts of chondroitin 4-sulfate, chondroitin 6-sulfate, and heparan sulfate. Glycosaminoglycans represent 0.1–0.5% of whole dried skin. The relative proportion of these different glycosaminoglycans varies not only among species and ages but also among the different dermal layers.

Glycosaminoglycan degrading enzymes are most suitable for identification. Three types of chondroitinase that are eliminases and produce unsaturated disaccharides from chondroitin sulfate are recommended for the analysis of dermatan sulfate–chondroitin sulfate hybrid structure (Table 2.3).

The method for isolation of glycosaminoglycan (GAG) from tissue, in brief, consists of 1) beta-elimination in cold 0.5N NaOH for 24 hr; 2) adjusting the pH

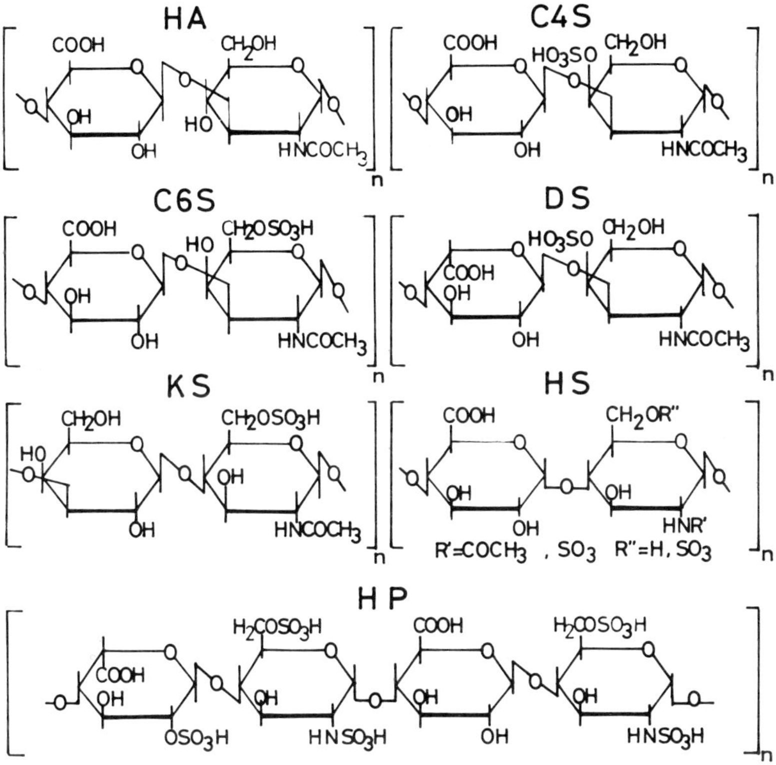

Figure 2.1 Repeating disaccharide units of glycosaminoglycans and typical oligosaccharide structure of heparin. HA, hyaluronic acid; C4S, chondroitin 4-sulfate; C6S, chondroitin 6-sulfate; DS, dermatan sulfate; KS, keratan sulfate; HS, heparan sulfate; HP, heparin.

to 7.0 with HCl, and heat denaturation of the protein in boiling water for 10 min; 3) digesting the protein in 0.05M Tris–HCl buffer pH 8.0 with pronase for 24 hr; 4) removing peptides by centrifugation in the presence of 10% trichloroacetic acid in the cold; 5) dialyzing the supernatant against water and lyophilizing. The products are identified as GAGs by the following methods: 1) carbazol reaction for uronic acid, Morgan-Elson reaction for N-acetylhexosamine, and determination of glucosamine and galactosamine using amino acid analyzer; 2) detection of each component on cellulose acetate membrane by electrophoresis before and after an enzyme digestion; 3) determination of the unsaturated disaccharide units on paper or thin-layer chromatography from the products by each glycosaminoglycan-degrading enzyme.

Table 2.2 Components of Glycosaminoglycans in Connective Tissues

	Major component sugars	Linkage	Location of sulfate	Distribution
Hyaluronic acid	GlcNAc	ß-1,4	—	Vitreous humor, skin
	GlcUA	ß-1,3		Synovial fluid, cartilage, umbilical cord
Chondroitin	GalNAc	ß-1,4	—	Cornea
	GlcUA	ß-1,3		
Chondroitin 4-sulfate	GalNAc	ß-1,4	4	Cartilage, cornea, bone
(chondroitin sulfate A)	GlcUA	ß-1,3		Ligamentum nuchae, aorta
Chondroitin 6-sulfate	GalNAc	ß-1,4	6	Cartilage, tendon, skin
(chondroitin sulfate C)	GlcUA	ß-1,3		Umbilical cord
Dermatan sulfate	GalNAc	ß-1,4	4	Skin, tendon, heart valve
(chondroitin sulfate B)	IdUA	α-1,3	2	Ligamentum nuchae, aorta
Heparan sulfate	GlcN	α-1,4	6	Aorta, lung, kidney
	GlcNAc	α-1,4		Basement membrane
	GlcUA	ß-1,4		Cell membrane
	IdUA	α-1,4	2	
Heparin	GlcN	α-1,4	3,6	Lung, liver
	GlcUA	ß-1,4		
	IdUA	α-1,4	2	
Keratan sulfate	GlcNAc	ß-1,3	6	Cornea, cartilage
	Gal	ß-1,4	6	

GENERAL STRUCTURE OF PROTEOGLYCANS

Sulfated glycosaminoglycan chains are linked to the core protein at their reducing terminal sugars and exist as proteoglycans in the connective tissues. Three types of carbohydrate–protein linkages have been recognized in the connective tissue proteoglycans: 1) an O-glycosidic linkage between D-xylose and the hydroxyl group of serine, 2) an O-glycosidic linkage between N-acetylgalactosamine and the hydroxyl groups of threonine or serine, and 3) a N-glycosylamine linkage between N-acetylglucosamine and the amide group of asparagine. In addition,

Table 2.3 Properties of Chondroitinase ABC, AC, and ACII

Enzyme	Chondroitinase ABC 4.2.2.4[a] *Proteus vulgaris*	Chondroitinase AC 4.2.2.5 *Flavobacterium heparinum*	Chondroitinase ACII 4.2.2.5 *Arthrobacter aurescens*
Optimal pH and buffer	8.0 Tris-HCl	7.3 Tris-HCl	6.0 Acetate
Relative activity			
C4S	100	100	100
C6S	100	65	110
C0S	20	110	195
DS	40	0	0
HA	2	12	320
HS	0	0	0
KS	0	0	0
HP	0	0	0
Activator		Mn^{2+}, Mg^{2+}, Ca^{2+}, Ba^{2+}	Ca^{2+}, Co^{2+}, Mg^{2+}, Ba^{2+}
Inhibitor		DS, HP, HS, KS Zn^{2+}, Fe^{2+}, Cu^{2+}	DS Pb^{2+}, Cu^{2+}, Fe^{2+}, Sn^{2+}

[a] EC number.

the positions of sulfated glycosaminoglycans are each linked at their reducing end to a tetrasaccharide unit, glucuronosyl–galactosyl–galactosyl-xylose. The xylose–serine linkage is unique to the connective tissue proteoglycans and has not been found in any other mammalian glycoconjugates. Whereas keratan sulfate (KS) I (corneal KS) is bound to core protein via the N-glycosylamine linkage between N-acetylglucosamine and asparagine, the N-acetylgalactosamine-reducing terminus of KS II (cartilage, bone) attaches to the threonine or serine residue of the protein.

STRUCTURE OF PROTEOGLYCANS IN SKIN

Two families of proteoglycans, chondroitin sulfate proteoglycans (CS-PG) and dermatan sulfate-containing proteoglycans (DS-PG), have been isolated from skin. Although CS-PGs in cartilage, aorta, and tendon have the hyaluronic acid-binding region at the N-terminus of the core proteins and are able to form large aggregates with hyaluronic acid, CS-PG in skin does not bind to hyaluronic acid. The amino acid composition of the core protein from CS-PG in skin is similar to that of the large aggregating CS-PG in cartilage but it lacks cystine and methionine located in the hyaluronic acid-binding region. The CS-PGs consist of a core protein with a molecular weight (MW) of 50 kDa and 50 CS chains each with a MW of about 20 kDa. Another non aggregating large CS-PG found in newborn rat skin displays a MW of more than 1000 kDa by Sepharose CL-2B and is composed of two different-sized (480 kDa and 520 kDa) core proteins. The tryptic peptide pattern from these core proteins is identical.

Large aggregating CS-PG with a MW of 240 kDa core protein is found on the cell surface of human melanoma (M21). Relatively large amounts of DS-containing PGs are also isolated from the skin. The whole molecule is 70–100 kDa in molecular size with a protein core of 38–55 kDa (Fig. 2.2). The glycosaminoglycan chain varies in size (15–45 kDa) and iduronic acid content (35–85% of total uronic acid). This molecule may have one or two DS chains. These variations in length and in number of chains and in molecular size of the core protein might be either due to differences related to age or to species. The amino acid composition of the core protein of DS-PG in skin is essentially similar in different species. Partial amino acid sequences of DS-PG from bovine skin have been determined as DEASGIGPEEHFPEVPEIEPMGPV and N-terminal

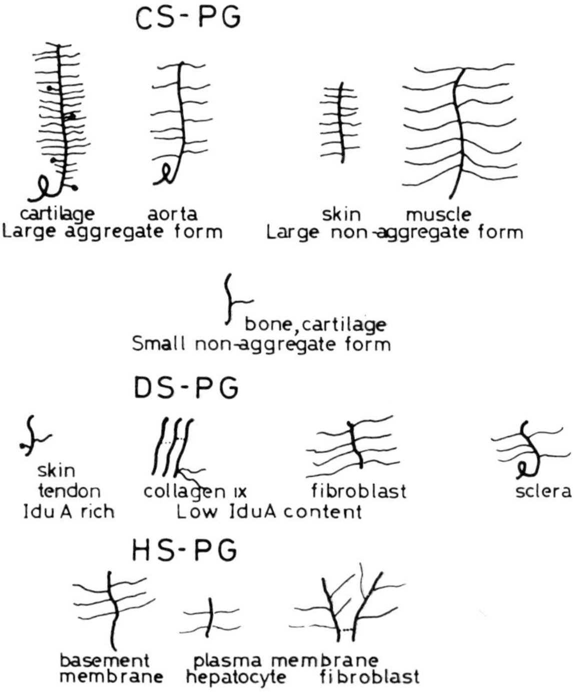

Figure 2.2 Schematic structure of the main proteoglycans. CS-PG, chondroitin sulfate proteoglycan; DS-PG, dermatan sulfate proteoglycan; HS-PG, heparan sulfate proteoglycan. The thick and the thin lines show the core proteins and glycosaminoglycans, respectively. The Mark (—●) identifies N-linked oligosaccharide unit.

sequence in the first 14 amino acids was identical with that from DS-PG from bovine tendon [5]. The skin DS-PG has three O-linked oligosaccharides and one N-linked complex type oligosaccharide per molecule [6]. Either a DS chain or an O-linked oligosaccharide probably binds to serine residue at position 4 of the core protein. The small DS-PGs from sclera and tendon show immunologic identity and have similar peptides. These immunologic identities and peptide patterns are also found in small PGs of bone and cornea that contain CS chain with no iduronic acid. The other DS-PG from cartilage (DS-PG I) that has a low iduronic acid content shows similarities with DS-PG of skin in overall size and core protein. Another DS-containing PG, originally called PG-Lt and found in cartilage [7], has now been identified as type IX collagen, which is composed of three α-chains and one or two DS chains. Human skin fibroblasts produce the small DS-rich PG and a large glucuronic acid-rich PG, which are associated with the cell and can bind to hyaluronic acid. The small DS-PG is associated with collagen fiber when fibroblasts are cultured on the collagen gel [8]. Guinea pig skin fibroblasts secrete into culture medium mainly the small DS-PGs composed of two different molcular-size core proteins (53 and 55 kDa) [9]. DS-PG coexisting in collagen fiber at the D band in the gap zone is observed in rat tail tendon collagen by electron microscopy [10]. Since DS-PG from tendon inhibits fibrillogenesis of type I and type II collagen in vitro, it may play a key role in the regulation of collagen fibril assembly and in the biomechanical strength of collagen fibrils. A glucuronic acid-rich small DS-PG is also found in cornea and related to corneal transparency. The interfibrillar spaces are abnormally extended in the opaque cornea scar and the glucuronic acid-rich DS-PGs are substituted for unusual large proteoglycans that contain normal-size glucuronic acid-rich chains and without KS-PG. When the scar heals, the normal-sized PGs reappeared together with KS-PG. DS-PG also may be related to the process of atherosclerosis, since DS-PG from pig aorta forms an insoluble complex with low-density lipoprotein [11].

HEPARAN SULFATE PROTEOGLYCANS

DS-PG, CS-PG, and KS-PG exist in extracellular matrices, whereas heparan sulfate (HS) PG is known as one component of cell membranes and of basement membranes. A cell surface HS-PG of liver cell is composed of a core protein with a MW of 30 kDa and four HS chains with a MW of 140 kDa. The entire molecule of HS-PG of fibroblasts has a MW of 300–400 kDa and consists of two core proteins linked by disulfide bonds and four to six HS chains with a MW of 20 kDa. Each core protein is composed of an HS-binding domain, an oligosaccharide-containing domain, and a non glycosylated region. This PG is considered to be identical with the transferrin receptor of the fibroblasts. Cultured epithelial cell from skin also synthesizes HS-PG and CS-PG and secretes them into the medium. The HS chain has the capacity for self-association. This self-association may be related to the interactions of cell surface PG and HS-PG in basement membrane. The HS-PGs from glomerular basement membranes have four to five HS chains with a MW of 130–250 kDa and show core proteins with MW of 90–170 kDa after digestion with heparitinase. Other HS-PGs are isolated from Engelbreth-Holm-Swarm (EHS) tumor and PYS-2 mouse teratocarcinoma cell line, which produce basement membrane components such as type IV collagen, laminin, and nidogen. Two different molecules can be separated by CsCl-density gradient centrifugation from EHS tumor. The low-density HS-PG ($\zeta = 1.3$–1.4) is composed of four to five HS-chains with a MW of 43 kDa and a core protein with a MW of 450 kDa. The high-density HS-PG ($\zeta < 1.6$) has a small core protein (5–12 kDa) and three HS chains of MW 29 kDa. PYS-2 cells produce HS-PG with an apparent MW of 400 kDa. The HS-PG is composed of 10 HS chains with a MW of 25 kDa and a core protein with a M of 150 kDa.

The antibodies against the core protein of HS-PG from EHS tumor react with basement membrane of human, calf, rat, and mouse and with cell surface of cultured cell that synthesizes HS-PG [12]. It indicates that genetically identical epitopes are present among the core proteins of the HS-PG families.

HYALURONIC ACID

Also called hyaluronate or hyaluronan, this glycosaminoglycan is not connected to a polypeptide. It is synthesized in many types of cells by a specific hyaluronan synthetase. The enzyme, bound to membranes, displays a rapid turnover. It is regulated by growth factors probably via protein kinase C [13]. Hyaluronate is secreted by the cells and perhaps remains connected to the membrane. Its large molecular size (on the order of 1 million kDa) and its extensive hydration do not allow it to diffuse except after degradation. Degradation is performed by hyaluronidase.

Many types of cells display surface receptors that allow them to respond to changes in the concentration of hyaluronate. This property is probably involved in several aspects of morphogenesis. Embryonic tissues are very rich in hyaluronate.

PREPARATION OF SKIN PGs

The PGs are isolated from skin by a method, which consists in brief, of extraction using 0.15–1.0M NaCl, 4M guanidinium chloride, or 6M urea (60°C) under neutral pH containing protease inhibitors (EDTA, 10–100 mM, benzamidine hydrochloride, 1–10 μM; N-ethylmaleimide, 1–5 μM; phenylmethane sulfonyl fluoride, 0.1–1 mM, pepstatin, 1–10 μM; L-*trans*-epoxysuccinic acid, 10 μM); separation from collagen using diethylaminoethyl (DEAE) ion exchange chromatography; segregation from acidic protein under dissociative condition (4M guanidinium chloride) by CsCl density gradient centrifugation; affinity chromatography on a concanavalin Sepharose CL-4B column and gel chromatography using Sepharose CL-4B gel.

The PGs obtained or the core proteins after digestion with chondroitinase ABC can be used to produce antibodies.

BIOSYNTHESIS OF PGs

Synthesis of the entire molecule of the core protein is required before elongation of the GAG chain. The formation of the core protein of PG is thought to be similar to that established for glycoprotein synthesis. The core protein enters the endoplasmic reticulum and the assembly of N-linked high-mannose-containing oligosaccharides starts from a dolichol diphosphate intermediate oligosaccharide that is transferred via an N-glycosidic bond to asparagine on the core protein. The high-mannose oligosaccharide is converted to the sialic-acid-containing complex-type oligosaccharide in the Golgi. The first glycosyl transfer reaction for several PGs is the transfer of xylose from UDP–xylose to serine hydroxyl groups in their core proteins. Since xylosyltransferase is tightly bound to the membrane of the endoplasmic reticulum, xylosylation of the core protein may occur before the Golgi. Even if the synthesis of the core protein of CS-PG is inhibited by cycloheximide or puromycine, which does not affect the GAG elongation enzymes, the CS chain, which has a β-xylose at the reducing end, is synthesized and increases in length. Completion of the carbohydrate–protein linkage region is effected by three additional glycosyltransferases, two galactosyltransferases, and one glucuronosyltransferase. Galactosyltransferase I interacts with a certain degree of specificity with the chain-initiation of xylosyltransferase and appears to be dependent on phospholipids for activity. When a microsomal pellet from chick embryonal cartilage is digested with phospholipase C, about 75% of the activities is lost. Galactosyltransferase II transfers to UDP-galactose to galactosyl–xylosyl–serine. The final step in the formation of carbohydrate–protein linkage region is the transfer of glucuronic acid to the second galactose residue by a glucuronosyltransferase, which is different from that involved in the formation of the repeating disaccharide units. The glycosaminoglycan chains are synthesized from sugar nucleotides. The repeating disaccharides of chondroitin sulfate are formed by alternating transfer of N-acetylgalactosamine and glucuronic acid to the nonreducing terminus of the elongating chain. This process is driven by two distinct enzymes: an N-acetylgalactosaminyltransferase and a glucuronosyltransferase. Sulfated as well as non sulfated oligosaccharides with terminal glucuronic acid residues serve as acceptors for N-acetylgalactosaminyl transfer. Glucuronosyltransferase II catalyzes transfer to nonreducing terminal N-acetylgalactosamine residues of oligosaccharides of chondroitin, chondroitin 6-sulfate. The 4-sulfated pentasacchride is not an acceptor for glucuronosyl transfer. These results suggest that sulfation may occur after the addition of a glucuronic acid residue. The different sulfotransferases catalyze transfer of sulfate from 3′-phosphoadenyl 5′-phosphosulfate (PAPS) to the specific site on the GAG. Sulfation and glycosaminoglycan polymerization probably take place simultaneously during the chain elongation in the Golgi apparatus. As with the biosynthesis of dermatan sulfate, it follows the same pathway that has been established for the chondroitin sulfate, and the formation of the iduronic acid residues takes place as in heparin and heparan sulfate synthesis, by conversion of glucuronic acid residues already incorporated into the elongating chain. The C5-epimerization of glucuronic acid residues to produce L-iduronic acid residues in DS chain is tightly coupled to the sulfation process. These biosynthetic processes are summarized in Figure 2.3.

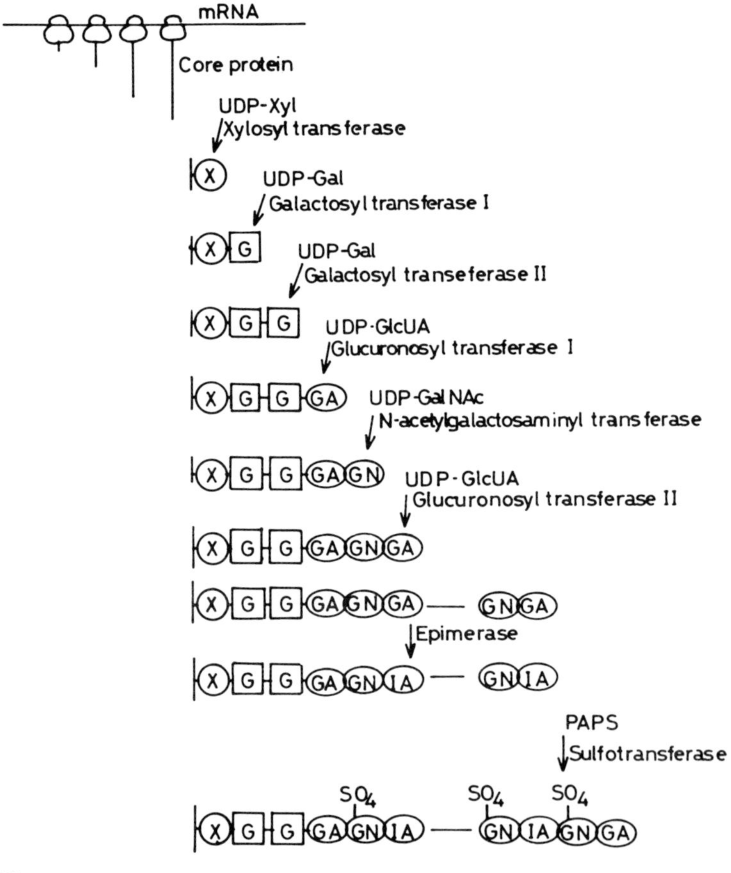

Figure 2.3 Biosynthesis of proteoglycan. X, xylose; G, galactose; GA, glucuronic acid; GN, N-acetylgalactosamine; IA, iduronic acid; PAPS, 3′-phosphoadenosine-5′phosphosulfate.

DEGRADATION OF PGs

When DS-PG labeled on DS-chain and core protein is incubated in a culture of fibroblasts, the intact core protein molecule cannot be detected in the medium in the cell. There is no evidence for the degradation of glycosaminoglycans in extracellular spaces, although almost all core proteins of PGs are probably degradated in the extracellular space by neutral metalloproteoglycanase.

The half-life in vivo of HA, CS, and DS is considered to be from 2 days to 2 weeks. About 3–6 mg/day GAGs are excreted into urine in the normal human adult. Urinary GAGs are characterized as equal amounts of chondroitin 4-sulfate (C4S) and chondroitin 6-sulfate (C6S) as major components and HS and DS as minor ones. The amount of HA in urine is not sufficient to account for the normal metabolic flux. Testicular hyaluronidase, which is an endo β-N-acetylhexosaminidase, cleaves β-linked N-acetylglucosaminyl groups HA, chondroitin, C4S, and C6S. This enzyme produces the tetrasaccharide, GlcUA β1,3-GlcNAc β1,4-GlcUA β1,3-GlcNAc as the major end products with small amounts of N-acetylhyalobiuronic acid, GlcUA β1,3 GlcNAc and hexasaccahride upon exhausive digestion of hyaluronic acid. A similar enzyme has been found in rat skin. This enzyme is a β-N-acetylhexosaminidase that acts as a transglycosylase, although it differs from testicular hyaluronidase, producing hexasaccharide as a major product and larger products with no disaccharide.

Glucuronic acid moieties located at the nonreducing terminal end of the desulfated oligosaccharides derived from the degradating products of GAGs by glycosaminoglycan-lyases will be removed by β-glucuronidase. However, the two disaccharides from hyaluronic acid and chondroitin sulfates, GlcUA β1,3-Glc NAc and GlcUA β1,3-GalNAc, are resistant to the enzyme. A terminal N-acetylhexosamine on the remaining oligosaccharide can in turn be removed by N-acetylhexosaminidases if it is non-sulfated. The presence of a limited number of glucuronic acid residues in dermatan sulfate chain suggests that some depolymerization has occurred at these points by hyaluronidase. DS may therefore be sequentially degraded by β-glucuronidase, N-acetylgalactosamine 4-sulfate sulfatase, β-N-acethylhexosaminidase, iduronate sulfatase, and α-L-iduronidase, which acts only as exoglycosidase, as shown in Figure 2.4. Furthermore, removal of galactose residue from Gal-Gal-Xylose-Serine in the linkage region can occur after release of the oligosaccharide chain from serine residue of the linkage region.

PGs AND GAGs IN DISEASES

Examples of diseases resulting from altered synthesis or degradation are numerous and varied, as illustrated here by a few examples.

A deficiency of the core protein of the small DS-PG has been observed in a

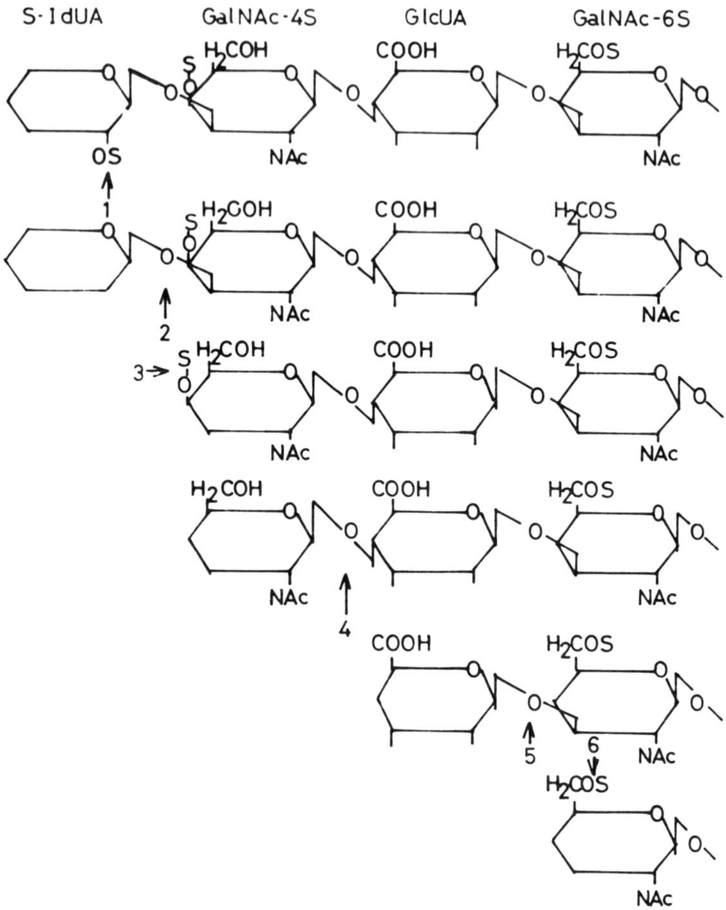

Figure 2.4 Degradation process of dermatan sulfate. 1, α-L-iduronosulfatase; 2, α-L-iduronidase; 3, N-acetylgalactosamine 4-sulfate sulfatase; 4, ß-N-acetylgalactosaminidase; 5, ß-glucuronidase; 6, N-acetylgalactosamine 6-sulfate sulfatase.

variant from of Ehlers-Danlos syndrome. Fibroblasts from patients with this disorder can synthesize DS chain only when beta-xyloside is added in the culture medium as an initiator [14].

Coffin-Lowry syndrome is a disorder characterized by mental retardation with skeletal abnormalities and thick soft skin. The cultured fibroblasts of one patient with this disorder produced abnormal DS-PG by an increase in molecular and a high iduronic acid content [15].

The Lowe syndrome (oculocerebrorenal syndrome), characterized by a low sulfate content in CS, is based on the increased degradation of PAPS due to the acceleration of nucleotidopyrophosphatase activity [16]. Low sulfate content in CS is also found in one form of spondyloepiphyseal dysplasia. This undersulfation results from the deficiency of the sulfotransferase that donates sulfate from PAPS. In the case of the brachymorphic mouse, there is evidence for undersulfation of CS and deficiency of PAPS synthesis due to defects of adenosine 5′-phosphosulfate kinase and adenosine triphosphate sulfurylase [17].

Defect of one or more of the degradative enzymes of GAGs leads to GAG storage diseases (the genetic mucopolysaccharidoses).

REFERENCES

1. Esko JD. Genetic analysis of proteoglycan structure, function and metabolism. Curr Opin Cell Biol 1991; 3: 805–16.
2. Scott JE. Proteoglycan: collagen interactions and subfibrillar structure in collagen fibrils. Implications in the development and ageing of connective tissue. J Anat 1990; 169: 23–35.
3. Ruoslahti E. Proteoglycans in cell regulation. J Biol Chem 1989; 264: 13369–72.
4. Hardingham TE, Fosang AJ. Proteoglycans: many forms and many functions. FASEB 1992; 6: 861–70.
5. Pearson CH, Winterbottom N, Facker DS, Scott PG. The amino acid sequence of bovine-skin proteodermatan sulfate. J Biol Chem 1983; 258:15101–4.
6. Nakamura T, Matsunaga E, Shinkai H. Isolation and some structural analyses of a proteodermatan sulphate from calf skin. Biochem J 1983; 213: 289–96.
7. Noro A, Kimata K, Oike Y, Shinomura T, Maeda N, Yano S, Takahashi N, Suzuki S. Isolation and characterization of a third proteoglycan (PG-Lt) from chick embryo cartilage which contains disulfide-bonded collagenous polypeptide. J Biol Chem 1983; 258: 9323–31.
8. Gallagher J, Gasiunas N, Schor SL. Specific association of iduronic acid-rich dermatan sulphate with the extracellular matrix of human skin fibroblasts cultured on collagen gels. Biochem J 1983; 215 107–16.
9. Honda T, Matsunaga E, Katagiri K, Fujiwara S, Shinkai H. Small dermatan sulphate proteoglycans in cultured fibroblasts from guinea-pig skin. Biomed Res 1987; 8:175–83.
10. Scott JE, Orford CR. Dermatan sulphate rich proteoglycan associates with rat tail tendon collagen at the d band in the gap region. Biochem J 1981; 197: 213–16.
11. Wegrowski J, Moczar M, Robert L. Proteoglycans from pig aorta. Comparative study of their interactions. Biochem J 1986; 235: 823–31.
12. Hayman EG, Oldberg A, Martin GR, Ruoslahti. Codistribution of heparan sulfate proteoglycan, laminin, and fibronectin in the extracellular matrix of normal rat kidney cells and their coordinate absence in transformed cells. J Cell Biol 1982; 94: 28–35.
13. Heldin P, Asplund T, Ytterberg D, Thelin S, Laurent TC. Characterization of the molecular mechanism involved in the activation of hyaluronan synthetase by platelet-derived growth factor in human mesothelial cells. Biochem J 1992; 283: 165–70.

14. Fushimi H, Kaneyama M, Shinkai H. Deficiency of the core proteins of dermatan sulfate proteoglycans in a variant form of Ehlers-Danlos syndrome. J Int Med 1989; 226: 409–16.
15. Beck M, Glossl J, Ruter R, Kresse H. Abnormal proteodermatan sulfate in three patients with Coffin-Lowry syndrome. Pediat Res 1983; 17: 926–9.
16. Yamashina I, Yoshida H, Fukui S, Funakoshi I. Biochemical studies on Lowe's syndrome. Mol Cell Biochem 1983; 52: 107–24.
17. Pennypacker JP, Kimata K, Brown KS. Brachymorphic mice (bm/bm): a generalized biochemical defect expressed primarily in cartilage. Dev Biol 1981; 81: 280–7.

3

Elastic Fibers

Jouni Uitto, Michael Fazio, and Veli-Matti Kähäri

Jefferson Institute of Molecular Medicine, Thomas Jefferson University, Philadelphia, Pennsylvania

Although elastic fibers are only a relatively minor component of the extracellular matrix in normal human skin, accounting for approximately 2–4% of dry weight in sun-protected dermis, it is clear that these fibers play a major role in providing elasticity and resilience to the skin. Recent studies have elucidated the complexity of the elastin gene structure and the biosynthetic events involved in the production and metabolic turnover of elastic fibers. Also, aberration of the elastic fiber network has been noted in a number of both acquired and inherited cutaneous diseases (for reviews on elastin biology and pathology, see [1–4]).

The elastic fibers of human skin can be visualized by special histopathologic staining techniques, such as Verhoeff–van Gieson or orcein stains. The elastic fibers are thickest in the reticular dermis where they are oriented parallel to the surface of the skin, intertwined among the collagen bundles. In the papillary dermis, the elastic fibers, known as elaunin, are organized in an arcadelike arrangement. In the most superficial papillary dermis, even thinner elastic fibers known as oxytalan fibers ascend vertically to terminate just below the dermal–epidermal junction.

Examination of elastic fibers by transmission electron microscopy has revealed that these fibers consist of two distinct components. The major component is elastin, a well-characterized connective tissue protein. Surrounding the elastin core, there are less well characterized electron-dense structures, known as elastic-fiber associated microfibrils. Although the precise composition of the microfibrils is currently unknown, recent studies have suggested that fibrillin, another extracellular matrix protein, may be an integral part of the microfibrillar structure.

THE GENE STRUCTURE AND BIOSYNTHESIS

Elastin is initially synthesized as a polypeptide of ~70 kDa (Fig. 3.1). The protein is coded by a single copy gene located in the long arm of chromosome 7 in the human genome [5]. The human elastin gene contains 34 exons separated by relatively large intervening sequences (introns) (Fig. 3.2A). The size of the total gene is ~45 kilobase pairs (kb) [6]. During the early stages of elastin gene expression, the nucleotide sequence in the gene is transcribed to a large messenger RNA (mRNA) precursor. This precursor molecule is then subjected to posttranscriptional modifications, including constitutive splicing, which remove the in-

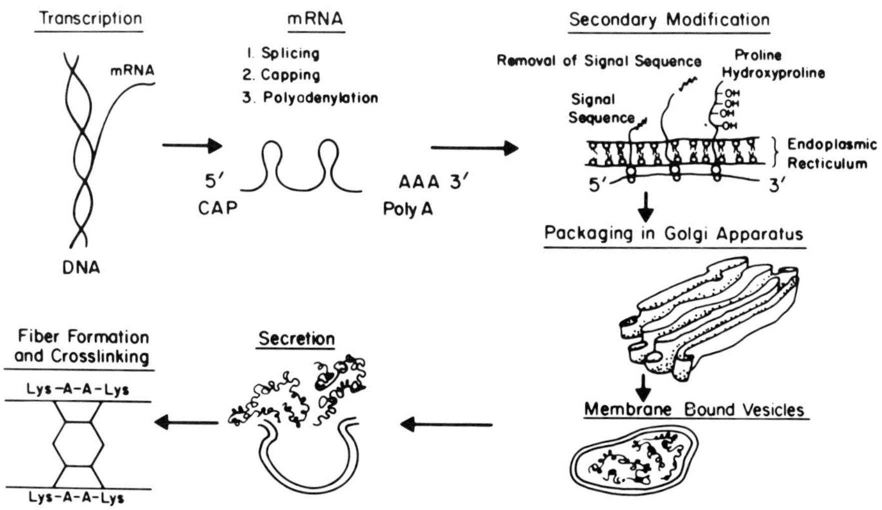

Figure 3.1 Schematic representation of the elastin biosynthetic pathway. The elastin gene, which is located on the long arm of chromosome 7 and is ~45 kb in size (see Fig. 3.2A), is transcribed to a messenger RNA precursor. After transcription, several intranuclear reactions participate in the processing of the primary mRNA transcript, including alternative splicing. The mRNA then serves as a template for translation, and the newly synthesized polypeptide is subject to several posttranslational modifications. The elastin polypeptides are then packaged in Golgi vesicles before being transferred to the extracellular space. After secretion, the individual elastin polypeptides align into the fiber structure that is stabilized by the formation of covalent cross-links, demosines, and isodesmosines (see Fig. 3) (from [1] with permission).

tron sequences, resulting in mature elastin mRNAs (Fig. 3.1). An unusual variation of constitutive splicing, noted in the processing of elastin mRNAs, is that some exon sequences are alternatively spliced (alternative splicing), thus resulting in the synthesis of mRNA molecules with slightly differing primary sequences [6]. The significance of the alternative splicing is currently unknown, but it could provide a mechanism that would result in the synthesis of elastin molecules of slightly different physiological properties. This might explain some tissue-specific differences of elastic fibers noted in morphologic studies.

The elastin mRNAs are ~3.5 kb in size and contain an ~2.2 kb translatable region that encodes a polypeptide of ~750 amino acids (Fig. 3.2B) [4,6]. Following translation of the elastin mRNAs on the ribosomes of the elastin-synthesizing

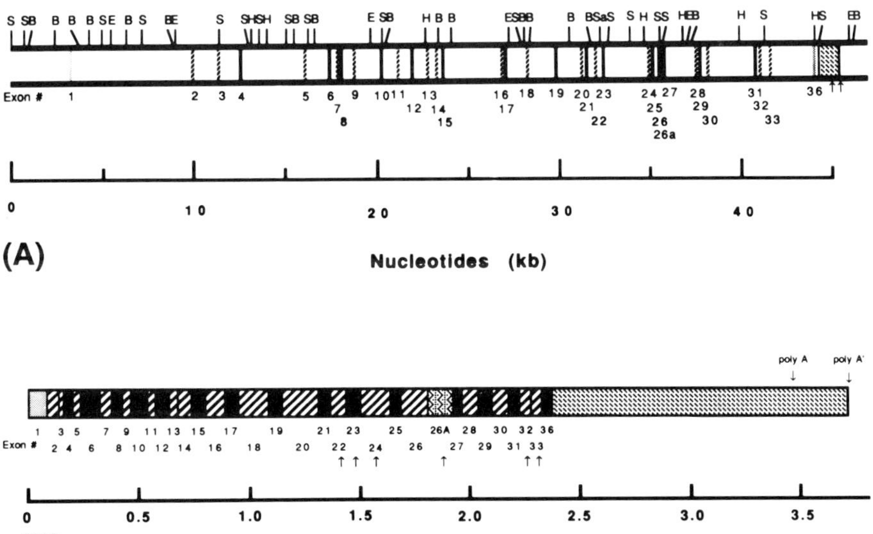

Figure 3.2 Schematic representation of the human elastin gene (A) and the corresponding cDNA (B). A. The exons are numbered starting from the 5′-end of the gene and correspond to those shown in the cDNA (see B). Restriction endonuclease cleavage sites are noted: BamHI (B), EcoRI (E), HindIII (H). Small arrows (↑) mark the positions of polyadenylation sites (modified from [10] with permission). B. The cDNA, which is ~3.5 kb in size, is divided into separate exons numbered from 1 to 36 and drawn to scale. The arrows (↑) indicate the exons that have been shown to be subject to alternative splicing. The two potential sites for polyadenylation of the messenger RNAs in the 3′-untranslated portion of the cDNA are indicated by arrows (↓) (from [10] with permission).

cells, such as human skin fibroblasts, the newly synthesized polypeptides are secreted into the extracellular space (Fig. 3.1).

FIBRILLOGENESIS

In the extracellular space, the individual elastin polypeptides align into a fiber structure. It has been postulated, on the basis of electron microscopic observations, that the microfibrillar component of the elastic fibers may act as a scaffold onto which the elastin polypeptides assemble (Fig. 3.1). Since the elastin polypeptides contain two uniquely conserved cysteine residues at the carboxy terminus, it has been postulated that the microfibrillar component, which is rich in cysteine, may interact with elastin through disulfide bonding [4].

The elastin fiber assembly is stabilized by the formation of unique cross-link compounds, called desmosines (Fig. 3.3). The tropoelastin polypeptides contain specific cross-link domains consisting of paired lysyl residues separated by two or three amino acids, frequently alanines. Certain lysyl residues are oxidatively deaminated to the corresponding aldehydes (allysines), in a reaction catalyzed by lysyl oxidase, a copper-dependent enzyme. Three of the allysines and an unmodified ϵ-amino group of a fourth lysyl residue spontaneously fuse to form a stable covalent cross-link, desmosine, or its isomer, isodesmosine (Fig. 3.3). The relative concentration of desmosines in normal human elastic fibers is constant, ~1.5 residues per 1000 amino acids and, consequently, assay of desmosines can serve as a quantitative index of the amount of cross-linked elastic fibers in tissues.

REGULATION OF GENE EXPRESSION

Several lines of evidence suggest that the elastin gene expression in normal situations is controlled at the transcriptional level. The elastin mRNA levels correlate, in general, with the amount of elastin polypeptides being synthesized and, therefore, the elastin mRNA steady state levels reflect the rate of elastin synthesis in tissues or cell cultures. For example, human skin fibroblasts, which actively express the elastin gene, have been used as a model system to study the modulation of elastin gene expression. These studies have demonstrated that elastin gene expression, which is activated during early stages of fetal development, remains at a relatively constant level through several decades. However, after the fourth decade of life, the elastin gene expression precipitously declines (Fig. 3.4). This observation may have relevance to the innate cutaneous aging characterized by loss of functional elastic fibers in the skin [7].

The 5′-flanking region is important in the transcriptional regulation of the elastin gene. The entire human elastin gene, including the 5′-flanking (promoter)

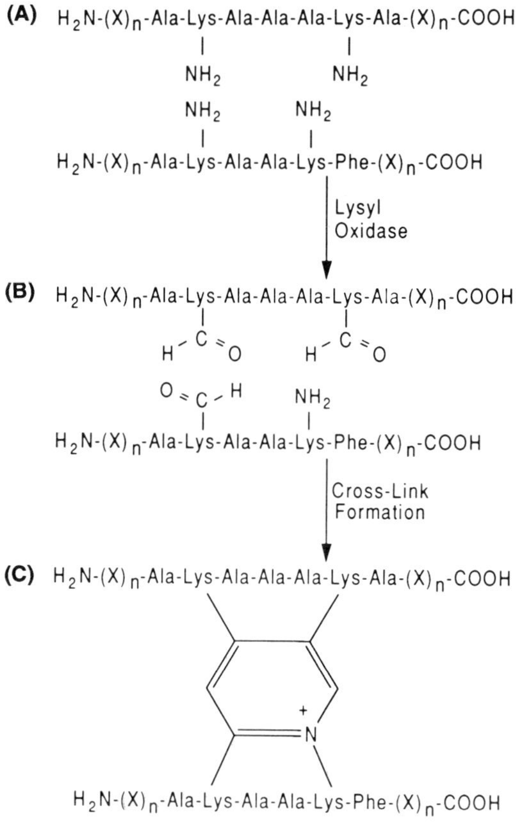

Figure 3.3 Schematic representation of the formation of intermolecular cross-links, desmosine and isodesmosine, between two tropoelastin polypeptides. A. Amino acid sequences of a potential cross-link region within the tropoelastin polypeptides. Note the ϵ-amino group (NH_2) of the four contributing lysyl residues. B. Three of the lysyl residues undergo oxidative deamination catalyzed by lysyl oxidase to yield corresponding aldehyde derivatives, allysines. C. Three of the allysines and the fourth unmodified lysyl residue, still containing an ϵ-amino group, fuse into a stable desmosine cross-link (from [3] with permission).

sequences, has recently been cloned and characterized [8,9]. Analyses of the 5′-flanking region of the human elastin gene revealed several unusual features that suggest that transcriptional regulation of the elastin gene is complex. There are multiple transcription initiation sites, while no canonical TATA box was identified. Extensive deletion analyses of the 5′-flanking region of the human elastin gene have delineated several *cis*-acting regulatory elements, including putative responsive elements for glucocorticoids, cAMP, and 12-O-tetradecanoylphorbol-

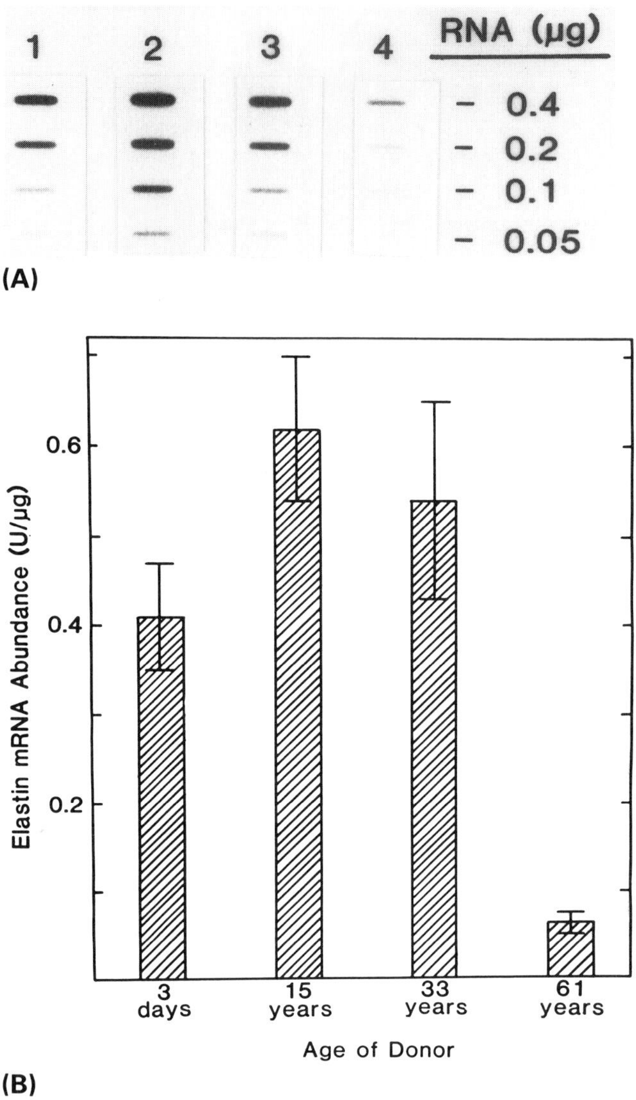

Figure 3.4 Elastin mRNA steady state abundance in skin fibroblast cultures established from individuals of varying ages. A. Slot-blot hybridizations. Poly(A)$^+$RNA was isolated, dotted onto nitrocellulose filters in varying amounts (0.4–0.05 μg), as indicated at right side, and hybridized with a ^{32}P-labeled human elastin cDNA. The figure shows the autoradiogram of ^{32}P-labeled cDNA/mRNA hybrids. Lanes 1–4 represent RNA isolated from fibroblast cultures established from individuals with ages of 3 days, 15 years, 33 years, and 61 years, respectively. B. Quantitation of elastin mRNA levels. The

13-acetate. The recent construction of elastin promoter/chloramphenicol acetyltransferase (CAT) plasmids provides a means to study transcriptional modulation of elastin gene expression by a variety of exogenous agents, as well as in cutaneous diseases [9].

DEGRADATION

Elastases make up a family of proteolytic enzymes capable of degrading elastic fibers. Although the metabolic turnover of connective tissue proteins, especially elastin, is relatively slow, it is clear that a portion of elastic fibers is continuously degraded and replaced during early stages of development. In addition, degradation of elastic fibers is markedly increased in a variety of pathologic conditions, such as some forms of cutis laxa [3,6].

The most powerful elastolytic enzymes are synthesized by polymorphonuclear leukocytes, and these enzymes presumably initiate elastin degradation in inflammatory processes. The activity of these serine proteases can be inhibited by serum factors, such as α1-antitrypsin and α2-macroglobulin.

In addition to serine elastases, the presence of elastase-like metalloproteases has been recently demonstrated in human serum and in different cells. These enzymes are not particularly active against insoluble elastin, but they are capable of degrading soluble elastin, as well as the oxytalan and elaunin fibers. Thus, these enzymes may contribute to the overall degradation of the elastic fiber network. Furthermore, some of the elastin-like metalloproteases have been suggested to play a role in the degradation of elastic fibers in patients with various cutaneous diseases [3].

PATHOLOGIC MANIFESTATIONS

The complexity of gene expression and metabolic turnover of elastin can introduce errors into the biosynthetic pathway of elastic fibers in a manner that these abnormalities may manifest as a clinical disease. In fact, abnormalities in the elastic fiber network have been detected in various diseases affecting the skin (Table 3.1). The mechanisms leading to elastic fiber pathologic conditions can occur at one of several different levels of elastin metabolic pathway. For example,

---

abundance of elastin mRNA was quantitated from the slot-blot hybridizations, shown in A, by scanning densitometry. The values are expressed as densitometric units (U)/μg of poly(A)$^+$RNA dotted, and corrected for the ß-actin mRNA levels in the same preparations, as determined by parallel hybridizations with a ^{32}P-labeled human ß-actin cDNA. The values represent mean ± SEM of three to five determinations in the linear range of the mRNA hybridization curve in triplicate cultures of the same cell strain (from [11] with permission).

Table 3.1 Heritable Diseases with Abnormal Elastic Fibers

Disease	Inheritance
Pseudoxanthoma elasticum	AR, AD
Buschke-Ollendorff syndrome	AD
Cutis laxa	AD, AR, XR
Ehlers-Danlos syndrome type IX	XR
Menkes syndrome	XR
Marfan syndrome	AD
Elastoderma	?

AD, autosomal dominant; AR, autosomal recessive; XR, X-linked recessive
Source: Modified from [3].

the elastin gene may have aberrations in the primary structure, or the rate of elastin gene expression may be altered in heritable cutaneous disorders [1,3,10]. As an alternative, posttranscriptional or posttranslational modifications could alter the structure of elastin, or the rate of degradation of the elastic fibers could be altered. These diseases can now be studied by biochemical and molecular biological approaches that have been developed during the past few years [2]. For example, highly specific and sensitive radioimmunoassays or enzyme-linked immunoabsorbent assays (ELISAs) are available for the quantitation of desmosines in tissues. Computerized morphometric analysis can be used to provide correlation between the histopathologic observations of elastic fibers and biochemically determined elastin concentration. Finally, the availability of human sequence specific elastin cDNAs allows for quantitation of elastin gene expression in tissues and cell cultures [2]. These techniques can now be utilized for the precise elucidation of the underlying molecular defects in both heritable and acquired diseases affecting the elastic fibers [2,7,10]. Further elucidation of specific abnormalities in molecular diseases of elastin will provide better understanding of the role of different domains of this protein in normal tissue physiology.

ACKNOWLEDGMENTS

The authors thank Charlene D. Aranda and Eileen O'Shaughnessy for expert secretarial help.

The original studies by the authors were supported, in part, by USPHS, NIH grants AR28450 and T32-AR7561. Dr. Kähäri was the recipient of a Dermatology Foundation Fellowship.

REFERENCES

1. Rosenbloom J. Biology of disease. Elastin: relation of protein and gene structure to disease. Lab Invest 1984; 51:605–23.
2. Uitto J, Olsen DR, Fazio MJ. Extracellular matrix of the skin: 50 years of progress. J Invest Dermatol 1989; 92: (Suppl. 1) 61–77s.
3. Uitto J, Fazio MJ, Olsen DR. Heritable connective tissue diseases of the skin. In: Alper JC, ed. Genetic disorders of the skin. St. Louis, Mosby: Year Book Medical Publishers, 1991, pp. 287–319.
4. Uitto J, Fazio MJ, Bashir M, Rosenbloom J. Elastic fibers of the connective tissue. In: Goldsmith L, ed. Physiology, biochemistry and molecular biology of the skin. New York: Oxford University Press, 1991, pp. 530–557.
5. Fazio MJ, Mattei M-G, Passage E, Chu M-L, Black D, Solomon E, Davidson JM, Uitto J. Human elastin gene: new evidence for localization to the long arm of chromosome 7. Am J Hum Genet 1991; 48:696–703.
6. Indik Z, Yeh H, Ornstein-Goldstein M, Kucich U, Abrams W, Rosenbloom JC, Rosenbloom J. Structure of the elastin gene and alternative splicing of elastin mRNA: implications for human disease. Am J Med Genet 1989; 34:81–90.
7. Uitto J, Fazio MJ, Olsen DR. Molecular mechanisms of cutaneous aging: age-associated connective tissue alterations in the dermis. J Am Acad Dermatol 1989; 21 (Suppl) 614–22.
8. Bashir MM, Indik Z, Yeh H, Ornstein-Goldstein N, Rosenbloom JC, Abrams W, Fazio M, Uitto J, Rosenbloom J. Characterization of the complete human elastin gene: delineation of unusual features in the 5′ flanking region. J Biol Chem 1989; 269:8887–91.
9. Kähäri V-M, Fazio MJ, Chen YQ, Bashir MM, Rosenbloom J, Uitto J. Deletion analyses of 5′-flanking region of the human elastin gene: evidence for a functional promoter and regulatory *cis*-elements. J Biol Chem 1990; 265:9485–90.
10. Fazio MJ, Olsen DR, Uitto J. Skin aging: lessons from cutis laxa and elastoderma. Cutis 1989; 43:437–44.
11. Fazio MJ, Olsen DR, Kuivaniemi H, Chu M-L, Davidson JM, Rosenbloom J, Uitto J. Isolation and characterization of human elastin cDNAs and age-associated variation in elastin gene expression in cultured skin fibroblasts. Lab Invest 1988; 58:270–7.

4

Cutaneous Basement Membranes

David T. Woodley
Northwestern University, Chicago, Illinois

Yves Sarret
Hôpital Edouard-Herriot, Lyon, France

Basement membranes are thin, extracellular, connective tissue structures that usually serve as morphologic divisions between dissimilar tissues [1]. In the skin, for example, there are two prominent basement membranes: one around dermal blood vessels and skin appendages that delineates these structures from dermal connective tissue and a second one separates the dermis from the epidermis, a zone that has been defined as the dermal–epidermal junction (DEJ) [2].

Basement membranes are often present at the interface between tissues whose origins from the primordial germ layers (ectoderm, mesoderm, endoderm) are different. In the skin, for example, the basement membrane zone (BMZ) within the DEJ lies between an ectodermal tissue (epidermis) and a mesodermal tissue (dermis). Therefore, BMZs are sites of interactions between ectoderm and mesoderm and between epithelial cells and extracellular matrix.

The importance of BMZs in the structure and function of skin has been recently reviewed by several authors [1–5] and encompasses both theoretical implications directed to the ultimate understanding of cutaneous biology to the more practical considerations of understanding the pathomechanisms of blistering diseases of the skin and wound healing. In brief, BMZs are important to the understanding of cutaneous biology for at least three reasons: They serve as a permeability barrier, they influence cell behavior (e.g., division and locomotion), and, they are critical for dermal–epidermal adherence.

ULTRASTRUCTURE

Until the late 1970s, basement membrane in the skin was largely described only by light and electron microscopy. A comprehensive and still largely current description of skin BMZ can be found in a review by Briggaman and Wheeler [2]. On light microscopic examination, vertical sections of skin stained with a periodic acid Schiff stain (PAS) labeled the BMZ lying between the epidermis and dermis a light pink color [2]. It is still unclear exactly what ultrastructural components or molecular species are localized within the PAS-positive basement membrane or exactly what is and is not labeled by the PAS stain. When this zone, the so-called epidermal-dermal junction (DEJ), was examined with the electron microscope, four distinct components were defined (Figs. 4.1, 4.2). The first of these was the **plasma membrane of the basal keratinocyte** juxtaposed to the BMZ proper. The plasma membrane of the keratinocyte is much more complex at sites of the hemidesmosomes. In this region, tonofilaments composed of cytokeratins converge on an electron-dense thickened area within the plasma membrane called the attachment plaque, which is about 15 nm in diameter [2]. Although variable from specimen to specimen, usually one sees retractions within the plasma membrane of the basal keratinocytes in which small amounts of amorphous material appear to be accumulated. These retractions have been called pinocytotic vesicles [2]. Their composition, nature, and function are not known. It is not clear what induces or modulates pinocytotic vesicles. However, Hay and colleagues [6] demonstrated that juxtaposition of epidermal cells with matrix molecules (collagens I–IV, laminin, fibronectin) would decrease the number of epidermal cell projections and blebs within the plasma membrane when compared to a nitrocellulose matrix coated with albumin, IgG, hyaluronic acid, or proteoglycans [6].

The next ultrastructurally defined component of the BMZ beneath the basal cell plasma membrane is the **lamina lucida**. This is an electron-lucent zone approximately 35 nm in diameter. In areas immediately beneath hemidesmosomes a few very delicate fibrils can be seen in a parallel array that is perpendicular to the hemidesmosomes. These fine fibrils that cross the lamina lucida zone have been termed anchoring filaments [2]. The biochemical nature and function of anchoring filaments have not been determined.

The biochemical composition of the lamina lucida region is discussed below. One of the interesting aspects of the dermal–epidermal junction is that the lamina lucida zone appears to be the area that is the most readily fractured [2, 7]. When skin blisters are induced by suction, friction, or freezing, the split within the dermal–epidermal junction occurs within the lamina lucida space. The same phenomenon is seen *in vitro* when various laboratory procedures (such as trypsinization, salt incubation, or warming) are used to fracture the dermal–epidermal junction [7]. The lamina lucida space could be regarded as the Achilles heel of the dermal–epidermal junction.

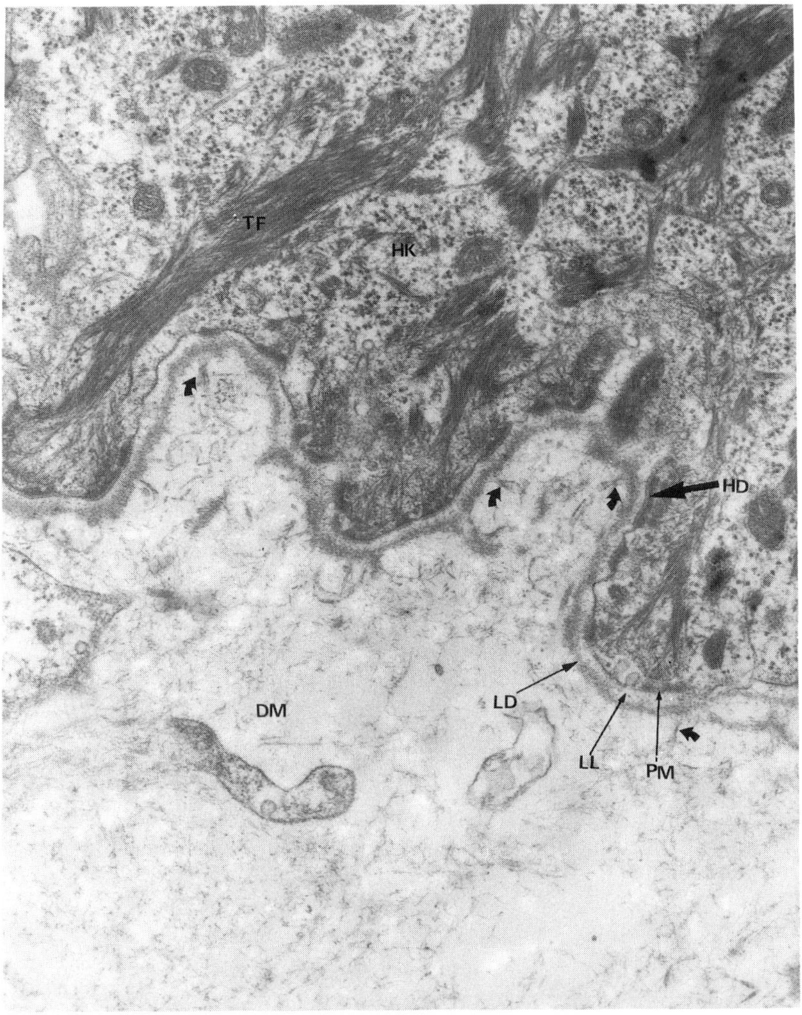

Figure 4.1 Electron micrograph of the basement membrane zone (BMZ) of human skin. The epidermal–dermal junction is formed by the basal human keratinocytes (HK) apposed to the dermis (DM). This junction has a complex structure when viewed with the electron microscope and consists of the plasma membrane (PM) of the basal HK, an electron lucent zone called the *lamina lucida* (LL), a 35–50 nm electron dense zone called the lamina densa (LD), and a sub-lamina densa fibrillar zone containing single collagen fibrils, microfibrils, and 50–250 nm ''wheat stack''-shaped structures aligned perpendicularly to and touching the LD called anchoring fibrils (short, curved arrows). Within the basal human keratinocyte (HK), tonofilaments (TF) can be seen converging toward hemidesmosomes (HD) (× 31,000).

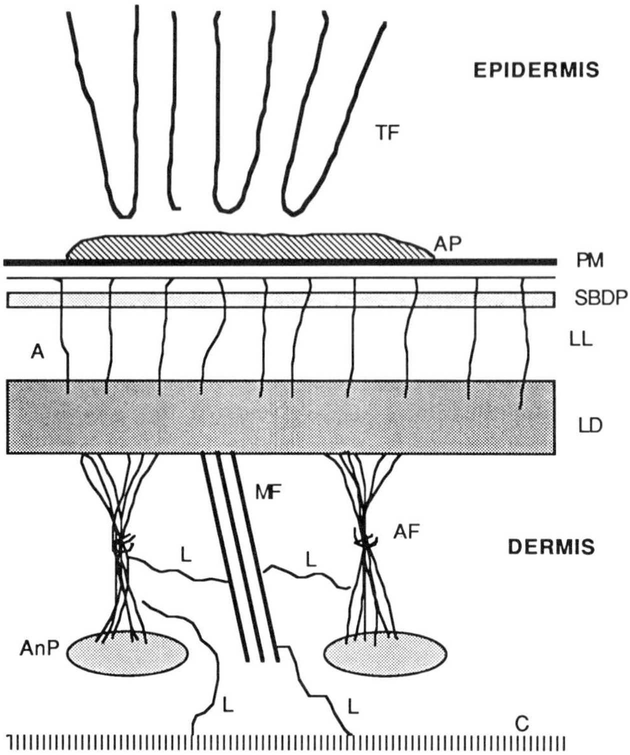

Figure 4.2 Schematic diagram of the ultrastructural components of the dermal–epidermal junction. Within the basal keratinocytes, tonofilaments (TF) converge toward the attachment plaques (AP), which are components of hemidesmosomes. PM, plasma membrane of basal keratinocyte; SBDP, sub-basal dense plaque of hemidesmosome; LL, lamina lucida; A, anchoring filaments; LD, lamina densa; MF, microfibrils; AF, anchoring fibrils; L, linkin; AnP, anchoring plaque; C, single dermal collagen fibers.

Beneath the lamina lucida space is the **lamina densa**, an electron-dense zone that is 35–50 nm in diameter. Some authors consider the lamina densa the basement membrane proper and others have called this structure the *basal lamina* rather than lamina densa. We prefer to use the term *lamina densa* because it is easy to remember, and the term has a certain logical symmetry with the term *lamina lucida*. Although the lamina densa is rich in basement membrane collagen (see below) it does not appear fibrillar when viewed with the electron microscope. Rather, it appears somewhat amorphous and granular. Some investigators have liken its appearance to that of a felt tip pen [1]. The lamina densa is a very stable structure, but occasionally gaps and reduplications of the structure may be seen in normal skin [2].

Beneath the lamina densa is a rather complex, less well defined zone called the **sub-lamina densa fibrillar zone**. The three main fibrillar structures are anchoring fibrils, microfibril bundles related to elastic fibers, and single collagen fibers [2]. In addition to these three main components, the sub-lamina densa fibrillar zone is rich in a newly described, noncollagenous matrix molecule called **linkin** that is a protein associated with microthread-like fibers that stain with ruthenium red [8].

Anchoring fibrils are shaped like sheaves of wheat bundled together in the middle. Anchoring fibrils are between 50 and 200 nm in length, and their gathered middle portion has a cross-banded appearance [2, 9, 10]. The majority of anchoring fibrils are found apposed or nearly apposed to the lamina densa at one end and hang perpendicularly off the lamina densa [2, 9, 10]. It must be remembered, however, that this apposition to the lamina densa when viewed ultrastructurally depends upon a good vertical cut of the tissue with minimal effacement. Some anchoring fibrils are seen in normal skin that are not connected to the lamina densa but appear to be lying loose in the upper papillary dermis. Some of these loose anchoring fibrils may be from reduplications of the lamina densa or the natural remodeling of the BMZ. As an alternative, some of these ''loose'' anchoring fibrils may actually be in contact with BMZ lying behind the plane of the cut section and not ''loose'' at all from BMZ.

In addition to the discovery of linkin (see above), another newly described component of the sub-lamina densa fibrillar zone is the anchoring plaque [10]. The anchoring plaque was first described by Keene and colleagues [10] and appears as amorphous, electron-dense, oval blobs beneath the lamina densa [10]. The size of a single anchoring plaque is approximately 200 × 170 nm. The distance from the lamina densa is variable and also depends upon what tissue is examined. In human neonatal foreskin, the average distance of the anchoring plaque from the lamina densa is 341 nm [10]. Anchoring plaques have not yet been isolated and purified, so their exact biochemical nature is unknown. However, immunologic labeling studies have shown that they contain both type IV and type VII collagen [10]. It appears that anchoring plaques are connected to the lamina densa by anchoring fibrils [10]. In other words, anchoring fibrils form a bridge between the lamina densa and anchoring plaques. This connection may play a role in ''anchoring'' the lamina densa to the papillary dermis.

BIOCHEMICAL COMPOSITION

Until the late 1970s very little information was known about the biochemical nature of skin BMZ. Since that time there has been a proliferation of knowledge and many of the major BMZ components have been defined. An updated, detailed review of the structure and biological activity of BMZ proteins has recently been published by Timpl [4]. The components discussed herein include the bullous pemphigoid antigen, laminin, entactin (also called nidogen), type IV collagen, the heparan sulfate proteoglycans, the epidermolysis bullosa acquisita (EBA) antigen (type VII collagen), and linkin (Fig. 3).

The Bullous Pemphigoid Antigen

Patients with the subepidermal blistering disease, bullous pemphigoid (BP), have IgG and complement deposits within the dermal–epidermal junction [11–15]. These patients have a circulating autoantibody in plasma that binds to a normal constituent of human skin basement membrane that has been termed the bullous pemphigoid antigen (BPAg). For many years, the nature of this component was totally unknown. Holubar and colleagues [11] and Schaumberg-Lever and colleagues [12] found that the IgG deposits in the skin of patients with BP were localized to the lamina lucida zone of the DEJ. More recently, Mutasim et al. [13], Regnier et al. [14], and Westgate et al. [15] demonstrated that there is

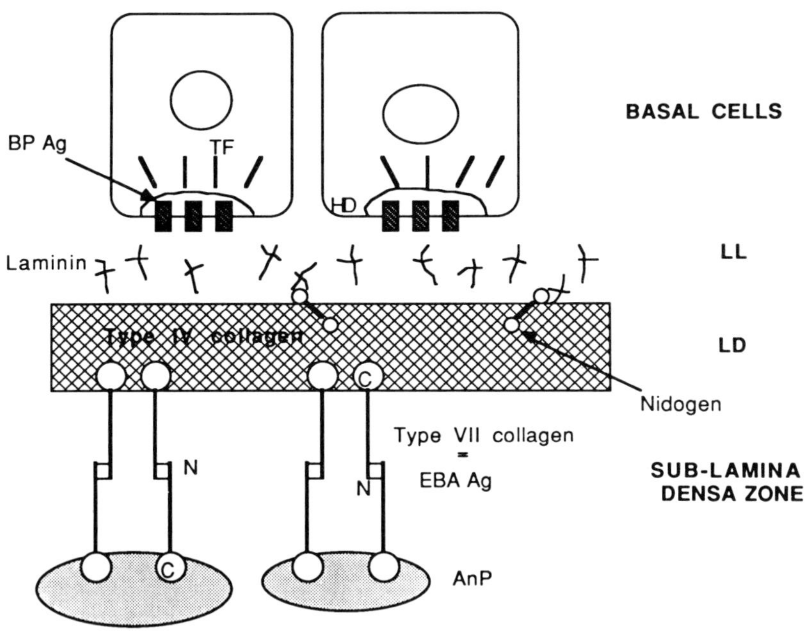

Figure 4.3 Biochemical components of the dermal–epidermal junction. BPAg, bullous pemphigoid antigen; HD, hemidesmosome; LL, lamina lucida; LD, lamina densa; EBA Ag, epidermolysis bullosa acquisita antigen (type VII "anchoring fibril" collagen); AnP, anchoring plaque; C, carboxyl terminus of type VII collagen; N, amino terminus of type VII collagen; TF, tonofilaments converging on the hemidesmosome of the basal keratinocytes.

also an intracellular pool of BP antigen associated with the basal keratinocyte hemidesmosome. It is likely that the BP antigen is a transmembrane glycoprotein with both intracellular and extracellular domains. Human and murine keratinocytes in culture synthesize the BP antigen [16–18]. In culture, the number of keratinocytes expressing BP antigen is almost identical to the number of basal keratinocytes in the cultures [18]. When keratinocyte cultures are labeled with [^{35}S]methionine or other radioactive amino acids and the cell layer extracted with nonionic detergent and neutral buffer, the BP antigen can be immunoprecipitated with anti-BMZ autoantibodies in the serum of patients with BP. The precipitated proteins have a molecular weight of 230,000 daltons and are noncollagenous proteins [17]. An identical protein can be extracted from isolated human epidermis and detected by a Western immunoblot labeled with BP antibodies [19]. In addition to the major 230,000 dalton BP antigen, another band between 160,000 and 180,000 daltons is labeled by some BP sera [20]. The 230 kDa BP antigen has been termed bullous pemphigoid antigen 1 (BPAG1) and the 180 kDa BP antigen [20] has been termed bullous pemphigoid antigen 2 (BPAG2) [21]. Both antigens have been shown to be localized within hemidesmosomes of basal keratinocytes [22–24]. However, BPAG1 and BPAG2 have both been cloned [22, 27–29] and are clearly distinct constituent components of the hemidesmosome. The gene for BPAG1 is localized to the short arm of chromosome 6 (locus 6p11–12) [29] while the gene for BPAG2 is localized to the long arm of chromosome 10 (locus 10q24.3) [30]. Moreover, both BP antigens have been cloned and the deduced amino acid sequences show no sequence homology. Although BP antigen was originally thought to be noncollagenous in nature, recent cloning data reveal nucleotide sequences within the BPAG2 gene that encode for Gly-X-Y sequences typical for helical collagen chains [26, 30]. Morrison and co-workers [31] have shown that the 180 kDa BP antigen is the target for autoantibodies in patients with herpes gestationis.

Laminin

Laminin is a large, noncollagenous protein within all BMZs [1–5]. Laminin is localized in the lamina lucida space within skin BMZ [32] and the lamina densa space in kidney BMZ [33]. Approximately 10–15 % of the molecular mass of laminin is carbohydrate [4]. Its overall molecular size is about 900 kDa, and it has a cruciate shape when viewed by rotary shadowing electron microscopy [4]. When denatured, reduced, and electrophoresed on sodium dodecyl sulfate (SDS) polyacrylaminde gels, (SDS-Page) laminin is identified by two characteristic broad bands (MW, 400,000 and 200,000, respectively). The bands correspond to the single, large A chain (400 kDa) flanked by two smaller B chains (200–230 kDa). These three chains are held together in a cruciate structure by disulfide bonds at the center of the molecule [1–5]. The amino acid sequence of the three chains have been determined, and it appears that the three chains are linked together at their globular carboxyl termini [4]. The B chains are aligned in parallel with the A chain, which they flank for about half the length of the A chain and then diverge away from it at right angles. This forms the cruciate structure, and the "short arms" are actually the amino termini of the three chains [4]. There are two globular domains near the ends of each of the chains that have been identified both by rotary shadowing and sequence data. The overall length of the laminin is about 80 nm and each arm is about 37 nm long. The tertiary structures of the three chains are varied with globular structures, alpha helical segments, rod-like segments, and cyteine-rich repeat areas [4].

Laminin has a variety of biological functions [4, 34]. One of its most important functions is the promotion of BMZ assembly [4]. Laminin has discrete domains that specifically adhere to other BMZ matrix molecules [4, 34, 35]. Laminin binds to type IV collagen by one of the globular domains on the short arms and this affinity may be mediated by nidogen (see below) [4]. Laminin also binds to heparin and basement membrane heparan sulfate proteoglycan [4] by the globular domain on the carboxyl terminus of the A chain linked to the two B chains as well as by domains in the center of the cross and on the short arms [4]. These areas of specific affinity could serve to organize multiple macromolecules into a structural BMZ that has sites for cell attachment.

Laminin has multiple biological properties [4, 34–36] in addition to its role of linking other molecules together within the BMZ and cell attachment. Laminin has been shown to induce neurite outgrowth in cultures of neuronal cells [36, 37] and serve as a haptotactic molecule for a variety of cell types [36]. Both normal human keratinocytes and fibroblasts are capable of synthesizing laminin [38]. Laminin may serve as an attachment factor for certain epithelial cells and mediate cell attachment to basement membrane collagen [34, 36]. It was recently, found that melanoma cell metastasis may be influenced by the ability of the malignant cell to attach to laminin [39]. In the B-1 laminin arm, near its approximation with the A chain, there is an amino acid sequence of tyrosine–isoleucine–glycine–serine–arginine = (YIGSR), which is the site within the laminin molecule recognized by the melanoma cell for attachment to laminin. When melanoma cells in suspension were first incubated in solutions of YIGSR peptide, the ability of the cells to metastasize to lung after injection into the tail vein of a mouse was markedly reduced [39]. The investigators hypothesized that this was due to a competitive inhibition for the laminin receptor site on the melanoma cell: YIGSR was thought to bind to the laminin receptor and thereby make the receptor unavailable or nonfunctional for binding to authentic BMZ laminin in the animal. This would render the cell unable to bind to the animal's BMZ and without attachment to BMZ within blood vessels, the malignant cells could not invade host tissues such as lung [39]. When the same melanoma cells were incubated with peptides with small changes in the YIGSR sequence, the inhibition of metastasis did not occur, suggesting that this specific sequence was necessary for the cell to recognize and bind through its cell receptor for laminin. This is an exciting and rapidly developing area in the possible prevention of cancer metastasis. Another RGD, "integrin" type of sequence has been found on the laminin molecule that also serves a role in cell attachment [40].

It has been found recently that human keratinocytes will migrate on fibronectin and collagen types I and IV, but that the addition of laminin will inhibit keratinocyte locomotion. While laminin appears to inhibit keratinocyte locomotion, it is not toxic to the cells and does not inhibit keratinocyte growth [41]. It may be that laminin has a role in re-epithelialization of wounds and is expressed when the wound has been covered by migrating keratinocytes, and now needs to be directed to stop migrating and establish a stable epithelium.

Nidogen/Entactin

Nidogen and entactin are synonyms for the same molecule [4]. Nidogen/entactin is a highly sulfated, noncollagenous glycoprotein found in all BMZs including those of skin. This matrix molecule is shaped like a small dumbbell with two globular ends separated by a short rod [4]. The length of the molecule is around 27 nm, with the central rod having a length of about 17 nm [4]. Like laminin, nidogen/entactin contains carbohydrate (about 5% of its weight), but unlike laminin, which only has N linked carbohydrates, the carbohydrate moieties are linked to nidogen/entactin by both N and O links [4]. On SDS-polyacrylamide gels nidogen/entactin migrates around 148–158 kDa. Nidogen/entactin has been cloned and found to have EGF-like repeats [4] within the central rod portion and the globular domain at the carboxyl end. It also has an RGD (arginine–glycine–D-aspartic acid) sequence in the central rod-like domain [4, 42]. Therefore, it is likely that nidogen/entactin either alone or complexed with laminin is biologically very active. Nidogen/entactin forms complexes with laminin and binds to laminin by one of its globular domains [4, 42]. The binding site on laminin for nidogen/entactin is near the central portion of one of the short arms [4]. It has been shown that nidogen/entactin has affinity for type IV collagen [4]. Therefore, nidogen/entactin may play a role in complexing laminin and type IV collagen together [4].

There are very few data available about the function of nidogen/entactin in human skin. Caughman and colleagues [43] have shown by immunoelectron microscopy that nidogen/entactin is localized in the lamina densa zone of human skin basement membrane.

Anchoring Filament Proteins

Beneath the hemidesmosomes of the basal keratinocytes, one observes with the electron microscope thin fibers called anchoring filaments that traverse the lamina lucida space. Recently, several laboratories have developed antibodies that label anchoring filaments and putative anchoring filament proteins [44–47]. These proteins have been called epiligrin [44], kalinin [45], BM600/nicein [46], and 19-DEJ-1 [47]. Kalinin and BM600/nicein are the same protein (unpublished information, Robert A. Burgeson). It is conceivable that epiligrin and 19-DEJ-1 are also identical or closely related to kalinin and BM600/nicein [48]. It is interesting that all of the components (whether identical or not) have been found to be absent in patients with severe junctional epidermolysis bullosa. Moreover, epiligrin and kalinin have been shown to support cell attachment in vitro, and epiligrin has been shown to be the main ligand for the $\alpha 3\beta 1$ integrin receptor. Therefore, it is very likely that these anchoring filament proteins are important for epidermal–dermal adhesion. Recently, two patients with a scarring, cicatricial pemphigoid-like disease have been identified who have circulating autoantibodies to epiligrin and BM600/nicein, which are, according to these authors, identical proteins [48].

Type IV Collagen

Type IV collagen is specifically found only in BMZs and is localized to the lamina densa region [1–5]. Its molecular shape is reminiscent of a hockey stick with a soft ball stuck on the end of the handle [1–5] (see Chap. 1). This globular end (called NC1) corresponds to the carboxyl terminus and the hockey stick blade corresponds to the amino terminus, which is highly resistant to collagenase and has been termed 7S collagen [1, 4]. Between the globular carboxyl terminus and the 7S terminus is a rod-like domain consisting of both typical alpha helix regions and nonhelical regions that are thought to give the molecule flexibility but also make it more susceptible to noncollagenase protease degradation. Human keratinocytes are capable of synthesizing type IV collagen [1, 49]. The composition of type IV collagen is two alpha 1 chains intertwined with one alpha 2 chain, which, when denatured and reduced for SDS-polyacrylamide gel electrophoresis, are identified as bands of 185 kDa and 170 kDa [1–5]. Type IV collagen molecules aggregate with one another by end-to-end links and by side-to-side aggregations [50] and form a "chicken wire-like" network [1, 4]. One of the main functions of type IV collagen is thought to be its role as a scaffold-like structure for other BMZ components and to provide structure and tensile strength to the BMZ. The helical domains are extremely stable and would provide stability and strength while the nonhelical domains would allow a degree of flexibility to the tissue [51].

Human keratinocytes cultured on a type IV collagen substratum migrate and form linear tracks [41]. A type IV collagen matrix also promotes keratinocyte attachment, growth, and spreading [52]. Human keratinocytes cultured on type IV collagen also exhibit enhanced collagenase synthesis when compared to laminin or tissue culture plastic substrata [53]. In addition to synthesizing type IV collagen, human keratinocytes in a migratory mode are capable of synthesizing a metalloprotease that specifically degrades type IV (basement membrane) collagen [54]. This may have implications in wound healing and in tissue invasion by keratinocyte-derived tumors. Type IV collagen in the skin may play other roles besides its structural role since it appears to be capable of modulating the biological behavior of human keratinocytes.

Heparan Sulfate Proteoglycans

Proteoglycans are macromolecules present in varying amounts in all connective tissues. They are primarily extracellular, although intracellular and cell membrane proteoglycans have been described. They are composed of polysaccharides (glycosaminoglycans) covalently attached to a protein core (see Chap. 2). Among them, heparan sulfate proteoglycans (HSPG) have been identified in basement membranes [1, 2, 4]. The cores of these proteoglycans are antigenically unique and can be differentiated from those of cell surface heparan sulfate proteoglycans [1]. Basement membrane heparan sulfate proteoglycans have been characterized from a variety of sources such as kidney glomerulus, aorta, cultured cells, and tumor cell lines [4]. Structural studies of heparan sulfate proteoglycans from the basement membrane-producing Engelbreth-Holm-Swarm tumor (EHS) have demonstrated a high-and a low-density form of the proteoglycan [4]. The HSPG is the most highly charged component in the basement membrane and is considered to be important in regulating the charge-dependent selective filtration properties of basement membranes [55]. Binding of the low-density proteoglycan to the end of the long arm of laminin and to two regions in the collagen IV triple helix (210 nm and 80 nm away from the NC1 domain) has been demonstrated by Laurie et al. [56].

Type VII Collagen/EBA Antigen

It is now clear that the EBA antigen and type VII collagen are synonymous [57]. However, it is likely that the most antigenic site on the type VII collagen molecule is the carboyxl globular domain (unpublished observation). Sakai and colleagues [58] showed that anchoring fibrils consist of type VII collagen. Keene et al. [10] showed by immunoelectron microscopy that type VII collagen aligned into anchoring fibrils forms a bridge between the lamina densa zone of BMZ and anchoring plaques (see above) localized within the upper papillary dermis. Type VII collagen chains are between 280 to 320 kDa, depending upon the tissue of origin and extraction conditions [41, 42]). Three chains form a helix and the size of the native molecule is around 900 kDa.

The shape of type VII collagen monomers is thought to be reminiscent of a baton with a ball stuck on one end, which would correspond to the noncollagenous carboxyl domain [10]. The noncollagen domain is approximately half the molecular mass since degradation of isolated type VII collagen chains with bacterial collagenase produces a 145 kDa species that is highly collagenase resistant [59]. Monoclonal antibodies have been made to the globular noncollagenous amino domain, and immunoelectron microscopic studies have shown that this end of the molecule is lodged within the lamina densa while the collagenous helical domain lies perpendicular to the lamina densa and projects down into the papillary dermis [13]. A second type VII collagen molecule is linked like-end to like-end by the carboxyl termini and projects further down into the papillary dermis, with its noncollagenous amino terminus at the most inward position lodged into an anchoring plaque [13]. It is also known that type VII collagen binds to the collagen-binding domain of fibronectin, a major dermal glycoprotein [60]. This complex conformation and complexing of lamina densa to anchoring plaques via an anchoring fibril bridge in addition to an interaction with fibronectin probably accounts for the extreme stability of this part of skin and firmly anchors the lamina densa to the papillary dermis.

Human keratinocytes and fibroblasts synthesize type VII collagen/EBA antigen in culture [61, 62]. The tissue of origin *in vivo* is unclear. It may be that under certain conditions type VII collagen/EBA antigen may be synthesized by keratinocytes while in another situation fibroblasts contribute to its synthesis. Another critical question is the relationship between type VII collagen detected by immunologic or biochemical methods and the formation of bona fide anchoring fibril structures as detected by electron microscopy and tested functionally by suction blistering times. We have shown recently that in certain wound healing situations, such as dermabrasion or burn wounds healed by the use of cultured keratinocyte autografts, type VII collagen synthesis can readily be detected when good ultrastructural anchoring fibrils have only minimally formed and are functionally deficient [63]. Anchoring fibrils are deficient in patients with recessive dystrophic epidermolysis bullosa (RDEB) [64]. In addition, certain epitopes of type VII collagen and other less well defined BMZ components have been found to be absent [65]. However, Rusenko and colleagues [66] have definitively shown that the amino domain of the type VII collagen molecule in these patients is present within the lamina densa and easily detected by immunofluorescent methods. In patients with RDEB, synthesis of type VII collagen is occurring but the formation of well-formed, functional anchoring fibrils is depressed, probably by rapid destruction or turnover of these structures.

Human skin collagenase has been shown to be increased in fibroblast cultures from patients with RDEB [67]. This collagenase is known to be concentrated within skin high in the papillary dermis where anchoring fibrils and anchoring plaques are located. Type VII collagen has been shown to be degraded by human skin collagenase [68], and it is conceivable that enhanced skin collagenase by some unknown mechanism is responsible for poorly formed anchoring fibrils in patients with RDEB, other bullous dermatoses, and early wound healing. Recently, it has been shown that human keratinocytes in culture synthesize significant quantities of collagenase (0.11 μg/10,000 cells/min) and that migration on collagen or stimulation with tetradecanoyl phorbol acetate (TPA) can boost collagenase synthesis by these cells [37, 69]. The role of keratinocyte-derived collagenase in the pathomechanisms of diseases such as RDEB or wound healing is yet to be determined.

There is good, albeit indirect, evidence that autoantibodies to the EBA antigen are pathogenic. First, Gammon and colleagues [70] have shown *in vitro* using organ cultures of human skin that DEJ separation can be induced when EBA antibodies, complement, and human neutrophils are added to the system. It has also been shown in vitro that EBA antibody complexed with EBA antigen and complement will induce human neutrophils to migrate to these complexes and line up along the BMZ [70]. Moreover, when patients with systemic lupus erythematosus (SLE), who are known to make autoantibodies to nuclear components and a variety of tissues, begin making autoantibodies to the EBA antigen, they very often begin to have a blistering skin eruption and their condition falls into the subclass of SLE called bullous SLE [71]. Although classic passive transfer experiments with EBA antibodies have not yet been accomplished, the data to date, taken together, would suggest that EBA antibodies are, in fact, pathogenic, meaning that they play a role in the disruption of epidermal–dermal function. However, the mechanistic details of how EBA antibodies, complexed with antigen within the BMZ, actually induce disadherence of the epidermis from the dermis are unclear. Since EBA patients may fracture their DEJ either below the lamina densa or within the lamina lucida, perhaps more than one mechanism is involved.

Linkin

Microthread-like fibrils that were first noted beneath rat tracheal epithelium [72] have recently been described in human skin [9, 10, 73]. The microthread-like fibrils are 80–90 nm in length, stain with ruthenium red, and appear as delicate strands that "link" various components within the BMZ and papillary dermis together, such as anchoring fibrils, microfibril bundles, anchoring plaques, and single collagen fibers [9, 10, 73]. A new monoclonal antibody has been shown by immunogold labeling and electron microscopy to label these delicate structures. When human skin BMZ proteins are extracted with urea or guanidine hydrochloride, separated by SDS-PAGE, transferred to nitrocellulose paper, and labeled with this new antibody (Western immunoblotting procedure), two protein bands are identified of 83 and 73 kDa. These newly identified proteins associated with microthread-like fibrils have been termed *linkin*. Linkin is synthesized by fibroblasts and is noncollagenous in nature. The role of linkin in human skin and disease states is only beginning to be defined. Recent preliminary data would suggest that linkin may be important during the reconstitution of dermis in wounds and the formation of dermis during gestation (unpublished data).

REFERENCES

1. Stanley JR, Woodley DT, Katz SI, Martin GR. The structure and function of basement membrane. J Invest Dermatol 1982; 79:69–72.
2. Briggaman RA, Wheeler CE. The epidermal–dermal junction. J Invest Dermatol 1975; 65:71–84.
3. Woodley DT. The importance of the dermal–epidermal junction and recent advances. Dermatologica 1987; 174: 1–10.
4. Timpl R. Structure and biological activity of basement membrane proteins. Eur J Biochem 1989; 180:487–502.
5. Uitto J, Olsen DR, Frzio MJ. Extracellular matrix of the skin—50 years of progress. J Invest Dermatol (suppl) 1989; 92:61s–77s.
6. Sugrue SP, Hay ED. Response of basal epithelial cell surface and cytoskeleton to solubilized extracellular matrix molecules. J Cell Biol 1981; 91:45–54.
7. Woodley DT, Sauder D, Talley MJ, Silver M, Grotendorst G, Qwarnstrom E. Localization of basement membrane components after dermo-epidermal junction separation. J Invest Dermatol 1983; 81:149–52.
8. Briggaman RA, Yoshiike, T, Woodley DT, Gammon WR, Cronce DJ. Linkin, a newly recognized component of extracellular matrix associated with microthread-like filamentous network beneath stratified squamous epithelium. J Cell Biol 1988; 107:590a.
9. Tidman MJ, Eady RA. Ultrastructural morphometry of normal human dermal-epidermal junction. The influence of age, sex, and body region on laminar and nonlaminar components. J Invest Dermatol 1984; 83:448–53.
10. Keene DR, Sakai LY, Lunstrum GP, Morris NP, Burgeson RE. Type VII collagen forms an extended network of anchoring fibrils. J Cell Biol 1987; 104:611–21.
11. Holubar K, Wolff K, Konrad K, Beutner EH. Ultrastructural localization of immunoglobulins in bullous pemphigoid skin. J Invest Dermatol 1975; 64:220–7.
12. Schaumburg-Lever G, Rule RA, Schmidt-Ullrich B, Lever WF. Ultrastructural localization of in vivo bound immunoglobulins in bullous pemphigoid: a preliminary report. J Invest Dermatol 1975; 64:47–9.
13. Mutasim DF, Takahashi Y, Ramzy LS, Anhalt GJ, Patel HP, Diaz LA. A pool of bullous pemphigoid antigen(s) is intracellular and associated with the basal cell cytoskeleton-hemidesmosome complex. J Invest Dermatol 1985; 84:47–53.
14. Regnier M, Vaigot P, Michel S, Prunieras M. Localization of bullous pemphigoid antigen in isolated human keratinocytes. J Invest Dermatol 1985; 85:187–90.
15. Westgate GE, Weaver AC, Couchman JR. Bullous pemphigoid antigen localization suggests an intracellular association with hemidesmosomes. J Invest Dermatol 1985; 84:218–24.
16. Woodley DT, Didierjean L, Regnier M, Saurat JH, Prunieras M. Bullous pemphi-

goid antigen synthesized in vitro by human epidermal cells. J Invest Dermatol 1980; 75:148–51.
17. Stanley JR, Hawley-Nelson P, Yuspa SH, Shevach EM, Katz SI. Characterization of bullous pemphigoid antigen: a unique basement membrane protein of stratified squamous epithelia. Cell 1981; 24:897–904.
18. Woodley DT, Saurat JH, Prunieras M, Regnier M. Pemphigoid, pemphigus, and Pr antigens in human keratinocytes grown on nonviable substrates. J Invest Dermatol 1982; 79:23–9.
19. Stanley JR, Woodley DT, Katz SI. Identification and partial characterization of pemphigoid antigen extracted from normal skin. J Invest Dermatol 1984; 82:108–11.
20. Labib RS, Anhalt GJ, Patel HP, Mutasim DF, Diaz LA. Molecular heterogeneity of the bullous pemphigoid antigens as detected by immunoblotting. J Immunol 1986; 136:1231–4.
21. Meyer LJ, Taylor MS, Kadunce DP, Zone JJ. Two groups of bullous pemphigoid antigens are identified by affinity-purified antibodies. J Invest Dermatol 1990; 94:611–6.
22. Diaz LA, Ratrie H, Saunders WS, Futamura S, Squiquera HL, Anhalt GJ, Giudice GJ. Isolation of a human epidermal cDNA corresponding to the 180 kD autoantigen recognized by bullous pemphigoid and herpes gestationis sera. Immunolocalization of this protein to the hemidesmosome. J Clin Invest 1990; 86:1088–94.
23. Klatte DH, Kurpakus MA, Jones JC. Immunochemical characterization of three components of the hemidesmosome and their expression in cultured epithelial cells. J Cell Biol 1989; 109:337–9.
24. Mutasim DF, Takahashi Y, Labib RS, Anhalt GJ, Patel HP, Diaz LA. A pool of bullous pemphigoid antigen is intracellular and associated with the basal cell cytoskeleton-hemidesmosome complex. J Invest Dermatol 1985; 84:47–73.
25. Stanley JR, Tanaka T, Mueller S, Klaus-Kovtun V, Roop D. Isolation of cDNA for bullous pemphigoid antigen by use of patient's autoantibodies. J Clin Invest 1988; 82:1864–70.
26. Giudice G, Squiquera HL, Elias PM, Diaz LA. Identification of two collagen domains within the bullous pemphigoid autoantigen, BP180. J Clin Invest 1991; 87:734–8.
27. Sawamura D, Li K, Nomura K, Sugita Y, Christiano AM, Uitto J. Bullous pemphigoid antigen (BPAG1): cDNA cloning, cellular expression, and evidence for polymorphism of the human gene. J Invest Dermatol 96:908–15.
28. Sawamura D, Li K, Chu M-L, Uitto J. Bullous pemphigoid antigen (BPAG1): amino acid sequences deduced from cloned cDNAs predict biologically important peptide segments and protein domains. J Biol Chem 1991; 266:17784–90.
29. Sawamura D, Normura K, Sugita Y, Mattie MG, Chu M-L, Knowlton R, Uitto J. Bullous pemphigoid antigen (BPAG1): cDNA cloning and mapping of the gene to the short arm of human chromosome 6. Genomics 1990; 8:722–6.
30. Li K, Sawamura D, Guidice GJ, Diaz LA, Mattei M-G, Chu M-L, Uitto J. Genomic organization of two collagenous domains and chromosomal assignment of human 180-kD bullous pemphigoid antigen (BPAG2), a novel collagen of stratified squamous epithelium. J Biol Chem–in press.

31. Morrison LH, Labib RS, Zone JJ, Diaz LA, Anhalt GJ. Herpes gestationis autoantibodies recognize a 180 kD human epidermal antigen. J Clin Invest 1988; 81:2023–6.
32. Foidart JM, Bere EW, Yaar M, et al. Distribution and immunoelectron-microscopic localization of laminin, a non-collagenous basement membrane glycoprotein. Lab Invest 1980; 42:336–42.
33. Laurie GW, Leblond CP, Martin GR. Localization of type IV collagen, laminin, heparan sulfate proteoglycan, and fibronectin to the basal lamina of basement membranes. J Cell Biol 1982; 95: 340–4.
34. Kleinman HK, Klebe RJ, Martin GR. Role of collagenous matrices in the adhesion and growth of cells. J Cell Biol 1981; 88: 473–85.
35. Woodley DT, Rao CN, Hassell JR, Liotta LA, Martin GR, Kleinman HK. Interactions of basement membrane components. Biochim Biophys Acta 1983; 761:278–83.
36. Kleinman HK, Cannon FB, Laurie G, Hassel JR, Aumailley M, Terranova VP, Martin GR, Dubois-Dalcq M. Biological activities of laminin. J Cell Biochem 1985; 27:317–25.
37. Engvall E, Davis GE, Dickerson K, Ruoslahti E, Varon M, Manthorpe M. Mapping of domains in human laminin using monoclonal antibodies: localization of the neurite-promoting site. J Cell Biol 1986; 103:2457–65.
38. Woodley DT, Stanley JR, Reese MJ, O'Keefe EJ. Human dermal fibroblasts synthesize laminin. J Invest Dermatol 1988; 90:679–83.
39. Iwamoto Y, Robey FA, Graf J, Sasaki M, Kleinman HK, Yamada Y, Martin GR. YIGSR, a synthetic laminin pentapeptide, inhibits experimental metastasis formation. Science 1987; 238:1132–4.
40. Gehlsen KR, Dillner L, Engvall E, Ruoslahti E. The human laminin receptor is a member of the integrin family of cell adhesion receptors. Science 1988; 241:1228–9.
41. Woodley DT, Bachmann PM, O'Keefe EJ. Laminin inhibits human keratinocyte migration. J Cell Physiol 1988; 136:140–6.
42. Mann K, Deutzmann R, Aumailley M, Timpl R, Raimondi L, Yamada Y, Pan T, Conway D, Chu M-L. Amino acid sequence of mouse nidogen, a multidomain basement membrane protein with binding activity for laminin, collagen IV and cells. EMBO J 1989; 8:65–72.
43. Caughman SW, Krieg T, Timpl R, Hintner H, Katz SI. Nidogen and heparan sulfate proteoglycan: detection of newly isolated basement membrane components in normal and epidermolysis bullosa skin. J Invest Dermatol 1987; 89:547–50.
44. Carter WG, Ryan MC, Gahn PJ. Epiligrin, a new cell adhesion ligand for integrin $\alpha 3\beta 1$ in epithelial basement membranes. Cell 1991; 65:599–610.
45. Rousselle P, Lunstrum GP, Keene DR, Burgeson RE. Kalinin: an epithelium-specific basement membrane adhesion molecule that is a component of anchoring filaments. J Cell Biol 1991; 114:567–76.
46. Verrando P, Hsi BL, Yeh C-J, Pisani A, Serieys N, Ortonne J-P. Monoclonal antibody GB3, a new probe in the study of human basement membranes and hemidesmosomes. Exp Cell Res 1987; 170:116–28.
47. Fine J-D, Horiguchi Y, Couchman JR. 19-DEJ-1, a hemidesmosome-anchoring filament complex-associated monoclonal antibody. Arch Dermatol 1989; 125:520–3.

48. Domloge-Hultsch N, Gammon WR, Briggaman RA, Gil SG, Carter WG, Yancey KB. Epiligrin, the major human keratinocyte (HK) ligand, is targeted by autoantibodies in patients with a form of cicatricial pemphigoid (CP). J Invest Dermatol 1992; 98(4):580 (abstract).
49. Petersen MJ, Woodley DT, O'Keefe EJ. Cultured human keratinocytes synthesize and secrete type IV procollagen. Clin Res 1988; 36:378A.
50. Yurchenco PD, Furthmayr H. Self-assembly of basement membrane collagen. Biochemistry 1984; 23:1839–50.
51. Sage H. Collagens of basement membrane. J Invest Dermatol 1982; 79:51–9s.
52. Woodley DT, Wynn KC, O'Keefe EJ. Type IV collagen and fibronectin enhance human keratinocyte thymidine incorporation and spreading in the absence of soluble growth factors. J Invest Dermatol (in press).
53. Petersen MJ, Woodley DT, Stricklin GP, O'Keefe EJ. Enhanced synthesis of collagenase by human keratinocytes cultured on type I collagen or type IV collagen. J Invest Dermatol 1990; 94:341–346.
54. Woodley DT, Kelebec T, Banes AJ, Link W, Prunieras M, Liotta L. Adult human keratinocytes migrating over nonviable dermal collagen produce collagenolytic enzymes that degrade type I and type IV collagen. J Invest Dermatol 1986; 86:418–23.
55. Farquhar MG, Courtoy PJ, Lemkin MC, Kanwar YS. In: Kuhn K, Shoene HH, Timpl R, eds. New trends in basement membrane research. New York, Raven Press, 1982: 9–29.
56. Laurie GW, Bing JT, Kleinman HK, Hassel JR, Aumailley M, Martin GR, Feldman JR. Localization of binding sites for laminin, heparan sulfate proteoglycan and fibronectin on basement membrane (type IV) collagen. J Mol Biol 1986; 189:205–16.
57. Woodley, DT, Burgeson RE, Lundstrum G, Bruckner-Tuderman L, Reese MJ, Briggaman RA. The epidermolysis bullosa acquisita antigen is the globular carboxyl terminus of type VII procollagen. J Clin Invest 1988; 81:683–7.
58. Sakai LY, Keene DR, Morris NP, Burgeson RE. Type VII collagen is a major structural component of anchoring fibrils. J Cell Biol 1986; 103:1577–86.
59. Yoshike T, Woodley DT, Briggaman RA. Epidermolysis bullosa acquisita antigen; relationship between the collagenase-sensitive and -insensitive domains. J Invest Dermatol 1988; 90:127–33.
60. Woodley DT, O'Keefe EJ, McDonald JA, Reese MJ, Briggaman RA, Gammon WR. Specific affinity between fibronectin and the epidermolysis bullosa acquisita (EBA) antigen. J Clin Invest 1987; 79:1826–30.
61. Woodley DT, Briggaman RA, Gammon WR, O'Keefe EJ. Epidermolysis bullosa acquisita antigen is synthesized by human keratinocytes cultured in serum-free medium. Biochem Biophys Res Commun 1985; 130:1267–72.
62. Stanley JR, Rubinstein N, Klaus-Kortun V. Epidermolysis bullosa acquisita antigen is synthesized by both human keratinocytes and human dermal fibroblasts. J Invest Dermatol 1985; 85:542–5.
63. Woodley DT, Peterson HD, Herzok SR, Stricklin GP, Burgeson RE, Briggaman RA, Cronce DJ, O'Keefe EJ. Burn wounds resurfaced by cultured epidermal autografts show abnormal reconstitution of anchoring fibrils. JAMA 1988; 259:2566–71.
64. Briggaman RA. Is there any specificity to defects of anchoring fibrils in epidermoly-

sis bullosa dystrophica, and what does this mean in terms of pathogenesis? J Invest Dermatol 1985; 84:371–3.
65. Bruckner-Tuderman L, Ruegger S, Odermatt B, Mitsuhashi Y, Schnyder UW. Lack of type VII collagen in unaffected skin of patients with severe recessive dystrophic epidermolysis bullosa. Dermatologica 1988; 176:57–64.
66. Rusenko KW, Gammon WR, Fine JD, Briggaman RA. The carboxyl-terminal domain of type VII collagen is present at the basement membrane in recessive dystrophic epidermolysis bullosa. J Invest Dermatol 1989; 92:623–7.
67. Bauer EA. Recessive dystrophic epidermolysis bullosa: evidence for an altered collagenase in fibroblast cultures. Proc Natl Acad Sci USA 1977; 74:4646–50.
68. Seltzer JL, Eisen AZ, Bauer EA, Morris NP, Glanville RW, Burgeson RE. Cleavage of type VII collagen by interstitial collagenase and type VII collagenase (Gelatinase) derived from human skin. J Biol Chem 1989; 264:3822–6.
69. Petersen MJ, Woodley DT, Stricklin GP, O'Keefe EJ. Production of collagenase by cultured human keratinocytes. J Biol Chem 1987; 262:835–40.
70. Gammon WR, Inman AO III, Wheeler CE Jr. Differences in complement-dependent chemotactic activity generated by bullous pemphigoid and epidermolysis bullosa acquisita immune complexes: demonstration by leukocyte attachment and organ culture methods. J Invest Dermatol 1984; 83:57–61.
71. Gammon WR, Woodley DT, Dole K, Briggaman RA. Evidence that anti-basement membrane zone antibodies in bullous eruption of systemic lupus erythematosus recognize epidermolysis bullosa acquisita autoantigen. J Invest Dermatol 1985; 84:472–6.
72. Wasano K, Yamamoto T. Microthread-like filaments connecting the epithelial basal lamina with underlying fibrillar components of the connective tissue in the rat trachea. Cell Tissue Res 1985; 239:485–95.
73. Yoshiike T, Briggaman RA, Woodley DT, Gammon WR, Cronce DJ. Identification and partial characterization of a microthread-like filamentous network beneath human skin basement membrane zone. J Invest Dermatol 1988; 90:620.

5

Fibronectin

Edward J. O'Keefe
University of North Carolina, Chapel Hill, North Carolina

Because it is a major protein of plasma and can be detected by different kinds of assays, fibronectin was discovered many times over more than 40 years in different laboratories and was known under several different names [1]. It is a large disulfide-linked protein of about 450–500 kilodaltons, depending on its source, and is made up of 2 similar polypeptide chains. It is found both in serum (at about 0.3 mg/ml) and in extracellular matrix. The extracellular matrix form of the protein is secreted by various types of cells, readily self-associates to form large multimers, and appears to be relatively insoluble when purified, whereas the form present in serum, which is secreted by the liver, is quite soluble [2]. As a cell-associated protein, fibronectin acts as an adhesion factor, enabling cells to attach to other proteins through a fibronectin linkage. Because it is a dimer, one arm can attach to cells and the other can attach to one of several other proteins. Furthermore, as a large multimer of many fibronectin molecules, cell-associated fibronectin can form a bridge between cells and numerous other molecules in connective tissue, in a wound, or at the base of a migrating tongue of healing epithelium.

Fibronectin appears to play an important role in both epidermis and dermis in the healing of wounds. Attempts to use fibronectin as a therapeutic agent have produced only modest results, however, and its utility in this respect has not been established. Detailed reviews regarding various aspects of fibronectin including its role in disease [3,4] and specifically in skin [5] have been published recently.

STRUCTURE AND FUNCTION OF THE MOLECULE

Fibronectin is composed of two identical subunits linked by disulfide bonds. Each subunit is organized into physical domains and has discrete binding sites for fibrin, heparin, collagen, DNA, and cells. These sites have been mapped by proteolytically cleaving fibronectin into fragments and then testing the ability of these fragments to bind or to inhibit binding to various proteins. Because the functional (binding) domains are identical with the physical domains produced by proteolytic cleavage, the proteolytic fragments remain functional. By comparing sequence data from complementary DNA clones with sequences determined from the proteolytic fragments, investigators have been able to determine where in the molecule particular binding fragments are located and have constructed the model shown in Figure 5.1. Both plasma and cellular fibronectin are derived from the same gene, an extended gene of as many as 48 exons, and the various fibronectins produced by different cells result from mRNA splicing to produce plasma or cellular fibronetin, which are then posttranslationally modified with sulfates, phosphates, and various carbohydrate chains [6–8]. These modifications presumably have important specific regulatory function but their significance is presently unknown.

The structure of fibronectin is distinctive in that it is composed of repeating homologous units of three types; these repeats, like beads of 10 kilodaltons or less on a chain, are organized into structural domains that give the protein its extended structure. The structural domains are in turn organized into binding sites for various proteins. The purpose of the heparin-binding site on fibronectin may be to bind heparan-containing proteoglycans in basement membranes and tissues. Fibronectin is known to be codistributed with collagen in some tissues and may form a scaffolding for the subsequent laying down of collagen in a

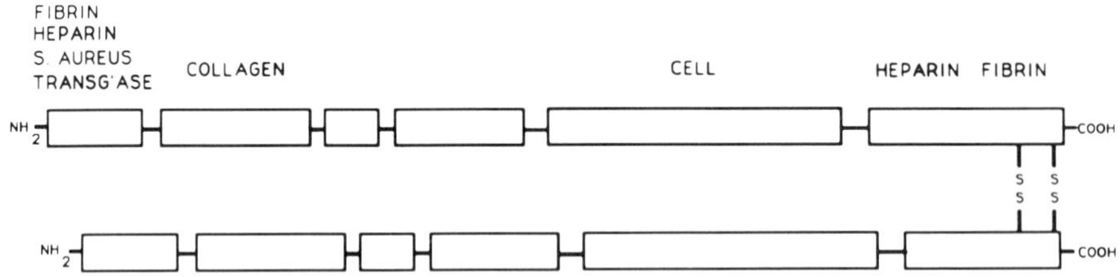

Figure 5.1 Structure of fibronectin. The domains of the molecule that bind other molecules such as cell surface proteins (integrins), matrix molecules (heparin, fibrin, collagen), soluble proteins (transglutaminase), or bacteria are shown, as are the two subunits of the disulfide-linked dimer.

healing wound [9]. Cross-linking of fibronectin to fibrinogen and fibrin presumably gives structural integrity to the fibrin thrombus [10].

Because of major interest in the nature of the cell-binding region of fibronectin, this region was isolated and cleaved into smaller fragments, and then selected regions were synthesized and tested for activity. The cell-binding activity was eventually localized to a tetrapeptide with the sequence Arg-Gly-Asp-Ser (RGDS). This sequence has subsequently been found in several proteins including vitronectin (also known as serum spreading factor or epibolin), fibrinogen, and von Willebrand factor, among others. This sequence binds to one of a family of protein receptors on cells known as integrins, of which the fibronectin receptor is a member. Integrins are composed of two integral membrane proteins, alpha and beta subunits. The variations in the structure of these receptors in different cells determine the specificity of the receptors for various RGDS-containing cell-binding proteins such as fibronectin [11].

The idea that the RGDS sequence is important for binding and biological function of fibronectin has been tested by using small synthetic peptides containing this sequence to try to inhibit biological phenomena such as spreading, attachment, and both in vitro and in vivo migration of cells. These functions have been inhibited in many types of cells in various experimental systems by the peptides, strongly supporting the biological role of the RDGS sequence. Furthermore, mutations in the RGDS-binding sequence of fibronectin obtained using recombinant DNA methods reduce activity by as much as 98%. It has been proposed that fibronectin may help to determine embryonic development by establishing paths for cellular migration required for correct organogenesis [12]; experimental support for this concept is strong. First, addition of RGDS peptide to early embryos triggers the process of compaction, a normal process in which a loose aggregate of cells is stimulated to form a more compact structurally defined architecture required for the development of somites [7]. Second, injection of RDGS peptides into chick embryos inhibits orderly migration of neural crest cells along the neural tube [12].

Extracellular fibronectin fibers appear to be connected to actin bundles in cells, forming a connection between extracellular matrix and the cytoskeleton [13]. This may provide a means for signaling from the environment to the interior of the cell, a means by which fibronectin may modify cellular behavior.

PHYSIOLOGICAL ROLE IN CELL–MATRIX ADHESION

After a wound is created in the dermis, the fibrin thrombus that forms can be shown to contain large amounts of fibronectin, some of which has been covalently cross-linked to fibrin by factor XIII, a transglutaminase present in plasma. Later, as the thrombus becomes organized, invading fibroblasts can attach to collagen by means of fibronectin deposited from serum and can also secrete more fibronectin for this purpose. In mature unwounded skin, fibronectin can be demonstrated throughout the dermis by immunofluorescence microscopy, although more dense staining is present near the basement membrane. In a wound, however, fibronectin staining is markedly enhanced, probably by fibronectin originating from serum, which floods the tissue and binds to collagen, and possibly also from fibroblasts. Fibronectin may also be involved in the recruitment of fibroblasts and inflammatory cells [5].

The action of fibronectin in epidermis also appears to be substantial. Fibronectin secreted into culture as insoluble matrix or as soluble fibronectin has multiple influences on cells; it has been shown to enhance attachment, spreading, migration, directional movement (chemotaxis), and growth of cells in vitro. The first studies were performed on skin fibroblasts, which showed that addition of fibronectin enhanced attachment to plastic surfaces coated with collagen. Later, cells were found to increase their movement, as demonstrated by first coating the surface with visible particles of colloidal gold and noting the paths of the cells through the bed of particles. If a gradient of fibronectin was laid down on a surface, fibroblasts would migrate along the gradient (haptotaxis).

The results of these studies varied according to the type of cell. In the case of epidermal keratinocytes, fibronectin is known to be secreted into the medium as a soluble protein and also deposited as an insoluble matrix [14,15]. Experiments showed that the cells attached and spread, had increased motility (Fig. 5.2), and also proliferated more rapidly on fibronectin-coated surfaces under the proper culture conditions [16–18].

The question of the role of fibronectin in epidermis remained unclear, however, since immunofluorescence studies indicated that there was no fibronectin in mature epithelium, although staining was enhanced in the dermis near the basement membrane region between dermis and epidermis. When a "skin equivalent" composed of collagen with fibroblasts (dermis) and cultured keratinocytes (epidermis) was assembled in vitro, it was shown using monoclonal antibody recognizing only keratinocyte fibronectin that the fibronectin in the region of the basement membrane is derived from the keratinocytes [19]. The epidermis therefore appears to play an active role in producing a fibronectin matrix, which may be important for maintaining attachment to the dermis during wound healing.

After epidermis is wounded, most keratinocytes probably are not able to interact with fibronectin immediately, since freshly obtained keratinocytes attach poorly to fibronectin. After several days, however, the receptor for fibronectin can be demonstrated [20, 21]. A similar phenomenon can be demonstrated in culture, when confluent cells lose the ability to bind to fibronectin until they are recultured at lower density. Emergence of fibronectin receptor function appears to be an important aspect of wound healing in the epidermis [21]. Transforming

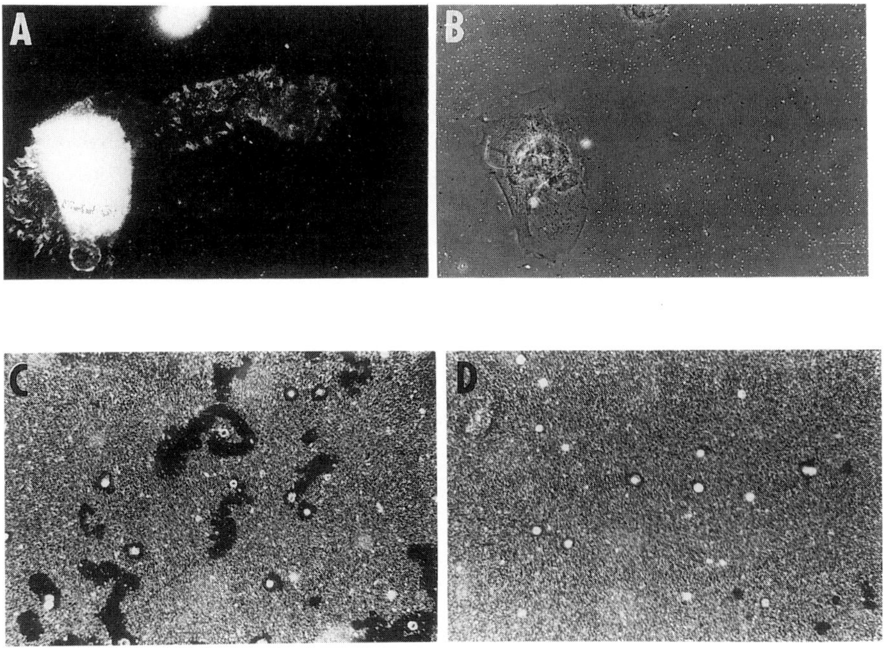

Figure 5.2 Motile keratinocytes lay down a path of fibronectin and are stimulated to move on fibronectin. A. A keratinocyte plated, fixed after 24 h, and stained by indirect immunofluorescence for fibronectin. A trail of fibrillar matrix left behind by the migrating cell is present. B. The same cell viewed under phase-contrast optics; the cell was plated on a bed of colloidal gold particles, which are visible. The particles have been removed from the coverslip by the motile cell in a path corresponding to the trail of fibronectin, indicating that the cell has moved over this area. When a coating of fibronectin was added to the gold particles (C), the keratinocytes were stimulated to move and displaced the gold particles after 24 h; only a few cells moved for short distances in controls (D) without fibronectin (dark-field optics after 24 h).

growth factor-beta, which inhibits keratinocyte growth, can increase synthesis of fibronectin substantially [22] and is the first agent shown to be a major regulator of fibronectin synthesis in keratinocytes.

Fibronectin either secreted or derived from plasma appears early in the establishment of an epidermal covering over a wound exposing the dermis and probably acts as an attachment factor for keratinocytes to dermal collagen. Fibronectin from serum, which is bound to the dermal connective tissue, provides a surface for keratinocyte attachment and, like collagen, provides a stimulus for movement. Once the epidermal covering is established, fibronectin provides a means of attaching the epithelial layer to the dermal tissue before other basement membrane antigens (laminin, type IV collagen, type VII collagen) are secreted by the epidermis and become localized between the epidermis and dermis (as can be demonstrated by immunofluorescence microscopy). Later, when these proteins are assembled into the characteristic structures demonstrated by electron microscopy (lamina lucida, lamina densa, anchoring fibrils, etc.), the fibronectin is largely removed.

OTHER ROLES

It has been proposed that plasma fibronectin, which has different solubility properties and some structural differences from cell-associated fibronectin and which is present in substantial concentration in plasma (about 300 μg/ml), has a unique biological role. Plasma fibronectin is an "opsonic," or coating, protein that facilitates phagocytic clearance by macrophages of particulate substances in blood including collagen, cell fragments, and fibrin. Unlike the opsonic functions of complement or immunoglobulin, which are directed primarily at bacterial substances, fibronectin may facilitate the clearance of nonbacterial debris by fixed macrophages in the liver, spleen, and bone marrow. In addition, fibronectin binds to numerous types of micro-organisms such as *Staphylococcus aureus* and some other bacteria including *Treponema pallidum*, to *Trypanosoma cruzi*, and to some yeasts. In contrast to its function as an opsonin in the case of nonbacterial substances, however, binding to fibronectin does not result in phagocytosis and killing of bacteria. The ability to bind fibronectin may be a mechanism evolved by the micro-organisms for their benefit, possibly to permit adherence to tissue.

In support of the notion that fibronectin may have a physiological role in plasma different from its role as a matrix protein, it has been found that sepsis, surgery, or injury may be associated with reduced ability to opsonize and remove particulate matter from the bloodstream and that this "opsonic deficiency" can be reversed with cryoprecipitate containing fibronectin or purified fibronectin. It has also been proposed that pulmonary vascular permeability experimentally produced in animals by challenge with bacteria is more severe if plasma fibronectin has been depleted (by injection of denatured collagen) and can be corrected by administration of fibronectin [23]. The therapeutic role of fibronectin in parallel clinical situations has not been established.

Plasma fibronectin may also participate in wound healing. For example, fibronectin fragments may mediate phagocytosis in wounds, since fragments of fibronectin, which may be generated in wounds as a result of proteolytic activity, have been shown to be chemotactic for monocytes and macrophages [24], but not for neutrophils. Also, factor XIIIa, plasma transglutaminase, can covalently cross-link fibronectin to fibrin, and may allow plasma fibronectin flooding a wound to remain fixed in the wound to provide a matrix for the subsequent organization of locally secreted collagen during healing (10).

Scleroderma fibroblasts produce increased amounts of fibronectin as well as collagen, but the pathophysiological role of this increase is not known. Since fibronectin fragments are chemotactic, generation of large amounts of such fragments could recruit fibroblasts to sites of scleroderma and further enhance matrix deposition [25]. The possible role of fibronectin in other rheumatic diseases, and the issue of the binding to fibronectin of the complement component C1q, which has a collagenous domain, have been discussed by Carsons et al. [25]. The use of antibody to the ''extra'' domains of fibronectin, which are present in the cellular but not the plasma form, should permit demonstration of the local rather than hepatocellular origin of fibronectin [6] in diseased or healing tissues, which is an issue in studies assessing the role of fibronectin in inflammation. In some cases, similar information should be obtained from examination of mRNA by in situ hybridization, since the complementary DNAs have been cloned.

Despite the potential contribution of fibronectin to healing and morphogenesis, only a modest therapeutic role for fibronectin has been established. Attempts to enhance healing by addition of exogenous fibronectin have not shown striking differences, possibly because of the large amounts of endogenous fibronectin in plasma and the ability of many types of cells to synthesize fibronectin. A preliminary report indicated that cutaneous ulcers may be helped by topical application of fibronectin [26], and experimental corneal lesions in rabbits may show more rapid healing. Contamination of fibronectin preparations with small amounts of potent growth factors has not been excluded, however, in these studies [3]. Because such large amounts of fibronectin are present in wounds, the addition of more may not have any therapeutic utility. Although a family with apparently dominantly inherited reduction of about 50 % in serum fibronectin has been described [27], there was no cosegregating disorder suggesting that the reduction had any consequences. The role of fibronectin in physiology has therefore not been elucidated by a mutant, suggesting that a complete lack of fibronectin may be a lethal mutation.

REFERENCES

1. Mosher DF. Physiology of fibronectin. Annu Rev Med 1984; 35: 561–75.
2. Ruoslahti E, Engvall E, Hayman EG. Fibronectin: current concepts of its structure and function. Coll Res 1981; 1: 95–128.
3. Mosher, DF, ed. Fibronectin, New York, Academic Press, Harcourt Brace Jovanovich, 1989.
4. Akiyama SK, Yamada KM. Fibronectin in disease. In: Wagner, BM, Fleischmajer R, Kaufman N, eds. Connective tissue diseases. Baltimore, Williams and Wilkins, 1983: 55–96.

5. Clark RA. Potential roles of fibronectin in cutaneous wound repair. Arch Dermatol 1988; 124:201–6.
6. Hynes RO. Molecular biology of fibronectin. Annu Rev Cell Biol 1985; 1: 67–90.
7. Yamada KM. Fibronectin domains and receptors. In: Mosher DF, ed. Fibronectin. New York, Academic Press, Harcourt Brace Jovanovich, 1989.
8. Petersen TE, Skorstengaard K, Vibe-Petersen K. Primary structure of fibronectin. In: Mosher DF, ed. Fibronectin. New York, Academic Press, Harcourt Brace Jovanovich, 1989.
9. Hedman K, Vaheri A. Fibronectin and the pericellular matrix. In: Mosher DF, ed. Fibronectin. New York, Academic Press, Harcourt Brace Jovanovich, 1989.
10. Mosher DF. Fibronectin. Prog Hemost Thromb 1980; 5: 111–51.
11. Hynes RO. Integrins: a family of cell surface receptors. Cell 1987; 48: 549–54.
12. Thiery J-P, Duband J-L, Dufour S, Savagner S, Imhof BA. Roles of fibronectins in embryogenesis. In: Mosher DF, ed. Fibronectin. New York, Academic Press, Harcourt Brace Jovanovich, 1989.
13. Singer II. Fibronectin-cytoskeleton relationships. In: Mosher DF, ed. Fibronectin. New York, Academic Press, Harcourt Brace Jovanovich, 1989.
14. O'Keefe EJ, Woodley D, Castillo G, et al. Production of soluble and cell associated fibronectin by cultured keratinocytes. J Invest Dermatol 1984; 82: 150–5.
15. Kubo M, Norris DA, Howell SE, et al. Human keratinocytes synthesize, secrete, and deposit fibronectin in the pericellular matrix. J Invest Dermatol 1984; 82: 580–6.
16. Clark RA, Folkvord JM, Wertz RL. Fibronectin, as well as other extracellular matrix proteins, mediates human keratinocyte adherence. J Invest Dermatol 1985; 84: 368–83.
17. O'Keefe EJ, Payne RE Jr, Russell N, et al. Spreading and enhanced motility of human keratinocytes on fibronectin. J Invest Dermatol 1985; 85: 125–30.
18. Gilchrest BA, Calhoun JK, Maciag T. Attachment and growth of human keratinocytes in a serum-free envirionment. J Cell Physiol 1982; 112: 197–206.
19. O'Keefe EJ, Woodley DT, Falk RJ, et al. Production of fibronectin by epithelium in a skin equivalent. J Invest Dermatol 1987; 88: 634–9.
20. Stenn KS, Milstone LM. Epidermal cell confluence and implications for a two-step mechanism of wound closure. J Invest Dermatol 1984; 83: 445–7.
21. Grinnell F, Toda K-I, Takashima A. Activation of keratinocyte fibronectin receptor function during cutaneous wound healing. J Cell Sci Supp 1987; 8: 199–209.
22. Wikner NE, Persichitte KA, Baskin JA, Nielsen LD, Clark RA. Transforming growth factor-beta stimulates the expression of fibronectin by human keratinocytes. J Invest Dermatol 1988; 91: 207–12.
23. Saba TM. Kinetics of plasma fibronectin: relationship to phagocytic function and lung vascular injury. In: Mosher DF, ed. Fibronectin. New York, Academic Press, Harcourt Brace Jovanovich, 1989.
24. Norris DA, Clark RA, Swigart LM, et al. Fibronectin fragment(s) are chemotactic for human peripheral blood monocyrtes. J Immunol 1982; 129: 1612–8.
25. Carsons S, Lavietes BB, Diamond HS. Role of fibronectin in rheumatic diseases. In: Mosher DF, ed. Fibronectin. New York, Academic Press, Harcourt Brace Jovanovich, 1989.

26. Wysocki AW, Baxter CR, Bergstresser PR, et al. Topical fibronectin therapy for treatment of a patient with chronic stasis ulcers. Arch Dermatol 1988; 124: 175–77,
27. Shirakami A, Shigekiyo T, Hirai Y, et al. Plasma fibronectin deficiency in eight members of one family. Lancet 1986; 1: 473–4.

6

Collagenase in Disease

Rosalind A. Grymes,* Annemarie Kronberger, and Eugene A. Bauer

Stanford University School of Medicine, Stanford, California

Collagen is the major structural protein of humans. It constitutes 70% of the dry weight of the dermis and 90% of the organic matrix of bone. Remodeling of collagen (in fetal development, wound healing, chronologic aging, tumor outgrowth and metastasis, and in genetic and acquired diseases of the skin and connective tissue) occurs following its specific cleavage by collagenase. Following the discovery of tadpole collagenase by Gross and Lapière [1] and their initial studies of this enzyme, it has become widely recognized that collagenases play a central role in both the normal and pathologic biology of collagen. In this chapter, we shall discuss collagenase from the perspective of its role in normal physiology and disease. This will include a review of collagenase in certain hereditary and/or congenital disorders of the skin and in aging, comparing normally aged cells with cells of progerias and progeroid diseases. Cancer also is included, since collagenase plays a central role in the invasion of normal stroma by tumor cells, and in the migration and implantation of metastatic cells.

Collagenase is centrally involved in connective tissue remodeling and degradation. In fact, it is likely that the principal role for these enzymes in normal postfetal physiology is during connective tissue remodeling in wound healing. The breakdown of matrix proteins by collagenase and related metalloproteases is also a hallmark of joint and periodontal diseases. Local secretion of cytokines

**Present affiliation.* NASA-Ames Research Center, Moffett Field, California and inflammatory factors attracts circulating immune cells, which augment the responses of resident immune cells and reactive gingival or synovial fibroblasts. Stimulation of these cell types results in the increased synthesis and secretion of collagenase, and in the further elaboration of cytokines to perpetuate the cycle.

The physiological control of collagenase expression is multifactorial and highly responsive to changes in the body's internal milieu. Many different cytokines affect collagenase biosynthesis, as can prostaglandins and hormones. In some cases, the responses of different types of fibroblasts differ. Chemical mitogens also affect the induction of collagenase in addition to their effects on cell proliferation. For changes in collagenase to occur, information must be transferred from the external environment of the cell to the nucleus. The induction of transcription from the human skin collagenase gene can be approached from several pathways and involves mediation by transcription factors, some of which are the products of proto-oncogenes or transforming viruses. The stimulation of collagenase expression following serum or mitogen application, as well as its inhibition by suppressive agents such as retinoids and glucocorticoids, are all mediated by nuclear factors and their binding to specific regulatory sequences.

In human skin, evidence indicates that collagenase is involved in the pathophysiology of recessive dystrophic epidermolysis bullosa (RDEB), an inherited disease characterized by extreme cutaneous fragility. Dermal fibroblasts of Werner's syndrome, an autosomal recessive progeroid disorder, show high levels of constitutive collagenase synthesis. Many of the clinical manifestations of Werner's syndrome primarily involve either the skin or other connective tissues, although the relevance of *in vitro* increases in collagenase expression remains to be elucidated. Collagenase has also been implicated in certain fibrotic diseases, in which decreased activity might be central to disease pathogenesis. Finally, it has been proposed that the matrix metalloproteases, including collagenase, are involved in the progression of malignancies in two ways. Factors are produced by some solid tumors that enhance the expression of these enzymes, presumably abetting the invasion of local stroma as the tumor grows and metastasizes. This effect is not limited to cutaneous cancers. Second, in systemic metastases, the breakdown of basement membrane barrier functions by collagenase type IV is important. Regulation of collagenase is thus central in the equation of containment as opposed to the spread of malignancies.

CHARACTERISTICS OF COLLAGENASE

The Enzyme

Human skin collagenase, as well as other animal collagenases, is synthesized and secreted as a pair of isoproenzymes. Details of the synthesis of this protease have been revealed by isolation and complete sequencing of a cDNA clone representing the full-size human skin collagenase mRNA. The protein consists of a 469 amino acid long preprocollagenase of molecular weight (M_r) 54,092 daltons. Prior to secretion, the 19 amino acid signal peptide is cleaved, yielding a protein of M_r 51,929. This represents the nonglycosylated form of the proenzyme, while the approximately 57 kDa isoproenzyme represents a partially glycosylated form. These proteins must undergo activation before achieving proteolytic potency. Experimentally defined mechanisms of activation include cleavage by tissue proteases (cathepsin, trypsin), the action of plasminogen activators, and autoactivation, which is an intramolecular autoproteolytic reaction. Chemical activation follows treatment with chaotropic ions or organomercurial compounds. For each collagenase form, the final product is a stable enzyme roughly 10 kilodaltons smaller than its precursor. Collagenase activation has also been observed to occur without a change to a lower-molecular-weight species, suggesting the importance of conformational changes in the creation of proteolytically active enzyme [2]. The enzyme is a neutral protease, which requires divalent zinc in the catalytic site, and calcium as both an enzyme activator and a stabilizer of tertiary structure [3].

Mechanism of Action

Collagenases cleave native, triple-helical collagen. Interstitial collagenase makes a single cut in the collagen molecule across all three chains approximately three-fourths of the length of the molecule from the amino-terminal end. Cleavage produces two fragments, termed TC-A and TC-B, the three-quarter and one-quarter length species, respectively. The cleavage site has been determined for both the alpha-1 and alpha-2 chains of type I collagen. A Gly-Ile bond (residues 775–776) is cleaved in the alpha-1 chains, and a Gly-Leu bond in the alpha-2 chain. Cleavage of type II and III collagens similarly results in the characteristic three-quarter and one-quarter length products and involves hydrolysis of Gly-Ile and Gly-Leu bonds [3].

Collagen types I, II, and III are all substrates for collagenase I with a nearly uniform Km of approximately 1 μM. Catalytic rates vary widely, so that with collagen monomers in solution at 25°C, type III collagen is cleaved 5 times faster than type I, while type II collagen is degraded at only 0.005 times the rate of type I [3]. Evidence suggests that there are multiple collagenases within the human organism and that these can and do differ in their collagen specificities. Biochemical analysis and molecular cloning demonstrate the existence of a family of matrix metalloproteases. One proposed nomenclature indicating these interrelationships is being applied at the gene level, as genetic loci are designated matrix metalloprotease (MMP).

Degradation is approximately 12 times slower on the solid form of the substrate than on the soluble form at the same temperature. The formation of intermolecular cross-links is associated with a decrease in collagenolytic activity. Collagenase activity measured by the degradation of collagen monomers in solution increases

15-fold with a 10°C increase in ambient temperature. The rate-limiting step in cleavage is hydrolysis of the peptide bond.

Matrix Metalloprotease Family

The gene for interstitial collagenase is located on the long arm of chromosome 11 (11q21–23). Other members of the matrix metalloprotease gene family have also been cloned. There is strong sequence homology between human interstitial collagenase and stromelysin, a protease of broad substrate specificity, including gelatin, proteoglycan, fibronectin, laminin, type IV collagen, type V collagen, and type VII collagen. Human stromelysin and interstitial collagenase are homologous to rat transin, an oncogene-inducible gene product. There is 46% homology of human interstitial collagenase with rat transin and 55 % homology with human stromelysin, whereas human stromelysin and rat transin share 75% homology. A third member of the gene family, the 72 kDa type IV collagenase, is also closely related, as are a 92 kDa type IV collagenase and a metalloprotease found in the pregnant uterus (so-called PUMP-1). Several laboratories have shown that expression of the 72 kDa type IV collagenase is linked to malignant transformation and to metastatic potential. The relationship and the genomic organization of the members of the matrix metalloprotease gene family are shown in Figure 6.1.

Natural Inhibitors

Collagenase proteolysis is controlled following secretion and activation by the action of naturally occurring inhibitors. The most significant of these is the tissue inhibitor of metalloproteinases (TIMP). It forms a tight complex with collagenase and is directly inhibitory with a stoichiometry of 1:1 [4]. Smaller inhibitors of metalloproteinases (IMPs) are also found in various cell types. Plasminogen activator inhibitor type 1 (PAI-1) acts on urokinase, or urinary plasminogen activator (u-PA) to preclude the activation of collagenase by this pathway [2]. Collagenolytic activity can also be blocked by the formation of a covalent com-

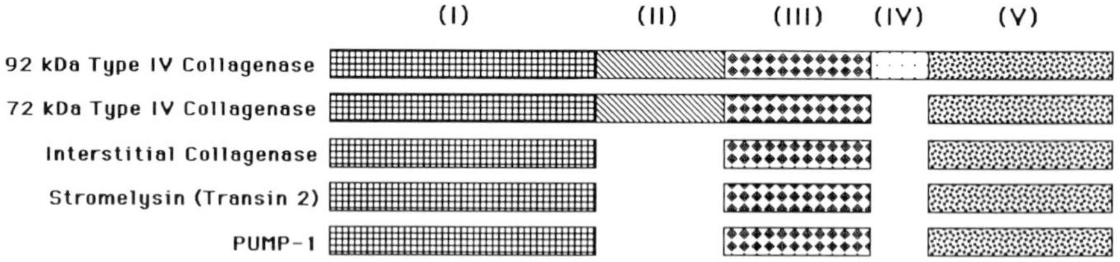

Figure 6.1 Genomic organization of the matrix metalloprotease gene family. I, NH_2 terminal domain; II, fibronectin-like collagen-binding domain; III, zinc-binding domain; IV, alpha-2 (V), collagen-like domain; V, hemopexin-like COOH-terminal domain.

plex between collagenase and various forms of mammalian alpha-2-macroglobulin. This direct interaction results in a specific limited proteolytic cleavage in the bait region of the macroglobulin molecule [5].

COLLAGENASE INDUCTION

Induction by Cytokines

Cells of different lineages may cooperate in connective tissue breakdown by synthesizing and secreting procollagenase, the zymogen form of the enzyme. The production of enzyme is influenced by inductive events (i.e., cytokines present following wounding), suppressive events (*in vitro* application of retinoids and corticosteroids), differentiated lineage, and by heritable alterations in collagenase regulatory or metabolic pathways.

Immune Cells

Polymorphonuclear cells (PMNs) and macrophages release a number of proteases, including collagenases types I and IV. Human peripheral blood monocytes/macrophages can release mononuclear cell factor (MCF), which stimulates collagenase production from both dermal and synovial fibroblasts. Synthesis and secretion of MCF are stimulated by treatment with concanavalin A or phytohemagglutinin, well-studied mitogens of PMNs [6, 7]. In inflammatory states, this source of collagenolysis is presumed to be particularly relevant. This factor is biochemically and biologically indistinguishable from interleukin (IL)-1. Pure preparations of IL-1, analyzed by high-pressure liquid chromatography (HPLC), stimulated collagenase production by dermal fibroblasts [8].

Dermal Cells

Dermal fibroblasts are the major source of skin collagenase, but keratinocytes can also synthesize and contribute to the cumulative levels of the enzyme. The cascade is expanded by the ability of keratinocytes to become activated in response to cytokines such as interleukin (IL)-3, IL-6, and granulocyte/macrophage colony stimulating factor (GM-CSF). The 'activated' keratinocyte can produce IL-1. Cell lysates from freshly prepared human epidermal cells increased the synthesis of collagenase and prostaglandin E2 (PGE2) from dermal fibroblasts. This inductive effect remained cell-associated for the first 2 days postculture, and was secreted into the growth medium by 4 days [8]. Extracts were also positive for thymocyte co-mitogenic activity, also known as lymphocyte-activating factor (LAF). All three activities (LAF, induction of PGE2, and enhanced synthesis of collagenase I) were contained in the same two fractions when analyzed by gel filtration and high-performance liquid chromatography (HPLC). The peaks were at 17 and 30 kDa, and are interpreted to be an IL-1-like molecule and its precursor. Thus, the elaboration of IL-1 in the skin can be traced to keratinocytes and to both local and recruited immune cells. The result of IL-1 interaction with receptors on dermal (or synovial) fibroblasts is an increase in the specific production of collagenase I [9, 10].

Keratinocyte-conditioned medium is a source both of immunoprecipitable procollagenase and TIMP. These activities are increased by 12-O-tetradecanoyl-phorbol-13-acetate (TPA), 6- to 34-fold and 3-fold, respectively [11]. TPA induction is abrogated by cycloheximide, an inhibitor of protein synthesis, indicating that the increased collagenase detected is not the result of release of stored enzyme [12]. In contrast to observations in dermal and synovial fibroblasts, IL-1 does not induce collagenase synthesis by keratinocytes [12]. Finally, keratinocytes growing in a dermal equivalent (a collagen lattice containing fibroblast cells) secrete collagenase that, over time, degrades the lattice. This effect is seen when the keratinocytes are grown in medium supplemented with delipidized serum, but not when the medium contains whole serum or retinoic acid, a well known inhibitor of collagenase synthesis *in vitro* [13]. The stimulation of cell–matrix contacts, as fibroblasts are grown in three-dimensional collagen gels, induces expression of the collagenase gene and results in enhanced proenzyme activation over monolayer culture [14].

Tumor necrosis factor (TNF) application stimulates collagenase and PGE2 production in human dermal fibroblasts [15], while treatment of the human diploid fibroblast cell line FS-4 resulted in the increased synthesis of both collagenase and stromelysin [16]. Similar experiments using the human fetal fibroblast cell line AF2 resulted in increased collagenase I transcription, a result shown by recombinant DNA techniques to be mediated by the AP-1 element (discussed below) [17]. In one set of experiments, IL-2 and GM-CSF had no effect on human adult dermal fibroblasts [15]. In contrast, recombinant interferons alpha, beta, and gamma (rIFN -α,-β,-γ) all increased the production of collagenase by human dermal fibroblasts [18]. rIFN-α and -β also inhibited glycosaminoglycan synthesis but had no effect on fibronectin. rIFN-γ increased both glycosaminoglycans and fibronectin.

Synovial Cells

Synovial fibroblasts are also stimulated by IL-1 to increase collagenase transcription, and to produce matrix metalloprotease 3 (MMP3), or stromelysin. Recombinant IL-1β induction of collagenase in human synovial fibroblasts was antagonized by retinoic acid and dexamethasone [10]. IL-1-stimulated increases in collagenase mRNA remain detectable for 48 hr, while the rate of transcription peaks at 6 hr postagonist, indicating considerable stability of the messenger molecules [19]. It is interesting that cycloheximide added up to 6 hr after treatment with IL-1 was able to inhibit collagenase I expression. Induction of Fos, an intermediate in the intracellular signaling pathway leading to collagenase expression (see below), is an early and transient event. Thus it is unlikely that induction in this system will be represented by Fos alone. While TNF stimulates synoviocytes to enhanced expression, as observed with dermal fibroblasts, the activity of PDGF is markedly different [20]. PDGF is a well-recognized stimulator of collagenase activity in fetal and adult dermal fibroblasts. However, it not only fails to stimulate synthesis in synovial fibroblasts but also blocks the increased synthesis associated with IL-1.

Bone

Although 90% of the organic matrix of bone is collagen, the role of collagenase in bone remodeling and resorption is still unclear. Osteoclasts are the main resorbing cells but do not produce collagenase [21]. Osteoblasts regulate the activity of osteoclasts and have been shown to produce collagenase in response to bone resorbing agents and hormones. This includes parathyroid hormone, retinoic acid, 1,25 $(OH)_2$ vitamin D3, epidermal growth factor, and monocyte-conditioned medium. IL-1 and catabolin are not inducers of collagenase synthesis in osteoblasts. TIMP synthesis is also induced by parathyroid hormone but not by the other agents mentioned. Il-1 can induce matrix metalloproteases and PGE2 in chondrocytes. At present, it seems that osteoblast-derived collagenase may be involved in the degradation of unmineralized bone and might remain active as the osteoclasts engage in acid proteolysis, at least until the pH drops below 5.5 [21].

Intracellular Signaling

The regulation of expression of the metalloprotease gene family has recently been illuminated. The collagenase I gene, in particular, lies at the confluence of many interconnecting transcription control pathways. The basic units of regulation are specific, conserved DNA sequences, termed response elements and/or enhancers. Transcription factors, many of which are nuclear oncoproteins, bind to these elements in an elegantly arranged system providing for signal amplification, feedback, and cross-talk.

The most important interaction related to the collagenase I gene occurs between the TPA response element (TRE) and its specific binding factor, AP-1 [22,23]. The major component of factor AP-1 is a heterodimer of the two nuclear oncoproteins, Fos and Jun. These proteins associate by a leucine-zipper motif and contact the DNA by creating a symmetrical recognition/binding site following dimerization [24,25]. Jun-Jun homodimers can also occur and may bind to TREs with different affinities [26]. Other Jun-and Fos-related proteins also participate in the formation of altered AP-1 molecules, enlarging the repertoire of gene modulation in both normal and abnormal states.

Fos and Jun are inducible proteins, transcribed from both cellular domains (c-fos and c-jun) and viral derivatives (v-fos and v-jun, in cells infected with the appropriate transducing retroviruses) [27]. The cellular homologs, c-fos and c-jun, are regulated by TREs and, in the case of c-fos, by additional sequences. C-fos is induced by serum, an effect mediated by serum response factor (SRF) binding to the serum response element (SRE), a 22 base pair dyad symmetry region [28]. Both the TRE and SRE are endpoints of the protein kinase C pathway of signal transduction [29,30]. C-fos is also induced by 3′-5′-cyclic adenosine monophosphate (cAMP) and other treatments that converge on the cAMP response element (CRE) through adenylate cyclase. Other genes contain TRE enhancers, notably the genes for tissue plasminogen activator (tPA) [31], an important element in the activation cascade of the zymogen form of collagenase to the active enzyme, and the TIMP gene [32]. The fine-tuning capacities of these systems reside in the capacity of the nuclear factors, singly and in combination, to modulate response by modulating binding specificities and affinities.

Fos is central to expression of collagenase I. It is a requisite of the induction pathway and is, itself, a protein subject to complex regulation. Fos binds as part of the AP-1 factor to the collagenase I gene TRE, as well as to the TREs of c-fos and c-jun. Levels of both Jun and Fos will control the nature and existence of heterodimeric AP-1, and thus the induction of collagenase. Intranuclear levels of these proteins depend on 1) expression (as discussed above), 2) mRNA and protein stability, 3) associable inhibitors, and 4) intranuclear transport. Fos is a highly labile phosphoprotein, and its mRNA precursor is unstable. Agents that block protein synthesis superinduce expression from the TRE. This is, in part, due to the absence of protein factors that associate with and inhibit AP-1 [33]. Another explanation is lack of transport of Fos and Jun into the nucleus. This movement is essential for intranuclear AP-1 activity. In the case of Fos, it is controlled by a labile transport inhibitor [34]. This inhibition is reversed by cAMP or by continuous stimulation of cells with serum. The transport mechanism does not act on v-fos proteins.

Cytokines can induce collagenase expression. TNF-α has been shown to stimulate both c-jun and the collagenase I gene through the TRE [17]. Il-1 probably also acts on the TRE of the collagenase gene through the mediation of AP-1. Platelet-derived growth factor (PDGF) utilizes the protein kinase C pathway, and thus the TRE [29]. However, evidence indicates that single stimulators and ligands can activate multiple intracellular pathways that may converge on one or a few genetic element(s), or may diverge and activate different nuclear systems. PDGF activity is such a case. Another is TPA-induced synthesis of c-fos, which is not wholly mediated by the TRE [29,30]. In addition, in synoviocytes c-fos is stimulated by PDGF, basic fibroblast growth factor (bFGF), and transforming growth factor (TGF)-β. However, increases in Fos levels are not translated as increases in collagenase transcription. In fact, collagenase production decreased in response to PDGF or TGF-β [20]. Collagenase I suppression by PDGF in these cells is directly opposite to the induction seen in dermal fibroblasts.

Inhibition of collagenase is also mediated by DNA regulatory sequences and nuclear transcription factors. Members of a superfamily of intracellular receptors transduce the suppressive effects of glucocorticoids and retinoid compounds. Just as the upregulation of steroid hormone responsive genes is the result of direct ligand-receptor binding to glucocorticoid response elements, it now appears that suppression is also mediated by direct ligand–receptor complex interaction [35]. Direct interaction between receptor–ligand complexes and Fos or Jun results in mutual inhibition of DNA-binding ability. The adenovirus gene product, E1a, also suppresses transcription of the collagenase gene. This effect is very specific: although E1a acts through the AP-1 complex the c-fos gene is not repressed by E1a [36].

ROLE OF COLLAGENASE IN AGING AND DISORDERS OF AGING

Data relating to the role of collagenase in aging derive from several sources: senescent cells in culture, chronologically aged cells (cultured from biopsies of older individuals), and cells isolated from patients with premature aging syndromes. Although these systems are not entirely uniform, the information generated is consistent. Before discussing this, we shall briefly recapitulate the place of collagenase in ontogeny. Collagenase production begins as early as the end of the embryonic stage of fetal development. Although the exact age at onset of expression is not known, collagenase is expressed in skin fibroblasts by 7 weeks of estimated gestational age. Concentrations of collagenase found in the culture medium of 29 week fibroblasts are approximately equal to those found in conditioned medium from cultures of adult dermal fibroblasts. At 7-8 weeks, measurements of collagenase immunoreactive material are only one-twentieth of adult levels. From 8 weeks until birth, the cell-rich mesenchyme of the developing embryo becomes the cell sparse, fibrous matrix of the fetus. At around 8 weeks, the matrix noticeably accumulates and large vessels demarcating the dermis from the subcutaneous tissue form, with small branches penetrating the dermis to join with capillaries. From 12 weeks, the papillary and reticular dermis become defined, and the dermis continues to remodel to permit the development of nerve and vascular networks, and appendageal structures [37].

It has been shown that late passage cells (those with greater than 80% of their lifespan completed) have basal levels of collagenase production 10–30 times higher than early passage cells (those with less than 40% of their lifespan completed) [38]. Based on results using immunofluorescence staining, only 1–6% of early-passage, compared to 35–77% of late-passage, cells expressed cellular collagenase [39]. RNA analysis demonstrated that late-passage cells have at least 10 times the amount of collagenase RNA of early-passage cells. Both early- and late-passage cells were responsive to collagenase induction by fibroblast extracellular matrix, fibroblast-conditioned medium, polypeptide growth factors, and phorbol esters. The induced levels were always higher in the late-passage cells.

Young (roughly equivalent to early-passage) and senescent (late-passage) cells were studied for their response to serum stimulation of collagenase production. Young cells that were serum starved in 0.5% fetal bovine serum (FBS) responded to 10% FBS with enhanced expression of both immunoreactive procollagenase and TIMP. This reaction was evident 4 hr after serum treatment. In contrast, senescent fibroblasts produced high basal levels of procollagenase even in low serum concentrations, and did not respond to increased serum with increase in procollagenase levels. They also made small amounts of TIMP, which did not increase following treatment with higher serum concentrations. To demonstrate that this phenomenon is not primarily related to growth inhibition, both exponentially growing and contact-inhibited young cells were examined [40].

Werner's syndrome is an autosomal recessive disorder characterized by premature aging, with major clinical manifestations in the connective tissue and skin. Our studies of these cells show that they have high constitutive levels of collagenase production and that this expression is unresponsive to most cytokines [41]. It is interesting that a cell strain isolated from the heterozygotic relative of a patient with Werner's syndrome showed constitutive collagenase concentrations that are intermediate between normal cells and those of the patient. These heterozygotic cells also respond partially to inductive cytokines. Several different Werner's syndrome cell strains that have been tested show normal patterns of collagenase suppression by hydrocortisone [42].

In a broad sense, aged or senescent cells seem to have high basal levels of collagenase production, both in hybridizing RNA and immunoreactive protein. In normal cells, these levels are inducible by matrix associations and cytokines. Cells derived from a heritable aging disorder have constitutively high levels of enzyme, but these are not inducible, although they can be suppressed with glucocorticoids.

ROLE OF COLLAGENASE IN CANCER

Tumorigenesis can be viewed as occurring in three steps involving tumor cell invasion and metastases [43]. The first step is attachment of tumor cells to the extracellular matrix through specific cell-surface receptors. In the second step, secretion of proteolytic enzymes produces local degradation of the matrix. The third step involves locomotion of tumor cells into the areas of degraded matrix. This movement is postulated to take place through the action of autocrine motility factor. There is abundant evidence that many tumor cells can produce enzymes that break down basement membrane collagens and gelatinized (denatured) collagens. There is, in fact, a high correlation between secretion of type IV collagenase and metastatic character. For example, H-*ras* transformed human bronchial epithelial cells (TBE-1) secrete a single major extracellular matrix metalloprotease of 72 kDa (in the proenzyme form) [44]. The substrate specificity of this enzyme is gelatin, type IV collagen, type V collagen, fibronectin, and type VII collagen, in that order. The enzyme does not degrade collagen types I/III or laminin. This type IV collagenase is identical to that of normal dermal fibroblasts, normal skin explants, and SV40-transformed human lung fibroblasts. In a second series of studies, when NIH 3T3 cells or rat embryo fibroblasts were transfected with the H-*ras* oncogene, all transfectants secreted high levels of type IV collagenase and were tumorigenic and metastatic *in vivo* [43]. Cells transfected with ras and the adenovirus E1a gene were tumorigenic but were not metastatic and did not secrete significant amounts of type IV collagenase. In another investigation of protease elaboration and metastases, type I collagenase activity from extracts of 11 squamous cell carcinomas was 9-fold higher, and type IV collagenase was 3-fold higher, than corresponding activity found in extracts of benign (seborrheic keratosis) lesions [45].

In addition to the elaboration of metalloproteases, tumor cells may stimulate collagenase production by cells of the surrounding stroma. Human basal cell carcinomas show increased collagenase levels *in vivo*. Dermal fibroblasts isolated from the surrounding stroma and grown in culture continue to exhibit this enhanced production of collagenase (34 times normal) for 10–14 mean population doublings and then lose the phenotype [46]. When extracts of tumor cells isolated free of stroma were applied to monolayers of adult dermal fibroblasts, there was an increase in both immunoreactive collagenase and collagenase activity of up to 10-fold in 24 hr [47]. The stimulatory activity, sized by gel filtration, was approximately 19 kDa. In addition, A431 cells, a human epidermoid carcinoma line, secrete an IL-1-like factor of 17 kDa [48]. This cytokine is able to stimulate collagenase and PGE2 production by fibroblasts, and to provide thymocyte comitogenic activity. LX-1 human lung carcinoma cells secrete a collagenase stimulatory factor of 58 kDa, which may be released into the medium by limited proteolysis as a 35 kDa product [49]. Immunofluorescence studies indicate that this protein is present on the cell membrane of LX-1 cells, but it is not found on normal fibroblasts.

The suppressive activity of retinoid compounds is also evident where collagenase production is tightly linked to metastatic potential. Four sublines of the human melanoma cell line A375 were treated with all-*trans* retinoic acid. Compared to untreated controls, these cells showed 10-40% less binding to a reconstituted basement membrane matrix. They also had both an impaired ability to penetrate Matrigel (a synthetic extracellular matrix equivalent) coated filters and a decreased activity in degrading collagen type IV. This correlated with very low levels of type IV collagenase RNA. The sublines also exhibited decreased tPA activity. Finally, these retinoic acid-treated sublines had a significant increase in the high-affinity metastasis-associated laminin receptor and high amounts of a cell surface receptor for motility factor [50]. The inhibitory effect of retinoic acid on the transcription of the collagenase gene (discussed above) clearly extends to a set of genes that can be co-operatively or independently regulated. This observation recalls the data on adenovirus E1a cotransfected cells, in which type IV collagenase was suppressed along with metastatic potential. Adenovirus E1a protein has been shown specifically to repress collagenase gene activity, while stimulating earlier events in the collagenase gene regulatory pathway.

ROLE OF COLLAGENASE IN OTHER PATHOLOGIC CONDITIONS

Recessive Dystrophic Epidermolysis Bullosa

The largest body of evidence relating to a role for collagenase in a pathologic skin condition is in recessive dystrophic epidermolysis bullosa (RDEB). This disease of autosomal recessive inheritance is characterized by extreme cutaneous fragility, leading to devastating blistering with subsequent healing and scar tissue formation. Patients also have a predisposition to squamous cell carcinomas. Skin obtained from friction blisters of patients with RDEB shows elevated levels of collagenase [51]. Both clinically uninvolved skin and blister fluids from a patient with RDEB likewise had collagenase and neutral protease values significantly higher than those of control normal skin and burn blisters [52]. When normal skin was cultured with blister fluid from this patient, the explant exhibited the dermal–epidermal separation characteristic of the disease [52].

In a large survey, human skin collagenase was quantitated by immunologic procedures in 40 patients with the 4 major categories of epidermolysis bullosa (EB) [51]. The results demonstrated elevated collagenase concentrations in all forms of EB, not an entirely unexpected development in view of the extensive and repetitive wounding and healing environment of patients with EB. The more impressive result was that collagenase levels were also higher in samples of clinically uninvolved skin from patients with RDEB. In addition, when dermal fibroblasts from the four major types of EB were placed in culture, only those from the genetic background of RDEB showed elevated collagenase levels as a seemingly stable phenotype. Although the kinetics of intracellular accumulation and secretion were enhanced, the rate of enzyme turnover was unaltered. Thus, the increased amount of collagenase must be ascribed to increased production. In a few individual patients, evidence for the existence of an aberrant form of the enzyme has been generated [53]. The activation state of the enzyme has also been implicated in disease pathogenesis [54]. Dermal fibroblasts were cultured from patients with RDEB, EB simplex, and controls (six individuals in each group) and tested for collagenase synthesis and activity. Fibroblasts from patients with both RDEB and EB simplex synthesized twice the amount of collagenase as controls. However, when collagenase activity was measured (in 4 lines per group), RDEB cells had 30% more activity than controls, and this value was unaffected by trypsin activation. In contrast, enzyme activity from EB simplex cells increased from 67 to 114% of control values following trypsin treatment. Both type I and type IV collagenases are able to cleave type VII collagen, the major structural protein of anchoring fibrils, which are critical for dermal–epidermal adhesion in the basement membrane zone of the skin. It is additionally essential to point out that not all patients with RDEB have the elevated collagenase phenotype. In one study, only one in four expressed the phenomenon [55].

Other Skin Diseases

Collagenase production has also been studied in other diseases of the skin. It has been found in above-normal quantities in patients with dermatitis herpetiformis, bullous pemphigoid, chronic bullous disease of childhood, and pemphigus vulgaris [56]. In one patient with nodular fibrosis of the skin, while collagen types I/III were considerably elevated, collagenase production was only one-fourth of normal [57]. This highlights the reciprocal nature of anabolic and catabolic functions in connective tissue homeostasis.

Arthritis

As discussed above, both synovial fibroblasts and chondrocytes produce collagenase. This enzyme probably assumes a major part in the complex interplay characteristic of arthritis. Degradation of the extracellular matrix distorts the function and structure of the affected joint(s), and the novel immunologic determinants revealed by collagen cleavage may stimulate immune cells to react against a "self" antigen. Infiltrating macrophages and monocytes can also produce collagenase, contributing to the progression of the disease. Although salicylates ease the pain of arthritis, and inhibit the production of prostaglandins associated with inflammation, they do not inhibit collagenase production, and thus do not alter the destructive course of the condition [58].

Periodontal Disease

It is widely thought that bacteria play a major role in periodontal disease, through their elaboration of bacterial collagenases and antigens that induce cytokine production, resulting in collagenase synthesis by gingival fibroblasts. Gingival fibroblasts are induced to make collagenase by recombinant TNF-α and IL-1, while TGF-β treatment strongly suppresses procollagenase [59,60]. A chemically modified tetracycline, with no antimicrobial activity, was able to inhibit collagenase both *in vivo* and *in vitro* [61]. *In vivo*, diabetic adult male rats showed markedly increased enzyme concentrations in the skin and gingiva. Treatment with the modified tetracycline reduced this excessive activity, and prevented loss of body weight, skin weight, and skin collagen mass. *In vitro*, collagenase activity from partially purified extracts of human rheumatoid synovial tissue was inhibited by the tetracycline analog. This points to a more direct role for cellular collagenase in the pathogenesis of periodontal disease and shows that production by bacteria is only part of the equation. It also has implications for the treatment of other disease conditions in which excess collagenase is a causative finding.

REFERENCES

1. Gross J, Lapière C. Collagenolytic activity in amphibian tissues: a tissue culture assay. Proc Natl Acad Sci 1962; 48: 1014–22.
2. He C, Wilhelm S, Pentland A, *et al.* Tissue cooperation in a proteolytic cascade activating human interstitial collagenase. Proc Natl Acad Sci 1989; 86: 2632–6.
3. Bauer EA, Goldberg GI, Eisen AZ, *et al. Collagenase*. New York: Oxford University Press, 1991.
4. Welgus HG, Stricklin GP. Human skin fibroblast collagenase inhibitor. J Biol Chem 1983; 258: 12259–64.
5. Sottrup-Jensen L, Birkedal-Hansen H. Human fibroblast collagenase–alpha-macroglobulin interactions. Localization of cleavage sites in the bait regions of five mammalian alpha-macroglobulins. J Biol Chem 1989; 264: 393–401.
6. Hauser C, Saurat J, Schmitt A, *et al.* Interleukin 1 is present in normal human epidermis. J Immunol 1986; 136: 3317–23.
7. Dayer J, Zavadil-Grob C, Ucla C, *et al.* Induction of human interleukin 1 mRNA measured by collagenase- and prostaglandin E2-stimulating activity in rheumatoid synovial cells. Eur J Immunol 1984; 14: 898–901.
8. Hauser C, Saurat J, Jaunin F, *et al.* Cultured human epidermis cells produce cell-associated interleukin 1-like prostaglandin E2-and collagenase-stimulating factors. Biochim Biophys Acta 1985; 846: 350–5.
9. Postlethwaite A, Lachman L, Mainardi C, *et al.* Interleukin 1 stimulation of collagenase production by cultured fibroblasts. J Exp Med 1983; 157: 801–6.
10. Saus J, Quinones S, Otani Y, *et al.* The complete primary structure of human matrix metalloproteinase-3. Identity with stromelysin. J Biol Chem 1988; 263: 6742–5.
11. Petersen M, Woodley D, Stricklin G, *et al.* Constitutive production of procollagenase and tissue inhibitor of metalloproteinases by human keratinocytes in culture. J Invest Dermatol 1989; 92: 156–9.
12. Petersen M, Woodley D, Stricklin G, *et al.* Production of procollagenase by cultured human keratinocytes. J Biol Chem 1987; 262: 835–40.
13. Bailly C, Dreze S, Asselineau D, *et al.* Retinoic acid inhibits the production of collagenase by human epidermal keratinocytes. J Invest Dermatol 1990; 94: 47–51.
14. Mauch C, Adelmann-Grill B, Hatamochi A, *et al.* Collagenase gene expression in fibroblasts is regulated by a three-dimensional contact with collagen. FEBS Lett 1989; 250: 301–5.

15. Duncan M, Berman B. Differential regulation of collagen, glycosaminoglycan, fibronectin, and collagenase activity production in cultured human adult dermal fibroblasts by interleukin 1-alpha and beta and tumor necrosis factor-alpha and beta. J Invest Dermatol 1989; 92: 699–706.
16. Lee T, Lee G, Ziff E, *et al*. Isolation and characterization of eight tumor necrosis factor-induced gene sequences from human fibroblasts. Mol Cell Biol 1990; 10: 1982–8.
17. Brenner D, O'Hara M, Angel P, *et al*. Prolonged activation of jun and collagenase genes by tumour necrosis factor-alpha. Nature 1989; 337: 661–3.
18. Duncan M, Berman B. Differential regulation of glycosaminoglycan, fibronectin, and collagenase production in cultured human dermal fibroblasts by interferon-alpha, -beta, and -gamma. Arch Dermatol Res 1989; 281: 11–8.
19. McCachren S, Greer P, Niedel J. Regulation of human synovial fibroblasts collagenase messenger RNA by interleukin-1. Arthritis Rheum 1989; 32: 1539–45.
20. Kumkumian G, Lafyatis R, Remmers E, *et al*. Platelet-derived growth factor and IL-1 interactions in rheumatoid arthritis. Regulation of synoviocyte proliferation, prostaglandin production, and collagenase transcription. J Immunol 1989 143: 833–7.
21. Eeckhout Y, Delaisse J. The role of collagenase in bone resorption. An overview. Pathol Biol 1988; 36: 1139–46.
22. Angel P, Baumann I, Stein B, *et al*. 12-O-tetradecanoyl-phorbol-13-acetate induction of the human collagenase gene is mediated by an inducible enhancer element located in the 5′-flanking region. Mol Cell Biol 1987; 7: 2256–66.
23. Lee W, Mitchell P, Tjian R. Purified transcription factor AP-1 interacts with TPA-inducible enhancer elements. Cell 1987; 49: 741–52.
24. Chiu R, Boyle W, Meek J, *et al*. The c-Fos protein interacts with c-Jun/AP-1 to stimulate transcription of AP-1 responsive genes. Cell 1988; 54: 541–52.
25. Neuberg M, Schuermann M, Hunter J, *et al*. Two functionally different regions in Fos are required for the sequence-specific DNA interaction of the Fos/Jun protein complex. Nature 1989; 338: 589–90.
26. Chiu R, Angel P, Karin M. Jun-B differs in its biological properties from, and is a negative regulator of, cJun. Cell 1989; 59: 979–86.
27. Miller A, Curran T, Verma I. C-fos protein can induce cellular transformation: a novel mechanism of activation of a cellular oncogene. Cell 1984; 36: 51–60.
28. Treisman R. Transient accumulation of c-fos RNA following serum stimulation requires a conserved 5′ element and c-fos 3′ sequences. *Cell* 1985; 42: 889–902.
29. Buscher M, Rahmsdorf H, Litfin M, *et al*. Activation of the c-fos gene by UV and phorbol ester: different signal transduction pathways converge to the same enhancer element. Oncogene 1988; 3: 301–11.
30. Hoeffler J, Deutsch P, Lin J *et al*. Distinct adenosine 3′,5′-monophosphate and phorbol ester-responsive signal transduction pathways converge at the level of transcriptional activation by the interactions of DNA-binding proteins. Mol Endocrinol 1989; 3: 868–80.
31. Feng P, Ohlsson M, Ny T. The structure of the TATA-less rat tissue-type plasminogen activator gene. Species-specific sequence divergences in the promoter predict differences in regulation of gene expression. J Biol Chem 1990; 265: 2022–7.

32. Alitalo R, Partanen J, Pertovaara L, *et al*. Increased erythroid potentiating activity/tissue inhibitor of metalloproteinases and jun/fos transcription factor complex characterize tumor promoter-induced megakaryoblastic differentiation of K562 leukemia cells. Blood 1990; 75: 1974–82.
33. Subramaniam M, Schmidt L, Crutchfield C, *et al*. Negative regulation of serum-responsive enhancer elements. Nature 1989; 340:64–6.
34. Roux P, Blanchard J-M, Fernandez A, *et al*. Nuclear localization of c-Fos, but not v-Fos proteins is controlled by extracellular signals. Cell 1990 63: 341–51.
35. Jonat C, Rahmsdorf H, Park K-K, *et al*. Antitumor promotion and antiinflammation: down-modulation of AP-1 (Fos/Jun) activity by glucocorticoid hormone. Cell 1990; 62: 1189–204.
36. Offringa R, Gebel S, van Dam H, *et al*. A novel function of the transforming domain of Ela: repression of AP-1 activity. Cell 1990 62: 527–38.
37. Bauer EA, Kronberger A, Stricklin G, *et al*. Age-related changes in collagenase expression in cultured embryonic and fetal human skin fibroblasts. Exp Cell Res 1985; 161: 484–94.
38. Sottile J, Mann D, Diemer V *et al*. Regulation of collagenase and collagenase mRNA production in early-and late-passage human diploid fibroblasts. J Cell Physiol 1989; 138: 281–90.
39. Millis A, Sottile J, Hoyle M, *et al*. Collagenase production by early and late passage cultures of human fibroblasts. Exp Gerontol 1989; 24: 559–75.
40. West M, Pereira-Smith O, Smith J. Replicative senescence of human skin fibroblasts correlates with a loss of regulation and overexpression of collagenase activity. Exp Cell Res 1989; 184: 138–47.
41. Bauer EA, Silverman N, Busiek D, *et al*. Diminished response of Werner's syndrome fibroblasts to growth factors PDGF and FGF. Science 1986; 234: 1240–3.
42. Grymes RA, Altman J, Chan J, et al. Induction and suppression of type I collagenase in a progeroid syndrome. Exp Cell Res submitted 1993.
43. Liotta L, Wewer U, Rao N, *et al*. Biochemical mechanisms of tumor invasion and metastases. Adv Exp Med Biol 1988; 233: 161–9.
44. Collier I, Wilhelm S, Eisen AZ, *et al*. H-ras oncogene-transformed human bronchial epithelial cells (TBE-1) secrete a single metalloprotease capable of degrading basement membrane collagen. J Biol Chem 1988; 263: 6579–87.
45. Tsuboi R, Yamaguchi T, Kurita Y, *et al*. Comparison of proteinase activities in squamous cell carcinoma, basal cell epithelioma, and seborrheic keratosis. J Invest Dermatol 1988; 90: 869–72.
46. Bauer EA, Uitto J, Walters R, *et al*. Enhanced collagenase production by fibroblasts derived from human basal cell carcinomas. Cancer Res 1979; 39: 4594–9.
47. Goslen J, Eisen A, Bauer EA. Stimulation of skin fibroblast collagenase production by a cytokine derived from basal cell carcinomas. J Invest Dermatol 1985; 85: 161–4.
48. Hauser C, Dayer J, Jaunin F, *et al*. Intracellular epidermal interleukin 1-like factors in the human epidermoid carcinoma cell line A431. Cell Immunol 1986; 100: 89–96.
49. Ellis S, Nabeshima K, Biswas C. Monoclonal antibody preparation and purification of a tumor cell collagenase-stimulatory factor. Cancer Res 1989; 49: 3385–91.

50. Hendrix M, Wood W, Seftor E, *et al.* Retinoic acid inhibition of human melanoma cell invasion through a reconstituted basement membrane and its relation to decreases in the expression of proteolytic enzymes and motility factor receptor. Cancer Res 1990; 50: 4121–30.
51. Bauer EA. Collagenase in recessive dystrophic epidermolysis bullosa. Ann NY Acad of Sciences 1986; 460: 311–20.
52. Takamori K, Naito K, Taneda A, *et al.* Increased neutral protease and collagenase activity in recessive dystrophic epidermolysis bullosa. Br J Dermatol 1983; 108: 687–94.
53. Bauer EA. Recessive dystrophic epidermolysis bullosa: evidence for an altered collagenase in fibroblast cultures. Proc Natl Acad Sci 1977; 74: 4646–50.
54. Oakley C, Priestley G. Collagen synthesis and degradation by epidermolysis bullosa fibroblasts. Acta Derm Venereol 1985; 65: 277–81.
55. Winberg J, Gedde-Dahl T, Bauer EA. Collagenase expression in skin fibroblasts from families with recessive dystrophic epidermolysis bullosa. J Invest Dermatol 1989; 92: 82–5.
56. Oikarinen A, Zone J, Ahmed A, *et al.* Demonstration of collagenase and elastase activities in the blister fluids from bullous skin diseases. Comparison between dermatitis herpetiformis and bullous pemphigoid. J Invest Dermatol 1983; 81: 261–6.
57. Bauer EA, Uitto J, Santa Cruz D, *et al.* Progressive nodular fibrosis of the skin: altered procollagen and collagenase expression by cultured fibroblasts. J Invest Dermatol 1986; 87: 210–5.
58. Pettipher E. Pathogenesis and treatment of chronic arthritis. Sci Prog 1989; 73: 521–34.
59. Meikle M, Atkinson S, Ward R, *et al.* Gingival fibroblasts degrade type I collagen films when stimulated with tumor necrosis factor and interleukin 1: evidence that breakdown is mediated by metalloproteinases. J Periodont Res 1989; 24: 207–13.
60. Overall C, Wrana J, Sodek J. Independent regulation of collagenase, 72-kDa progelatinase, and metalloendoproteinase inhibitor expression in human fibroblasts by transforming growth factor-beta. J Biol Chem 1989; 264: 1860–9.
61. Golub L, McNamara T, D'Angelo G, *et al.* A non-bacterial chemically-modified tetracycline inhibits mammalian collagenase activity. J Dent Res 1987 66: 1310–4.

7

Connective Tissue Protein Receptors

Monika Borchert
University of Munich, Munich, Germany

Connective tissue in the skin can be classified into two compartments based on the major type of extracellular matrix proteins found in each. The interstitial connective tissue of the dermis consists primarily of the fibrillar collagens I and III, collagen VI microfibrils, fibril-associated collagens XII and XIV, fibronectin, vitronectin, and proteoglycans. The basement membrane, on the other hand, contains collagens IV and VII, laminin, and nidogen as well as proteoglycans.

In addition to their role in providing structural stability and flexibility for the connective tissue or serving as a physical barrier, these extracellular matrix proteins can influence many fundamental aspects of cell behavior such as migration, chemotaxis, attachment, differentiation, and biosynthesis. These cellular functions play an important role in such important phenomena as development, wound healing, and metastasis as well as in the maintenance of functional connective tissue. Increasing interest in the molecular mechanisms by which cells interact with their environment has developed in recent years and thus cell–matrix interactions have been the subject of previous reviews [1,2].

Several different classes of receptors for extracellular matrix components have been described to date, including integrins, cell surface proteoglycans, and anchorins (Fig. 7.1). In addition, other extracellular matrix receptors not belonging to any of these classes have been characterized and will be reviewed briefly. Subsequently, the role of matrix receptors with respect to cell–matrix interactions will be reviewed.

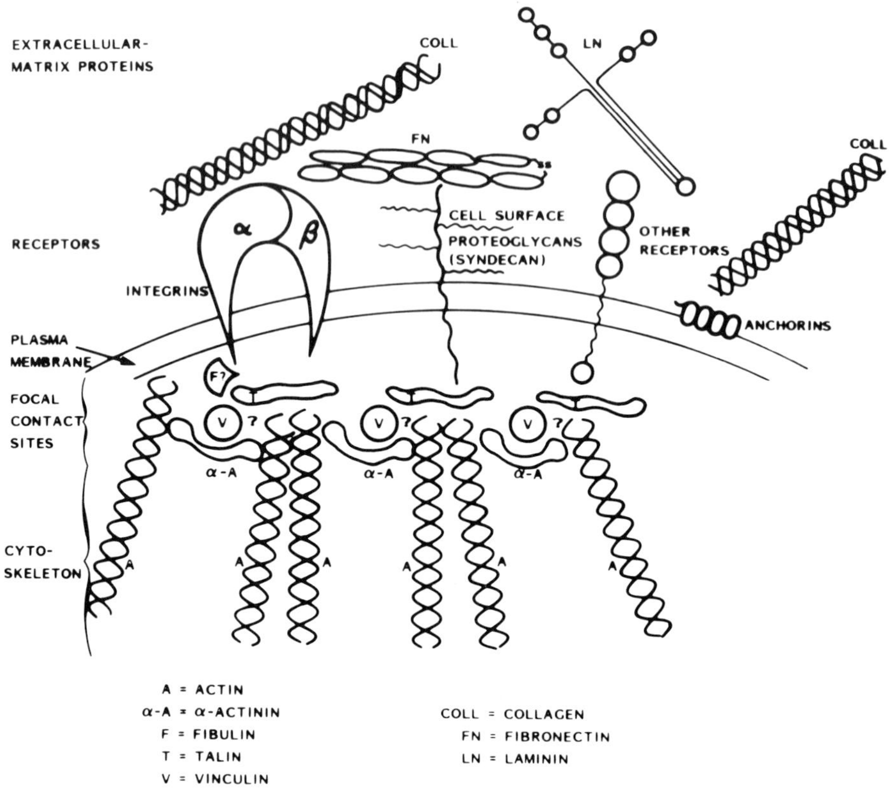

Figure 7.1 Schematic representation of four different classes of extracellular matrix receptors and their postulated role in the transmembrane linkage between the extracellular matrix and the cytoskeleton.

STRUCTURAL CHARACTERISTICS OF EXTRACELLULAR MATRIX RECEPTORS

Integrins

In the past several years a superfamily of structurally related extracellular matrix receptors has emerged that plays a key role in cell–matrix as well as cell–cell interactions. Termed integrins [1,3], these proteins are related immunologically and on the basis of protein and cDNA sequences. Furthermore, several of these receptors share the common ability specifically to recognize the tripeptide arg-gly-asp (RGD), which is found in many extracellular matrix proteins including fibronectin, vitronectin, collagens, laminin, nidogen, and thrombospondin, among others. The conformation of the peptide appears to be important in determining the binding specificity. Members of this family of receptors consist of heterodimers of noncovalently linked α and β subunits. In all cases described thus far both the α and β subunits are transmembrane glycoproteins with large extracellular and small intracellular domains (Fig. 7.2). The α subunits range from a molecular weight (M_r) of 90 to 180 kilodaltons. Several of the α subunits consist of two disulfide-linked peptides, a small membrane-spanning peptide of approximately 25 kD, and an extracellular peptide larger than 110 kD. Three or four potential metal-binding sites similar to the EF-hand motifs in calmodulin are located toward the N-terminus of the α subunits and are thought to bind divalent cations such as Ca^{2+}, Mg^{2+}, or Mn^{2+}, which are required for receptor function. The divalent cation specificity, however, appears to vary among the different integrins. The β subunits range in size from 95 to 205 kD. They are characterized by a high percentage of cysteine residues, in particular, four highly conserved tandem cysteine repeats in the extracellular domain. In addition, the cytoplasmic tail of the integrin β subunits shows a remarkably high homology to the intracellular domains of the EGF receptor, the insulin receptor, and the *neu* oncogene product.

Several lines of evidence indicate that families of integrin receptors contain unique α subunits, but share common β subunits. At least eight different yet homologous β subunits have been described to date, which each are able to pair with one or more different known α subunits. This chapter will review only those best characterized so far. Since information concerning members of the integrin family has originated independently in a large number of different laboratories, the nomenclature in this field is confusing. Hynes et al. [3] proposed a system of classification based on the common β subunits, which will be adopted in this review in introducing the individual integrin receptors.

The first group of integrin proteins, known as the β_1 family and primarily involved in cell–matrix interactions, includes the lymphocyte family of very late antigens (VLA) and the high-affinity fibronectin receptor (Table 7.1). The β_1 chain with a reduced M_r of 130 can associate with at least eight different known α subunits. These VLA antigens, which are also involved in cell–cell interactions, were originally described because of their appearance on T cells several days after stimulation with mitogens or alloantigens. Most of these β_1 integrins, however, are additionally expressed on a number of other cell types. VLA-1 containing the α_1 subunit exhibits a wide distribution and has been shown to serve as a receptor for collagens I and IV on melanoma cells. The VLA-2 complex with its α_2 (or α_c) subunit represents the major integrin collagen receptor. In addition to lymphocytes, platelets, endothelial, and epithelial cells, this heterodimer is expressed in most rapidly growing adherent cell lines and in most primary lung tumors. Its ligands include collagens I, II, III, IV, V, and VI. The VLA-3 α_3 is part of an integrin receptor binding to laminin, collagens I and VI, and fibronectin, albeit with low affinity to the latter. This RGD-dependent

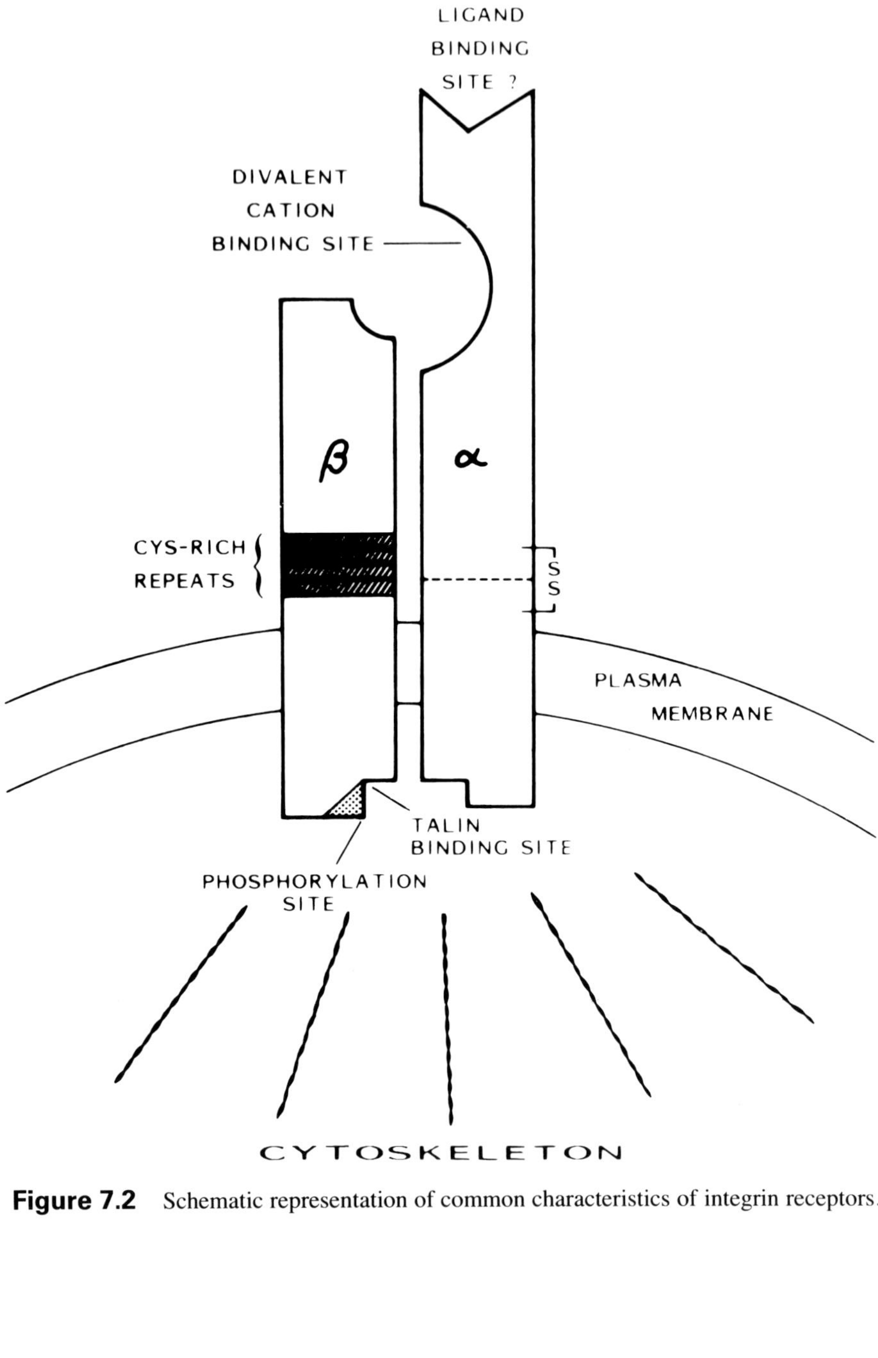

Figure 7.2 Schematic representation of common characteristics of integrin receptors.

polyvalent receptor also displays a wide distribution on different cell types. In contrast, α_4 from the VLA-4 protein is primarily expressed on suspension cells, where it is thought to be involved in cell–cell interactions. Recent evidence suggests that it also recognizes fibronectin, but at a site distinct from the RGD sequence. The fifth member of the β_1 integrins is the high-affinity fibronectin receptor consisting of the β_1 and α_5 (or α_F) subunits. The fibronectin receptor is identical to VLA-5 and is detected on a wide variety of adherent cell types as well as on platelets and myeloid cell lines. VLA-6 has been described as a laminin receptor on platelets and a large variety of adherent cells. The α_6 subunit is very similar in size to the α_5 subunit, which caused initial difficulties in its isolation and characterization. Finally, VLA-7 has just recently been described as the laminin receptor on myoblasts and melanoma cells. The β_1 subunit family also includes an RGD-dependent receptor for tenascin, but the specific α subunit conveying affinity for this developmentally regulated matrix molecule has not yet been identified.

Members of the β_2 group of integrin receptors are characteristically expressed on leukocytes and are primarily involved in cell–cell and cell–matrix adhesion-related functions. The reduced β_2 chain displays an M_r of 95 and can pair with the α_L subunit to form the lymphocyte function-associated antigen (LFA-1). This molecule is expressed on all leukocytes and, for example, mediates T-cell helping and killing by recognizing ICAM-1 and ICAM-2 on target cells. Mac-1, another member of this integrin class, is also referred to as the macrophage C3 receptor or OKM1 and consists of the α_M subunit paired with the β_2 subunit. As a receptor for complement C_3b_i, this protein is expressed primarily on macrophages as well as, to a lesser degree, on monocytes, granulocytes and lymphocytes. Furthermore, Mac-1 can recognize fibrinogen and blood coagulation factor X, but only after induction on activated cells. Until now, the specific ligand for the α_x subunit in p150/95, a further member of the β_2 group, has not been determined, although some evidence indicates that it also recognizes complement C_3b_i.

The third integrin family, the cytoadhesins, is again primarily involved in cell-matrix adhesion and includes the mammalian vitronectin receptor and platelet gp IIb/IIIa, which share the common 120 kD β_3 subunit and both recognize extracellular matrix ligands by an RGD-dependent mechanism. Whereas β_3 corresponds to gp IIIa, the α subunit of this polyvalent platelet glycoprotein has been named α_{IIb}. Its ligand specificity includes fibronectin, vitronectin, fibrinogen, von Willebrand's factor, and thrombospondin. The vitronectin receptor with its α_v subunit is more widely distributed and recognizes a similar range of ligands: vitronectin, fibronectin, von Willebrand's factor, and thrombospondin. Recent evidence suggests that the α_v subunit, unlike other α subunits described thus far, can also associate with a second, novel β subunit, β_5, (with a reduced M_r of 120) to form an integrin with affinity for vitronectin and fibronectin, but not fibrinogen or von Willebrand's factor. This newly described integrin is expressed

Table 7.1 Mammalian Integrin Receptor Family

ß Subunit	M_r (Reduced)	α Subunit	M_r (Reduced)	Ligands	Distribution
$ß_1$ (gpIIa)	130	α_1	210 (VLA-1)	Coll I,IV	Smooth muscle cells, skin fibroblasts, hepatocytes, melanoma cells
		α_2	165 (VLA-2)	Coll I,II,III,V Coll IV,VI	Platelets, hepatocytes, smooth muscle cells, skin fibroblasts, epithelial cells, most primary lung tumors, melanoma cells
		α_3	135 (VLA-3)	LN, FN, Coll I,VI	Wide distribution: epithelial cells, monocytes, transformed cell lines
		α_4	150 (VLA-4)	FN	Most suspension cells, thymocytes, peripheral blood lymphocytes, myelomonocytic lines
		α_5	140+25 (FN-R, VLA-5)	FN	Platelets, smooth muscle cells, skin fibroblasts, hepatocytes, myeloid cell lines, human osteosarcoma cells
		α_6	140+25 (LN-R, VLA-6)	LN	Platelets
$ß_2$	95	α_L	180 (LFA-1)	ICAM-1, ICAM-2	Leukocytes
		α_M	170 (Mac-1, OKM1)	C_3b_i, FBGN[a], F X[a]	Monocytes, macrophages, granulocytes, lymphocytes
		α_X	150 (p150/95)	C_3b_i (?)	Monocytes, macrophages, granulocytes, lymphocytes
$ß_3$ (gpIIIa)	120	α_{IIb}	110+25 (gp IIb)	FN, VN, FBGN, vWF, TSP	Platelets
		α_V	120+25 (VN-R)	VN, FN, vWF, TSP	Human osteosarcoma cells

[a] Inducible.

Coll, collagen; FN, fibronectin; LN, laminin; ICAM, intercellular adhesion molecule; FBGN, fibrinogen; F X, factor X; vWF, von Willebrand factor; TSP, thrombospondin.

on a carcinoma cell line. Its relationship to another recently characterized heterodimer consisting of α_v and a novel β subunit, which is expressed on fibrosarcoma, fibroblast, and endothelial cell lines, remains to be determined.

The β_4 integrin family has only one member as yet. The β_4 chain displays an unusually large M_r of 205 kD and associates with the 125 kD α_6 subunit. This $\alpha_6\beta_4$ heterodimer has only been found on normal and malignant epithelial cells and its potential ligands are still unknown.

Finally, human polymorphonuclear leukocytes exhibit an integrin receptor with M_rs of 130–140 and 110 for the α and β chains, respectively, which recognizes the RGD tripeptide and displays affinity for fibronectin, fibrinogen, vitronectin, von Willebrand factor, and collagen IV. This receptor, which belongs to neither the β_1 nor the β_2 integrin family and cannot be immunoprecipitated by an anti-β_3 monoclonal antibody, has been named leukocyte response integrin. Its ligand-binding activity in extracellular matrix-stimulated phagocytosis is rapidly destroyed by oxidants from the myeloperoxidase–hydrogen peroxide–halide system, suggesting an early role in the inflammatory response of polymorphonuclear leukocytes. Sequencing is required to determine the precise relationship of this heterodimer to the known integrin family members.

This brief summary of integrin receptors and their ligands only reflects those best characterized to date and unfortunately cannot be complete. New members of the integrin receptor family are currently being characterized and the ligand specificities and cell distribution of all integrins are being examined more closely.

Cell Surface Proteoglycans

Heparan sulfate proteoglycans can bind extracellular matrix proteins and are known to be found on the cell surface of most adherent cells. Saunders et al. [4] have recently described a 33 kD integral membrane core protein for a mouse cell surface proteoglycan bearing heparan sulfate and chondroitin sulfate, which they have called syndecan. This macromolecule binds collagens I, III, and V as well as fibronectin and thrombospondin with high affinity via its heparan sulfate chains [1]. Syndecan proteoglycans are expressed mainly on epithelial cells in mature tissues and can vary with respect to the number, type, and sequence of glycosaminoglycans chains [4].

Anchorins

Anchorins are a group of collagen-binding proteins that associate with the cell surface in a Ca^{2+}-dependent manner, but do not appear to contain a transmembrane domain. Anchorin CII is a 34 kD protein expressed in chicken chondrocytes and fibroblasts, which shows a higher affinity for collagen II than collagen I [1,2]. A similar 34 kD molecule, p34, has been isolated from human placenta and specifically binds collagens I and III [23]. It is expressed in a wide variety of adherent cell lines in addition to primary fibroblasts and keratinocytes. These proteins may be involved in the processing of collagen or fibrillogenesis.

Other Extracellular Matrix Receptors

In addition to integrins, syndecan, and anchorins, other receptor proteins have been characterized that also appear to play a role in cell-matrix interactions.

Collagen

Collagens constitute a major component of the extracellular matrix and can exert many effects on cell behavior. Consequently, a number of collagen-binding proteins have been detected. Three molecules with M_rs of 250, 70, and 30 kD from human osteosarcoma cells bind specifically to a collagen I affinity column and can be eluted with the synthetic peptide gly-arg-gly-asp-thr-pro (GRGDTP) [1]. In addition, a 40 kD type I collagen-binding glycoprotein on the acrosomal surface of ejaculated rabbit sperm was described early on. Chicken corneal epithelial cells express a 70 kD integral membrane protein recognizing collagen IV and denatured collagen I, which may mediate epithelial cell attachment to the underlying basement membrane. Colligin, a 47 kD heat shock protein, binds collagens I, III, and IV [5]. Its localization in the endoplasmic reticulum, however, suggests that it is involved in intracellular processing of procollagen molecules rather than in cell–matrix interactions.

Several platelet membrane collagen-binding proteins that may play a role in platelet activation during hemostasis have been characterized. In addition to the $\alpha_2\beta_1$ integrin receptor for collagen found on platelets, a 65 kD molecule binds collagen I [6]. Its relationship to a 61 kD protein with affinity to skin-insoluble collagens has not been clarified. Finally, glycoprotein IV, an 88 kD major platelet membrane glycoprotein, mediates platelet adhesion to collagen I.

Laminin

As one of the major components of the basement membrane, laminin interacts with a variety of cell types. Several investigators have described a 67 kD protein with a high affinity ($K_d = 2$ nM) for laminin [1]. This receptor appears to derive from a 37 kD precursor protein that binds laminin with high affinity and contains a membrane-associated domain [7]. Such laminin receptors have been detected in skeletal muscle, breast carcinoma cells, fibrosarcoma cells, melanoma cells, neuronal cells, and in chicken corneal epithelium [1]. Effects of laminin are also mediated by a 120 kD integral membrane protein known as cranin and found in neural tissue and fibroblasts [8]. Finally, cell surface galactosyltransferase promotes cell spreading on laminin by interacting with oligosaccharides on the laminin molecule [9].

Fibronectin

Cell interactions with the multifunctional glycoprotein fibronectin involve not only several integrin receptors and syndecan but also a class of cell surface proteins with M_rs of 45–47 kD [1,10]. In addition, fibroblasts express a 36 kD fibronectin-binding protein that also forms 72 kD dimers and does not recognize the RGD sequence.

Elastin and Hyaluronate

The extracellular matrix component elastin is found in the interstitial dermis and can be bound by a 67 kD cell surface glycoprotein with a binding efficiency (K_d) of 8 nM. This protein exhibits β-galactoside-binding activity [11], which has implications for its possible functions and will be discussed later. Hyaluronate, on the other hand, has been shown to be deposited in many basement membranes and between cells in stratified epithelia. Thus the 85 kD transmembrane hyaluronate receptor is a likely candidate to mediate effects of hyaluronate on epithelial cells.

FUNCTIONS OF EXTRACELLULAR MATRIX RECEPTORS

One of the strategies used to isolate several extracellular matrix receptors of the integrin family involves screening for monoclonal antibodies with the ability to perturb cell adhesion and then characterizing the antigen recognized by such antibodies. Evidence indicates that monoclonal antibodies directed against integrin receptors inhibit attachment and spreading of a variety of cells on matrix substrates such as fibronectin, vitronectin, and laminin [1,2,12]. In some cases RGD-containing peptides also have a similar effect [1,2]. Antibodies against the nonintegrin 67 kD laminin receptor also inhibit cell adhesion to laminin. Taken together, these studies demonstrate that connective tissue receptor proteins play an important role in mediating cell adhesion to components of the extracellular matrix.

Adhesion receptors are also involved in other aspects of cell–matrix interactions such as matrix assembly. Monoclonal antibodies directed against the α_5 and β_1 subunits cause decreased deposition of a pericellular fibronectin matrix in a concentration-dependent manner [12]. Retention of fibronectin at the cell surface appears to be impaired. Furthermore, the assembly of elastic fibers can be inhibited in cultured chondrocytes by the addition of lactose that binds to the 67 kD elastin receptor [11].

Chemotaxis and migration of cells on extracellular matrix substrates also appear to be mediated by adhesion receptors. Chemotaxis of 3T3 fibroblasts toward fibronectin can be blocked with a polyclonal antiserum against the $\alpha_5\beta_1$

fibronectin receptor. Akiyama et al. [12] have shown that in addition to inhibiting attachment and spreading, monoclonal antibodies against the β_1 subunit inhibit the migration of fibroblasts on fibronectin. Antibodies against the 67 kD laminin receptor inhibit chemotaxis to laminin, a major basement membrane component.

Recent data suggest that adhesion receptors also play a role in signal transduction. Binding of a monoclonal antibody directed against the integrin $\alpha_5\beta_1$ fibronectin receptor to rabbit synovial fibroblasts induces the expression of collagenase and stromelysin on protein and mRNA levels. Fibronectin fragments containing the RGD sequence and ranging in size from 6 amino acids to 120 kD, but not intact fibronectin, can also elicit such an induction. Thus the conformation of the ligand may determine whether gene expression of the two metalloproteinases is induced after binding to the receptor. In addition, receptor clustering appears to be required for the signal transduction.

Adhesion Receptor Distribution and Interaction with the Cytoskeleton

Interactions between extracellular matrix proteins, cell surface matrix receptors, and the cytoskeleton are dynamic. This is illustrated by the fact that matrix substrates influence the distribution of receptors on adherent cells and these receptors, in turn, induce rearrangement of cytoskeletal proteins. The ability of substrate components to modulate integrin receptor distribution has been illustrated. Culturing endothelial cells on a mixture of fibronectin and vitronectin resulted in the clustering of both fibronectin receptors and vitronectin receptors at focal contact sites. On a pure fibronectin substrate, however, only fibronectin receptors localized to the adhesion plaques whereas vitronectin receptors remained diffusely distributed on the cells. An analogous result was seen when cells were grown on vitronectin with vitronectin receptors alone clustering at the focal contacts. In all cases receptor clustering at adhesion plaques preceded association of vinculin with the focal contacts and stress fiber formation. Another group of investigators describe basically similar results and additionally observed that after 24 hr in culture fibronectin receptors are no longer exclusively located at the focal contact sites, but also colocalize with newly deposited fibronectin fibers [13]. In fact, substrates derivatized with RGD peptides are sufficient to induce focal contact formation on fibroblasts. Other integrin receptors, namely $\alpha_1\beta_1$ and $\alpha_2\beta_1$, also colocalize in adhesion plaques when human melanoma cells are cultured on collagen substrates [14]. The 67 kD laminin receptor, on the other hand, codistributes with laminin in adherent endothelial cells.

Not surprising is the finding that receptor distribution is different in motile cells. The 67 kD laminin receptor and the integrin fibronectin receptor become concentrated in the ruffling membranes of migrating cells. In the case of the fibronectin receptor it could be shown that the receptor is endocytosed and recycled to the leading edge of fibroblasts.

A number of different proteins including talin, vinculin, and α-actinin associate intracellularly to form specialized structures known as focal contacts or adhesion plaques, which serve to link the actin cytoskeleton to the plasma membrane (Fig. 1). Addition of the pentapeptide GRGDS to 3T3 fibroblast cultures causes rapid dissociation of α-actinin and vinculin from focal contact sites [15]. The tripeptide alone, in contrast to intact extracellular matrix molecules, does not appear to be able to maintain a stable adhesion plaque structure by binding to integrin receptors. This suggests that the binding state of the integrin receptors is important in the transmembrane effect on cytoskeletal organization.

The colocalization of matrix receptors at focal adhesion sites is thought to be due to direct association of the cytoplasmic receptor domain with one of the focal contact proteins or actin. Mouse cells are able to express hybrid integrin heterodimers containing a mutated form of the avian β_1 chain that lacks the cytoplasmic tail. Although these hybrid fibronectin receptors are exported to the cell surface and exhibit normal ligand affinity, they do not colocalize to adhesion plaques in response to fibronectin. This points to a role for the cytoplasmic domain of the β_1 chain in interactions between adhesion receptors and focal contacts. In fact, evidence suggests that the avian β_1 chain binds talin. Fibulin has now been shown by three different labs to be extracellular and a serum protein.

Mechanisms to regulate integrin receptor association with the cytoskeleton may include variant subunits with alternate splicing of the cytoplasmic tail. An example of alternate splicing has been described for the integrin β_3 chain. The 21 amino acid residues at the C-terminus can be replaced by a shorter, 13 amino acid tail. An equivalent splicing variation apparently exists for the β_1 chain, suggesting the potential importance of such a mechanism.

Several other extracellular matrix receptors colocalize with and associate either directly or indirectly with actin. These include syndecan [4], the 67 kD laminin receptor [1,2], and the 85 kD hyaluronate receptor.

Regulation of Adhesion Receptor Expression

Until recently not much was known about factors regulating the expression of cell surface receptors for matrix components. One of these factors has proven to be transformation. Fibronectin receptors on Rous sarcoma virus transformed chicken fibroblasts or transformed mammalian cells diffuse away from focal adhesion sites and appear to be shed into the medium to a greater extent [1, 2]. At the same time receptor binding to talin decreases [1]. Furthermore, levels of the $\alpha_5\beta_1$ fibronectin receptor and two other unidentified α subunits decrease, whereas levels of the $\alpha_3\beta_1$ receptor are unchanged [16]. Transformation of chicken fibroblasts with Rous sarcoma virus concomitantly causes increased phosphorylation of the β_1 subunit on a cytoplasmic tyrosine residue. Aside from redistribution of the receptor molecules to a more diffuse pattern, no change in the level of expression is seen as a direct result of the phosphorylation [1,2], but perhaps the affinity for talin is regulated in this manner. Phosphorylation of the fibronectin receptor decreases during the retinoic acid-induced differentiation of F9 teratocarcinoma cells, but again no change in receptor expression was observed.

Cytokines have also demonstrated the ability to modulate extracellular matrix receptor expression. Transforming growth factor $\beta 1$, which influences the expression of a variety of extracellular matrix components, increases the mRNA steady-state levels and protein expression of the $\beta 1$ integrin subunit and the α_1, α_2, α_3, and α_5 subunits in WI-38 lung fibroblasts. The posttranslational maturation of the $\beta 1$ integrin subunit concomitantly appears to be accelerated. Expression of members of the other integrin β families is also regulated by TGF-$\beta 1$. Higher levels of mRNA and protein for the $\alpha_v\beta_3$ vitronectin receptor and the intercellular leukocyte adhesion receptor LFA-1 ($\alpha_L\beta_2$) are found in fibroblastic cells in response to TGF-$\beta 1$.

The second cytokine regulating the expression of integrin receptors is interferon-gamma. Interferon-gamma decreases collagen synthesis and is purported to increase collagen deposition into the matrix. At the same time, levels of the integrin collagen receptor $\alpha_2\beta_1$ in fibroblasts increase under its influence.

Two further examples illustrate the dynamics of integrin receptor expression in response to changing external environments. A group of investigators was able to select a subpopulation of human osteosarcoma cells based on their ability to attach and grow in the presence of an RGD peptide. These cells overproduced fibronectin receptors whereas levels of vitronectin receptors remained unaffected. In addition, these overproducing cells grew more slowly and exhibited a different morphology. In contrast, human keratinocytes in unwounded skin apparently do not express significant levels of integrin fibronectin receptors. Although freshly isolated keratinocytes from skin lack fibronectin receptor molecules, keratinocytes in culture for 10 days show increased receptor expression, which is presumably induced by exposure to fibronectin substrates.

ROLE OF ADHESION RECEPTORS IN DIFFERENTIATION

During differentiation cells may undergo changes in their adhesive properties that are reflected by a regulation of the expression of their adhesion receptors. Murine erythroleukemia cells, for example, lose their ability to bind to fibronectin when they are induced to differentiate with dimethylsulfoxide in vitro, as do reticulocytes when they differentiate into erythrocytes in vivo [2]. This loss of adhesion to fibronectin correlates with loss of integrin fibronectin receptor expression in the differentiated erythrocytes.

A similar phenomenon is observed in thymocytes, which are precursors of a different type of circulating cell. Hematopoietic precursor cells migrate into the thymus where they proliferate and differentiate. Analysis of the thymocyte population in the thymus shows that integrin fibronectin receptors are preferentially expressed on immature thymocytes whereas mature, committed thymocytes express lower levels of this adhesion receptor.

The third example of extracellular matrix receptor regulation during differentiation involves the nonintegrin 85 kD hyaluronate receptor. This adhesion molecule is found in many epithelia, particularly in areas of active cell proliferation, such as in the basal layers of stratified epithelia and in the base of the crypts of Lieberkühn in the intestinal epithelium. This suggests that epithelial cell adhesion is modulated during differentiation.

ROLE OF EXTRACELLULAR MATRIX RECEPTORS IN DEVELOPMENT

Cell–matrix interactions are also fundamental during developmental processes. The importance of directed cell migration and attachment in normal embryogenesis has been investigated extensively and is beyond the scope of this chapter. However, a few examples can illustrate the critical role and precise temporal expression of adhesion receptors in development. Injection of RGDS peptides or monoclonal antibodies and hybridomas against avian β_1 integrins into the mesenchyme of developing chick embryos results in altered distribution of neural crest cells and can result in a malformed neural tube [1]. If anti-integrin hybridomas are injected into the body cavity of 3–4 day chick embryos, aberrant development of abdominal muscle tissue results. Thus the regulation of adhesion receptors is thought to allow for the temporal modulation of cell adhesion behavior and the disruption of cell–matrix interactions results in aberrant morphogenesis.

As a further example, syndecan expression in vitro is induced in mesenchymal cells only after induction by developing dental epithelium. Levels of syndecan on cells increase with time of contact to the dental epithelium, suggesting that the expression of this cell surface proteoglycan is regulated by epithelial–mesenchymal interactions. This evidence implicates the involvement of syndecan in the condensation and differentiation of dental mesenchymal cells.

Precise temporal and spatial regulation of 67 kD laminin receptor levels occurs in the developing mouse kidney. Like dental mesenchyme condensation, nephrogenesis also involves extensive epithelial–mesenchymal contacts. Steady state mRNA levels of the laminin receptor are temporally linked to the expression of laminin and collagen IV mRNA: receptor mRNA expression precedes the expression of laminin and collagen IV mRNA and subsequently subsides.

ROLE OF ADHESION RECEPTORS IN METASTASIS

Metastasis is a multistep process involving not only cell–cell but also cell–matrix interactions. The extent of tumor cell contact with the surrounding matrix can promote or inhibit metastasis depending to a large extent on the adhesive properties of the invasive cells. The ability of the peptide RGDS to inhibit experimental lung metastasis formation by murine B16 melanoma cells suggests that integrin receptors play a role in the invasive behavior of these cells [2]. The ability of two human melanoma cell lines and a glioblastoma cell line to penetrate the amniotic basement membrane and the underlying stroma in an in vitro invasion assay could also be inhibited by RGD-containing peptides in a dose-dependent manner [17]. In further experiments antibodies directed against a specific integrin receptor, the $\alpha_2\beta_1$ collagen receptor, and coupled to ^{125}I inhibited the growth of lung tumor lines in vitro.

LFA-1, an integrin of the β_2 family of leukocyte receptors, also appears to play a role in metastasis. Antibodies against LFA-1 inhibit invasion of hepatocyte cultures by a lymphoma cell line [18]. LFA-1 mutants lacking cell surface expression of the receptor complex were generated for further experiments. The mutant clones demonstrated a decreased invasive potential in hepatocyte and fibroblast cultures in vitro as well as in other tissues in vivo. Thus, LFA-1, which may mediate adhesion to the surface of cells in target tissues, is required for the efficient metastasis of some lymphomas.

Other studies have characterized the extracellular matrix receptors found on tumor cell lines. Melanoma cells, for example, express the 67 kD laminin receptor. The same cells utilize $\alpha_1\beta_1$ and $\alpha_2\beta_1$ heterodimers to bind to collagens I and IV [14], which represent interstitial and basement membrane collagens, respectively.

DISEASES INVOLVING ADHESION RECEPTOR DEFICIENCY

The physiological relevance of functional adhesion receptors is best demonstrated by the effects of a deficiency in these molecules. Several conditions have been described involving deficient expression of particular integrin adhesion receptors.

The first of these diseases is known as leukocyte adhesion deficiency (LAD). Patients with this autosomal, recessive affliction are characterized by recurrent bacterial infections, little or no pus formation, impaired wound healing, and other deficiencies in adhesion-dependent leukocyte functions [1]. On a molecular level, patients with this disease express mutant integrin β_2 subunits that vary in their ability to complex with α subunits. Since expression of the α_L, α_M, and α_x subunits depends on the coexpression of the β_2 subunit, patients with severely deficient β subunits express none of these adhesion receptors. Polymorphonuclear leukocytes from such patients are unable to undergo a normal respiratory burst in response to tumor necrosis factor when tested on polystyrene coated with fibronectin, vitronectin, fibrinogen, thrombospondin, or laminin [19]. The same effect was observed when polymorphonuclear leukocytes from healthy donors were incubated with a monoclonal antibody against the β_2 subunit. Thus the importance of the β_2 integrin family of receptors in adhesion-related leukocyte functions with respect to cellular immunity is clearly established.

Glanzmann's thrombasthenia is a heterogenous, autosomal, recessive bleeding disorder involving the multispecific platelet receptor gp IIb/IIIa ($\alpha_{IIb}\beta_3$). Patients exhibit normal platelet counts, but abnormal platelet aggregation and clot retraction, which result in prolonged bleeding times [1]. In vitro these deficient platelets adhere normally to collagen, but show decreased ability to bind to fibronectin, von Willebrand's factor, fibrinogen, and thrombospondin [20].

Another platelet disorder has been described in which the platelet count is normal, but platelets are largely deficient in the α_2 subunit of the integrin collagen receptor, gp Ia [21,22]. Although other physiological stimuli induce platelet activation in these patients, collagen does not induce aggregation of the deficient platelets [21] or only induces aggregation at unusually high doses and no clot retraction is observed [22]. Platelets from one of the patients were also unable to bind purified human collagen I [21], but platelets from another patient exhibited normal collagen I-binding properties [22]. The bleeding deficiency in the latter patient later spontaneously disappeared and levels of gp Ia, the integrin α_2 subunit, returned to normal. Hemostasis is thus another process that depends on well-coordinated cell–matrix interactions.

In conclusion, the concept of connective tissue proteins as passive support structures is changing to accommodate the increasing evidence for dynamic interactions between cells and their extracellular matrix environment. Recently characterized connective tissue receptors play an essential role in these interactions.

REFERENCES

1. Buck CA, Horwitz AF. Cell surface receptors for extracellular matrix molecules. Annu Rev Cell Biol 1987; 3: 179-205.
2. Juliano RL. Membrane receptors for extracellular matrix macromolecules: relationship to cell adhesion and tumor metastasis. Biochim Biophys Acta 1987; 907: 261–78.
3. Hynes RO. Integrins: a family of cell surface receptors. Cell 1987; 48: 549–54.
4. Saunders S, Jalkanen M, O'Farrell S, et al. Molecular cloning of syndecan, an integral membrane proteoglycan. J Cell Biol 1989; 108: 1547–56.

5. Saga S, Nagata K, Chen WT, et al. pH-dpendent function, purification, and intracellular location of a major collagen-binding glycoprotein. J Cell Biol 1987, 105: 517–27.
6. Chiang TM, Kang AM. Isolation and purification of collagen a1(I) receptor from human platelet membrane. J Biol Chem 1982; 257: 7581–6.
7. Castronovo V, Taraboletti G, Sobel ME. Functional domains of the 67-kDa laminin receptor precursor. J Biol Chem 1991; 266: 20440–6.
8. Smalheiser NR, Schwartz NB. Cranin: a laminin-binding protein of cell membranes. Proc Natl Acad Sci USA 1987; 84: 6457–61.
9. Runyan R, Versalovic J, Shur B. Functionally distinct laminin receptors mediate cell adhesion and spreading: the requirement for surface galactosyltransferase in cell spreading. J Cell Biol 1988; 107: 1863–71.
10. Urushihara H, Yamada KM. Evidence for involvment of more than one class of glycoprotein in cell interactions with fibronectin. J Cell Physiol 1986; 126: 323–32.
11. Hinek A, Wrenn DS, Mecham RP, et al. The elastin receptor: a galactoside-binding protein. Science 1988; 239: 1539–41.
12. Akiyama SK, Yamada SS, Chen W-T, et al. Analysis of fibronectin receptor function with monoclonal antibodies: roles in cell adhesion, migration, matrix assembly and cytoskeletal organization. J Cell Biol 1989; 109: 863–75.
13. Singer II, Scott S, Kawka DW, et al. Cell surface distribution of fibronectin and vitronectin receptors depends on substrate composition and extracellular matrix accumulation. J Cell Biol 1988; 106: 2171–82.
14. Kramer RH, Marks N. Identification of integrin collagen receptors on human melanoma cells. J Biol Chem 1989; 264: 4684–8.
15. Stickel S, Wang Y. Synthetic peptide GRGDS induces dissociation of alpha-actinin and vinculin from the sites of focal contacts. J Cell Biol 1988; 107: 1231–9.
16. Plantefarber LC, Hynes RO. Changes in integrin receptors on oncogenically transformed cells. Cell 1989; 56: 281–90.
17. Gehlsen KR, Argraves WS, Pierschbacher MD, et al. Inhibition of in vitro tumor invasion by arg-gly-asp-containing synthetic peptides. J Cell Biol 1988; 106: 925–30.
18. Roossien FF, de Rijk D, Bikker A, et al. Involvement of LFA-1 in lymphoma invasion and metastasis demonstrated with LFA-1-deficient mutants. J Cell Biol 1989; 108: 1979–85.
19. Nathan C, Srimal S, Farber C, et al. Cytokine-induced respiratory burst of human neutrophils: dependence on extracellular matrix proteins and CD11/CD18 integrins. J Cell Biol 1989; 109: 1341–9.
20. Nurden AT. Glanzmann's thrombasthenia. In: Nurden AT, Phillips DR, eds. Platelet membrane glycoproteins. New York: Plenum Press, 1985: 374–92.
21. Nieuwenhuis HK, Akkerman JW, Houdjik WP, et al. Human blood platelets showing no response to collagen fail to express surface glycoprotein Ia. Nature 1985; 318: 470–2.
22. Kehrel B, Balleisen L, Kokott R, et al. Deficiency of intact thrombospondin and membrane glycoprotein Ia in platelets with defective collagen-induced aggregation and spontaneous loss of disorder. Blood 1988; 71: 1074-8.
23. Von der Mark K, Pfäffle M, Hofman C, et al. Anchorin CII, a collagen-binding protein of the calpactin-lipocortin family. In: Mecham R, ed. Biology of the extracellular matrix. New York: Academic Press, 1991: 301–22.

8

Mechanical Properties of the Dermis: An Engineer's Nightmare

Christopher Edwards and Ronald Marks
University of Wales College of Medicine, Cardiff, Wales

The word skin is a deceptively simple word, composed of four letters linked in a straightforward linear fashion. If only the physical entity of skin were as simple. In fact, the properties of the dermis account for most of the mechanical properties of skin. The outward appearance of normal skin is also suggestive of a single, basic covering, like the skin of a fruit (a peach-like complexion, orange peel skin, apple cheeks). In reality, our skin performs many functions and has evolved into an extremely complex structure. It is many-layered with convoluted three-dimensional boundaries between layers; it is anisotropic (has different properties in different directions) in all dimensions. In addition its structure and appropriate function vary with body site. These factors make skin a mechanical testing nightmare. The fact that the properties of skin are also time dependent (they vary with the rate of application of stress, and with time for which stress or strain are maintained), are contaminated by all surrounding structures, and are influenced by ambient conditions, recent stress history and age turn the tester's nightmare into an extraordinarily difficult exercise. Having said all that, determination of the mechanical properties and function of the dermis is the only way that some kinds of information can be obtained and this approach to the biology of skin should be more used than it is.

Mechanical properties modeling, or any analytical interpretation of test results, requires either that the boundaries of the specimen are known or, for infinite (i.e., thick) specimens, that the properties are constant or predictable in the direction of the test. When skin is on the body, only its surface boundary is accessible, so none of the conditions for modeling or interpretation of results exists. Even with estimates or assumptions of the missing information ("a constant thickness of 1 mm is assumed," "taking skin as a parallel-sided flat slab") analytical solutions (those that calculate a basic property of the test specimen from the measured behavior) of in vivo tests are at best approximately true over a limited, often unrealistic, range of conditions, and, at worst, prove intractable. This is not to say that in vivo tests are useless. On the contrary, their function is different since they provide the only relevant clinical information. However, in terms of measuring the pure, basic mechanical properties, they would be considered by mechanical engineers to be imprecise, uncontrolled, and unorthodox, and therefore not the methods of first choice [1].

IN VITRO TESTING

If the skin is removed from the body, the requisite test conditions can be arranged and empirical equations proposed to describe the observed skin responses to loading. Numerical values for the coefficients and constants of these equations can be found from the measured data by curve-fitting techniques, resulting in very good agreement between the derived equation and the actual skin behavior [2]. The question of how relevant such data are is often raised but there is no straightforward answer. The in vitro results are estimates of properties assumed to be important influences on function in vivo.

In vitro tests can inform us about the basic mechanical properties of strength, elasticity, and density inherent in the architecture of skin. In vivo tests tell us about how the skin reacts to external forces of stretch [3–5], shear [6], torsion [7], compression [8] and indentation [9] when it is on the body. In vitro tests can be considered as once-only tests in that the specimen, once removed, cannot be further modulated in vivo. The serial testing of one site possible with nondestructive in vivo tests provide information on the *function* and the *kinetics* of change in mechanical properties. The numerical values given by in vitro tests usually exhibit a smaller spread than the results of in vivo tests, but in both cases objective data are available to support (or supplant) subjective assessments of the physical state of the skin.

ELASTIC PROPERTIES

Materials science, in particular metallurgy and mechanical engineering, has defined certain properties of solid and liquid substances that are useful for predicting the behavior of structures made from such materials [10,11]. The properties thus described are usually classified into elastic properties and strength properties, and both of these are also subdivided into linear and nonlinear regions. A brief definition of some linear elastic properties will serve to clarify some of the experimental data presented later in this section.

For small forces, and small extensions, the outer parts of the skin react in a linear fashion. This reaction is entirely reversible and is not time-dependent. This is known as the linear elastic region and is common to most solid materials, although the range of extension over which linearity holds for skin is at least 10 times that of most metals. Elastic moduli are defined for typical test methods and shapes of test specimens, and the first three can be regarded as being appropriate to one, two, and three dimensions respectively.

If a solid rod of uniform cross-sectional area A is pulled with a tensile force F the tensile stress, σ, is defined as:

$$\sigma = \frac{F}{A} \tag{1}$$

If as a result the rod increases its length from 1 to $1 + \Delta 1$, the fractional increase is called the linear strain, ϵ:

$$\epsilon = \frac{\Delta 1}{1} \tag{2}$$

Within the elastic limit, stress is proportional to strain (Hooke's law). The ratio, E, is defined as Young's modulus:

$$E = \frac{\text{linear stress}}{\text{linear strain}} = \frac{F/A}{\Delta 1/1} \tag{3}$$

A solid may be deformed by a sideways, or *shear force*. For a rectangle we may apply a *shear stress*, τ (force/area), across opposite faces. This must result in equal shear stresses τ along the orthogonally opposite pair of faces so the net couple is zero (or the solid would move). The rectangle is thus distorted through a small angle θ, the *shear strain*. Within the elastic region strain is proportional to stress and the ratio is defined as the rigidity modulus, n:

$$n = \tau/\theta \tag{4}$$

The third possibility is the three-dimensional case of deformation of a solid by hydrostatic pressure. If a pressure P changes the volume V of a solid by an amount $-\Delta V$ (the minus sign signifies a *compression*), the *volume strain* is $-\Delta V/V$, and is once again proportional to P. The ratio is known as the Bulk modulus, K:

$$K = \frac{P}{-\Delta V/V} \tag{5}$$

The reciprocal of K is the *compressibility*, β

If a body is extended in tension to give a linear strain ϵ_{lin}, it contracts in directions orthogonal to the direction of tension. The fractional contraction in the transverse direction, ϵ_{trans} is proportional to the linear strain, and the ratio is defined as Poisson's ratio:

$$\nu = \frac{\text{contractile strain}}{\text{linear strain}} = \frac{\epsilon_{trans}}{\epsilon_{lin}} \tag{6}$$

Note if $\nu = 0.5$, there is no volume change on compression or contraction: this is the case for natural rubber.

The preceding quantities are related to each other in many ways, for example:

$$n = \frac{E}{2(1 + \nu)} \tag{7}$$

and

$$K = \frac{E}{3(1 - 2\nu)} \tag{8}$$

Note that if $\nu = 0.5$, then $K = \infty$; that is, the material is incompressible.

The above are some of the elastic properties of solids often reported for skin. However, they are strictly only true for epidermis and stratum corneum over a restricted range of test stimuli, and are invariably different in different directions in the skin. The dermis is a more complicated structure, and must be measured and analyzed differently.

Viscoelastic Properties

The time dependence of the skin's reactions to mechanical forces is given by the viscoelastic or time-dependent properties. The two most useful parameters are *creep* and *stress relaxation*. Creep occurs when a specimen is stretched by a predefined load and instead of remaining at its initial stretched length, it stretches further with time. Stress relaxation, on the other hand, is the reduction in load required to maintain a constant stretched length. For skin, these are not simply inversely related.

The creep or relaxation of skin begins as soon as the loading or extension begins, making the initial behavior (in the transition between resting condition and application of full test stimulus) complicated. This can be minimized by rapid loading, but there will still be a measurable transition time for any tensile testing machine. As a rule of thumb, it is taken that the effects of initial load application are negligible after 10 times the transition period, but since transition times of about 1 sec are usual, the first 10 sec of data are complicated by the behavior of the skin sample in the first second. The slower the strain application, the lower the measured load. Since the relaxation process is exponential, the most rapid response to the test stimulus will be during and immediately after the initial stretching. To determine simple moduli a correction should be made for the effects of rate of loading, but this is at best very approximate, since for skin the relationships between stress, strain, and time are far from simple.

In vitro tensile tests involve removing the specimen from the body, isolating the area and tissue of interest, and attaching the test sample to the tensile testing machine. The first step in the procedure is to plan the whole experiment carefully, because time and specimen handling are important factors governing the measured tissue mechanical properties, and should be kept to an absolute minimum.

Skin is under tension when in situ, with the maximum stress usually along specific directions (Langer's lines) [12] but of varying magnitude, depending on, for example, the amount of flexion of a limb. Since skin exhibits a ''memory'' of recent stress history for a number of hours, it is important to ensure that specimens are taken from areas of similar prestress in such a way that additional stretching is avoided during removal. The site and orientation of the sample must be recorded and explicitly referred to in test results.

Once removed from the body skin will retract (more in the direction of the greatest in situ tension). If the skin surface is marked in some way, restretching the excised specimen to regain the same dimensions of surface marking will produce an approximation to the pre-stress condition. This is not always possible, for example, with isolated dermis, since the surface marks will not be visible, and distortion of the surface does not necessarily reflect the condition of deeper tissues.

Time and storage conditions after the removal of skin, as well as time since death for cadaver samples, are important variables. Best results will be obtained from freshest samples, but practical considerations of availability and preparation of samples often force overnight storage, for which a temperature of 4°C in a sealed container or in physiological buffer is usually recommended [13]. Longer storage requires freezing of the specimens, but inevitably this will introduce some unquantifiable changes depending on the exact freezing procedure, storage temperatures, and time.

ISOLATING THE TEST AREA

For tensile testing the dimensions of the specimen should be known. In particular the thickness is important since the strain is defined as force per unit cross-sectional area. It is unfortunate that the lower surface of most excised specimens is far from flat, so an approximation to the thickness is all that is possible. In addition, at high strains skin may be reduced in thickness, making the true cross-sectional area, and thus the true stress, at any particular strain very difficult to obtain.

For studies of individual compartments of the skin (stratum corneum, whole epidermis, dermis, whole skin without subcutaneous fat) the tissue(s) of interest must be isolated from other neighboring and often intimately intertwined tissues. Mechanical separation can stretch, shear, or compress the tissues causing unpredictable residual effects. Chemical separation probably alters the properties of tissues too, so that there is no ideal method. Subcutaneous fat is usually separated mechanically, with a scalpel used to cut or scrape. Epidermis can be carefully peeled from the dermis after being heated at 60°C for 5 min. Stratum corneum can be isolated after blisters are raised by suction or chemicals such as ammonia vapor [14]. Other examples include the use of trypsin or other proteases to separate epidermis [15], or canthadrin for stratum corneum removal [16].

Once the tissue of interest has been isolated it must be cut to the required shape and dimension and mounted in the jaws of the tensile testing machine. All of these operations may introduce new and unquantifiable strains to the tissue, which will exert effects for many hours. The best method of ensuring that the tissue specimen does not slip from the jaws is to use a glue (cyanoacrylate is probably best) and clamp the skin with smooth jaws or to use one of the many proprietary designs of self-locking jaws. Examples of the latter include the use of eccentric rollers, or bollard systems that enable the gripping pressure to be progressively increased with the tensile force.

The humidity and temperature of the test specimen and environment must be carefully controlled if repeatable and meaningful measurements are to be made. These two variables are by far the most influential on measured elastic properties of skin.

The procedures described for preparing a skin specimen from excision to a ready-to-measure state are unavoidably very time-consuming and require considerable planning, dexterity, and skill. Once in the tensile tester the skin specimen is very unlikely to be in the same biochemical state, or in the same mechanical state or physical environment as it was in situ. Small wonder, then, that in vitro test results are difficult to compare with in vivo results, and are difficult to compare with data from other experiments of the same kind from the same or other experimenters. However, the test regimens are easy to control, and the type and quality of data collection in commercial tensile testers are uniformly excellent. The variability in test results arises from the specimen sources (site, sex, age, orientation, time since death for cadaver specimens) and, most importantly, specimen preparation (effects of storage, separation, mounting, test ambient conditions). Thus, in spite of the theoretical advantages of in vitro testing, in practice the much less pure techniques of in vivo testing have as much, if not more, validity in answering questions of the mechanical properties of our live skins.

MEASUREMENT PROCEDURES

There are two basic ways to measure tensile properties. The first involves applying all the strain at once, with minimum time between the steady states of zero load and maximum load. This method is useful to study stress relaxation (the way the specimen alters its structure, dimensions, or properties in order to minimize the stress), but the instant application of load is difficult. Also, skin exhibits a rate-dependent resistance to applied stress, and if load is applied too fast it may rupture at stress levels much lower than the ultimate stress levels determined by other tests. The other method involves the application of load in very small increments, with time delays between successive load increases long enough for all stress relaxation to have ceased. This gives more consistent and reproducible results for the linear elastic portion of the skin response.

PROPERTIES OF SKIN MEASURED IN VITRO

Probably the largest comprehensive and complete study of in vitro properties of human skin has been undertaken by Vogel [17,18]. In these experiments, using an Instron tensile testing machine, the number of samples ranged from 250 to 350, covering ages from birth to 100 years, so the results and conclusions have some statistical weight. The site of samples was above the sternum, and all samples were punched into dumbbell shapes 4 mm wide in the central portion with the long axis longitudinal to the body axis. Time since death and postmortem storage conditions, however, are not given.

Results can be summarized into the five categories reviewed below.

Ultimate Values

These results were obtained from 348 autopsy specimens. The ultimate load ranged from about 20 to 250 Newtons (N). The mean value shows a sharp rise to a maximum of about 150 N at 17 years, then declines steadily to about 100 Newtons at 90 years. The tensile strength (ultimate load divided by cross-sectional area) ranged from 5 to 30 N/mm^2 with the mean showing a maximum of about 21 N/mm^2 at 8 years, declining to about 17 N/mm^2 at 95 years.

The ultimate modulus of elasticity (calculated from the end portion of the stress-strain curves) ranged from about 15 to about 150 N/mm^2. The mean gave a maximum value of about 70 N/mm^2 at age 11 years, with a shallow decline to about 60 N/mm^2 at 95 years.

The ultimate strain varied from about 35 to 115%. The mean value declined in a linear fashion from 75% at birth to 60% at 90 years.

Hysteresis

For these experiments 251 specimens were measured. The samples were extended at a rate of 20 mm/min by 20%, then the cross-head was immediately returned to its initial position with the same velocity. Then the process was immediately repeated in 10% extension increases up to rupture. The stress–strain curves for the extensions did not coincide with the curves for the return to zero, forming hysteresis loops. The area under the stress–strain curves represents the energy put into the system, and the difference in the loading and unloading curves represents the energy used or lost in the system. The relative amount of energy loss is a measure of the viscosity of the sample (a fat hysteresis loop represents a highly viscous material, while coincidence of the loading and unloading curves represents purely elastic behavior). In general, a steady decrease in the viscosity parameter from young to old age was seen.

The extension still present after each unloading cycle (the residual tension) indicates the plasticity of the specimens, and was not age-dependent. Approximate average values of residual tension were 6% after 20% stretch; 13% after 30% stretch; 22% after 50% stretch; 36% after 60% stretch. Other parameters indicating elasticity and typically strength showed increases during maturation and a plateau (at low extensions) or a reduction (at high extensions) during aging.

Relaxation

The skin sample was extended at a rate of 1000 mm/min by 20% (this is an attempt at instant loading). This extension was maintained for 5 min while the stress values were recorded. Then the sample was unstretched to 90% (i.e., to 118% of its original length) and the tension measured. The experiment was immediately repeated on the same specimen at 40% extension, and further repeated with extension increases of 20% until specimen failure. The relaxation phenomenon caused the stress values to drop with a roughly logarithmic rate after initial strain application, confirming the assumptions of other authors [19]. The loss of tension as a percentage of initial tension indicated a clear loss of plasticity with age. Other parameters showed a similar pattern to those found in the hysteresis experiments, in which the extension rates were slower.

Creep

The samples were loaded with either 200 or 500g and the extension measured over time. The skin showed an initial sudden extension followed by a slow and more or less continuous extension. At 200 g load, this final extension rate was about 0.03% min. For the 500 g load, the average rate declined from about 0.06% min for younger skin to about 0.03% per min for skin of 90 years. The extension after 1 hr, which included the initial extension, varied from about 36% in the youngest specimens to about 30% for the oldest with 200 g load, and about 63% and 48%, respectively, for the 500 g load. This again shows the loss of plasticity (viscosity) with age.

Biochemical Correlations

Broad analysis of samples used for the mechanical testing was undertaken for soluble and insoluble (in 0.15 mol NaCl, 0.5 mol NaCl, and in citrate buffer of pH 3.7) collagens, glycosaminoglycans, and elastin. A correlation between tensile strength and insoluble and total collagen was found. The collagen content was seen to decrease with age. Viscosity parameters correlated with glycosaminoglycans and/or soluble collagens. Elastin content was not correlated with any measured mechanical property.

From this and other in vitro studies, it can be clearly stated that skin shows extremely complicated viscoelastic behavior. In general, however, a summary of properties and their age variation can be given: young skin is less protective against large strains than older skin; young skin is more viscous, or plastic, than older skin; older skin has a proportionately greater elastic region in its stress–strain behavior than younger skin. It also seems reasonable to conclude that the strength and elastic properties of skin are determined by the collagen content (specifically the insoluble collagen content), and not the elastin or ground substance components. Viscoelastic properties do seem to correlate with the soluble collagen and glycosaminoglycans content. Since these substances probably contribute to the water-binding capacity of skin, and since viscoelastic properties arise largely from the fluid (blood, lymph) and water content of skin, the observed correlation is not unexpected.

IN VIVO TESTING

Assessing the mechanical properties of components of skin in vivo is an engineer's nightmare. In fact, from the purist's point of view it is impossible. What is frequently done is to test mechanical function of skin as a whole. Some form of mechanical stimulus is delivered to the skin surface and the way that the area stimulated responds is recorded. Two types of stimulation can be recognized. The first of these is the static test mode in which a discrete single stimulus is provided, and the other type is the dynamic test mode. The availability of suitable equipment and the analytical techniques have dictated that techniques employing the static test mode have greatly outnumbered dynamic tests.

The static tests described can be characterized as follows;

1. Uniaxial extensometry: The force required to extend the skin after and during application of strain along a single axis[3] is measured and recorded.
2. Biaxial extensometry: The force applied to the skin with this method is distributed over a broad area, reducing the contributions from skin strained inadvertently either side of the single axis in uniaxial tests [20]. In both uniaxial and biaxial extensometry tests it is also possible to preset the force and record the deformation.

3. Torsional tests: A twisting force is applied to the skin surface and the resultant angular displacement is recorded. As with extensometry, it is possible to deform the skin to a set angle and record the force required to achieve this[21].
4. Indentation: The deformation produced by a preset indenting force is recorded[22]. The reverse process has also been used in which the elevation produced by a preset pulling force on the skin surface is recorded[23]. Use of adhesives to attach a piston to the skin surface and suction have both been used to supply the pulling force. The latter has also been used to supply a biaxial extensometric assay[24].

Results obtained from these test systems should be interpreted with caution because of the following constraints and considerations. (1) When a force is applied to the skin surface, it is distributed over a much wider volume of skin than the exact points at which it was applied, so the data are inevitably contaminated. (2) It is uncertain what contributions are made to the data from adnexae, nerves, and blood vessels. Nor can it be determined with any certainty if the data obtained primarily stem from dermal or epidermal properties (or indeed from subcutaneous fat or stratum corneum). (3) Interpretation is possible only if the rate of delivery of the stimulus is known and standardized and the recent stress history of the part is known. The data from any test depend on the number of test cycles already performed, as accommodation occurs. (4) The attachment of the apparatus delivering the force is difficult and subject to slippage. In addition, the shape and size of the "feet" influence the response obtained. (5) As discussed above, skin is anisotropic and the accurate orientation of the test is extremely important. (6) The ambient temperature and humidity influence the findings: not as much as they do when tests of the stratum corneum are considered, but sufficient to merit control as much as possible.

The dynamic test modes used have included the following.

1. In ballistometric test systems the wave forms generated by an impact are recorded and analyzed [25]. The recorded response will inevitably contain contributions from an undetermined volume of skin, plus the underlying structures of fat, muscle, or bone.

2. Elastic wave propagation systems have, in the main, concentrated on the measurements of shear wave velocities and the rate at which they are dissipated during their passage in the skin [26]. The application of the mechanical stimulus producing these vibrational waves (in which propagation is effected by the sideways movement of one layer of the medium being transmitted via viscous coupling to the next layer) has been via a vibrating stylus or a piezoelectric element. Detection of the resultant wave is also achieved by a separate stylus or element. This method represents a uniaxial dynamic test method, the axis defined by the line between transmitter and detector of the shear waves.

3. With dynamic suction methods a circular suction cup is applied to the skin and cyclical suction is applied. The height to which the skin is raised on each cycle is recorded either from the position of the skin surface or, in a more sophisticated design, by using M-mode ultrasound [27] to visualize the movement of different skin layers throughout the suction cycle. This method isolates a defined area of skin, and the ultrasound visualization allows individual layer responses to be observed. Of course these layers are still connected to adjacent tissue, so their response is not due entirely to their inherent tissue properties.

4. Mechanical impedance methods measure the resistance that the skin shows when forced into motion. It varies with the frequency of the applied force, the state of stress of the tissues, and the mechanical properties of the tissues. Sensitive instruments such as the electrodynamometer [28] accurately measure the force on and displacement of a vibrating head attached to the skin. This arrangement results once again in measurement of an undetermined volume of skin, but regional differences in skin mechanical properties are obvious.

The interpretation of all of these dynamic in vivo tests is difficult, and no successful analytical solution to any test is presently available. Since each method described above, and often each implementation of the method, utilizes subtle differences in attachment to the skin or frequency and form of application force, comparisons of results between methods is impossible. Nevertheless, each method will show changes of some mechanical properties of the skin tissues and thus may be of use in the evaluation of state of disease, treatments, and interindividual variations.

CLINICAL APPLICATIONS

There is an inherent reluctance on the part of dermatologists to employ instrumental adjuncts to diagnosis and clinical assessment. This probably stems from the view inculcated into them from the moment they start training that sufficient information about a skin disorder can be obtained by use of the senses, particularly the eyes. However, the sensory information this approach provides is subjective (and potentially prejudiced) and not quantitative (making it difficult to assess significance or collate or compare a collection of observations). Furthermore, the senses may not detect minor abnormalities and wrongly assess abnormal appearance, which may show relatively few faults either structurally or functionally.

Nowhere are these issues more apparent than when one in dealing with the mechanical properties of the skin. It is just not possible, for example, to assess the degree of abnormality present, the amount of progress made with treatment, or the deterioration in areas affected by scleroderma. The same is true of scars or areas affected by long-term treatment with potent corticosteroids.

It would be impossible to describe all the instruments that have been applied and their use. However three (clinician friendly) devices that have been employed in the clinic are the in vivo uniaxial extensometer, the twistometre (sic), and the tonometric device developed by Pierard.

Uniaxial extensometric tests are easy to apply and give a relatively simple force–extension measurement output. Such tests have been used extensively to study the aging of skin, in which an increase in stiffness, loss of elasticity, and reduced ability to accommodate after stretching are common compared to younger skin [29]. Studies of mechanical changes due to radiation therapy [30], psoralen/ultraviolet A(PUVA) [31], and steroids [32] have been undertaken, and it has been shown that uniaxial extensometry can yield parameters that directly relate to disease severity in the gravitational syndrome [19].

Skin aging has also been studied with torsional testing [33]. Such tests (together with skin thickness measurements) have been proposed as the most useful parameters in the study of the progression of (and, by implication, of the effects of treatment on) scleroderma, both the localized morphea and the systemic varieties [34]. Mechanical differences between different racial groups have been demonstrated using torsional testing [35], although these differences are mainly related to the increased photoprotection afforded by darker skin. The vertical displacement tonometric device developed by Pierard was used to study aging [36] and other conditions, with some impressive results obtained using cluster analysis of the data [37].

These brief examples of the uses of some devices for obtaining data of clinical interest illustrate the potential of mechanical testing in vivo. It is hoped that such devices will find a wider use in the clinical setting.

REFERENCES

1. Payne PA, Marks R, Guibarra EJ. International standards for instruments, measurement methods and units for determination of physical properties and function of skin. In: Marks R, Payne PA, eds. Bioengineering and the skin. Lancaster: MTP Press, 1981:9–11.
2. Ridge MD, Wright V. A rheological study of skin. In: Kenedi RM, ed. Proceedings of a symposium on biomechanics and related bioengineering topics. Oxford: Pergamon Press, 1965: 165–75.
3. Gunner CW, Hutton WC, Burlin TE. The mechanical properties of skin in vivo—a portable hand-held extensometer. Br J Dermatol 1979; 100: 161–3.
4. Wijn P. The alinear viscoelastic properties of human skin in vivo for small deformations. Thesis, University of Nijmegen 1980.
5. Brody GS, Peng TJ Landel RF. The rheological properties of human skin and scar tissue. In: Marks R, Payne PA, eds. Bioengineering and the skin. Lancaster: MTP Press, 1981: 147–58.
6. Escoffier CE, de Rigal J, et al. Age-related mechanical properties of human skin: an in vivo study. J Invest Dermatol 1989; 93: 353–7.

7. Agache P, Monneur C, Leveque JL, de Rigal J. Mechanical properties and Youngs modulus of human skin in vivo. Arch Dermatol Res 1980; 269: 221–32.
8. Dikstein S, Hartzshtark A. In vivo measurement of some elastic properties of human skin. In: Marks R, Payne PA, eds. Bioengineering and the skin. Lancaster: MTP Press, 1981: 45–53.
9. Thompson DE, Hussein HMG, Perritt RQ. Point impedance characterisation of soft tissues in vivo. In: Marks R, Payne PA, eds. Bioengineering and the skin. Lancaster: MTP Press, 1981: 103–11.
10. Higgins RA. Properties of engineering materials. Sevenoaks, UK: Hodder and Stoughton Educational, 1977.
11. Titcomb GRA. Fundamentals of engineering science. London: Hutchinson Educational, 1970.
12. Langer K. (trans. Gibson T). On the anatomy and physiology of the skin. III. Br J Plast Sur. 1978; 31:185–99.
13. Al-Haboubi AM. Effect of different aqueous solutions on the physical and mechanical properties of connective tissues. Master's Thesis, University of Strathclyde, Glasgow, 1977.
14. Vinson LJ, Kochler WR, Lehman MD, Masurat I, Singer EJ. Basic studies in percutaneous absorption. Semi-annual report No. 7 Army Chemical Centre, Edgewood, MD. Sec. 3, 1964.
15. Park AC, Baddiel CB. Rheology of stratum corneum. I. A molecular interpretation of the stress-strain curve. J Soc Cosmet Chem 1972; 23: 3–12.
16. Wildnauer RH, Bothwell JW, Douglass AB. Stratum corneum biomechanical properties. I. Influence of relative humidity on normal and extracted human stratum corneum. J Invest Dermatol 1971; 56: 72–8.
17. Vogel HG. Age dependence of mechanical and biochemical properties of human skin. Part I: stress–strain experiments, skin thickness and biochemical analysis. Bioeng Skin 1987; 3(1): 67–91.
18. Vogel HG. Age dependence of mechanical and biochemical properties of human skin. Part II: Hysteresis, relaxation, creep and repeated strain experiments. Bioeng Skin 1987; 3(2): 141–76.
19. Mourad MM, Edwards C, Marks R. Skin extensibility in the gravitational syndrome. Bioeng Skin 1988; 4(3): 199–215.
20. Cook TH. An in plane method for determining the two dimensional stress-strain behaviour of living human skin. Proc. 29th ACEMB, 43, 1979.
21. Finlay B. The torsional characteristics of human skin in vivo. J Biomed Eng 1984; 6:567–73.
22. Hendley A, Marks R, Payne PA. Measurement of forces for point indentation of the stratum corneum in vivo. Bioeng Skin Newsletter 1982; 3: 234–40.
23. Dikstein S, Hartzhtark A. In vivo measurement of some elastic properties of human skin. In: Marks R, Payne PA, eds. Bioengineering and the skin. Lancaster: MTP Press, 1981: 45–53.
24. Cook FH, Alexander H, Cohen M. Experimental method for determing the two-dimensional mechanical properties of living human skin. Med Biol Eng Comp 1977; 15: 381–90.

25. Tosti A, Campagno G, Fazzini MC, Villardita S. A ballistometer for the study of the plasto-elastic properties of the skin. J Invest Dermatol 1977; 69: 315–7.
26. Potts RD, Chrisman DA, Buras EM. The dynamic mechanical properties of human skin in vivo. J Biomech 1983; 16: 365–72.
27. Breitbart EM, Hicks R, Rehpenning W. Möglichkeiten der Ultraschall diagnostik in der Dermatologie. Z Hautkr 1986; 61(8): 522–6.
28. Hargens CW. The gas bearing electrodynamometer (GBE) applied to measuring mechanical changes in the skin and other tissues. In: Marks R, Payne PA, eds. Bioengineering and the skin. Lancaster: MTP Press, 1981: 113–22.
29. Wijn P, Brakkee AJM, Kuioer JP and Vendrik AJH. The alinear viscoelastic properties of human skin in vivo related to sex and age. In: Marks R, Payne PA, eds. Bioengineering and the skin. Lancaster: MTP Press, 1981: 135–45.
30. Hutton WC, Ranu HS, Burlin TE. An apparatus for measuring th effects of radiotherapy on the elastic properties of human skin in vivo. Med Biol Eng 1975; 13:584.
31. Gunner CW, Williams EW, Greaves M, Hutton WC, Burlin TE. Effects of treatment with prednisolone and PUVA on the mechanical properties of human skin in vivo. In: Marks R, Payne PA, eds. Bioengineering and the skin. Lancaster: MTP Press, 1981: 31–43.
32. Burton JL, Shuster S. A rapid increase in skin extensibility due to prednisolone. Br J Dermatol 1973; 89: 491.
33. Leveque J-L, Corcuff MS, de Rigal PD, Agache MD. In vivo studies of the evolution of physical properties of the human skin with age. Int J. Dermatol 1984; 5:322–9.
34. Kalis B, de Rigal J, Leonard F, Leveque J-L, Riche O, Le Corre Y de Lacharriere O. In vivo study of scleroderma by non-invasive techniques. Br J Dermatol. 1990; 122: 785–91.
35. Berardesca E, de Rigal J, Leveque J-L, Maibach HI. In vivo biophysical characterisation of skin physiological differences in races. Dermatologica 1991; 182:89–93.
36. Pierard GE. Investigating rheological properties of skin by applying a vertical pull. Bioeng. Skin 1980; 2(3): 31–6.
37. Pierard GE, Lapierre CM. Physiopathological variations in the mechanical properties of skin. Arch Dermatol Res 1977; 260: 231–9.

9

The Family of Stromal Cells

Giulio Gabbiani and Marie-Luce Bochaton-Piallat
University of Geneva, Geneva, Switzerland

Like all connective tissues, the dermis is composed of small vessels, a complex extracellular matrix, and histiocytic or fibroblastic cells. Fibroblasts are responsible for most of the synthesis of extracellular components. They replicate and become contractile during wound healing, and it appears more and more clear that they produce compounds collectively termed cytokines, capable of inducing or repressing activities of neighboring cells, including epithelial cells. In this chapter, we shall limit our discussion to stromal fibroblastic cells. We will review their morphologic and biochemical features, as well as the modulations of these features during physiological and pathologic conditions.

NORMAL FIBROBLAST

Development, Morphology, and Biochemical Features

The general morphologic features of fibroblasts are presently well known [1, 2]. The nucleus is generally large and contains one or more nucleoli. The most prominent cytoplasmic organelle is rough endoplasmic reticulum, which consists of a series of interconnected saclike or tubular structures present throughout the cytoplasm. The content of the cisternae is relatively dense and sometimes finely filamentous. Ribosomes form large aggregates on the membranes [1]. Some aggregates of ribosomes are also found free within the cytoplasm. The Golgi apparatus is generally prominent and has no preferred location. It consists of stocks of flattened lamellae and vesicles (Fig. 9.1a). Peripheral vesicles and vacuoles may be related to the process of pinocytosis or to the excretion of cell products. Abundant mitochondria are present throughout the cytoplasm. They have regular cristae and a relatively dense matrix. A few cytoplasmic microfilaments (40–70 Å) and some intermediate filaments (80–110 Å in diameter) may be seen in fibroblasts of adult animals or humans, particularly close to the plasmalemma. Microfilaments are more common in embryonic and fetal fibroblasts. Other rare components of the fibroblast cytoplasm are centrioles, cilia, multivesicular bodies, and lipid droplets (particularly in old fibroblasts). In normal tissues of adult animals, there are no contacts between fibroblasts. However, contacts can be seen between embryonic and fetal fibroblasts, as well as between fibroblasts of newborn animals. It is now accepted that fibroblasts are the main source of collagen fibers, proteoglycans, and collagenases.

In certain organs, such as the mammary gland or the intestinal mucosa, fibroblastic stromal cells have been shown to interact with epithelial cells in order to coordinate the development of the organ. It has been suggested that interactions between mesenchymal and epithelial components continue through postfetal life and are important in the development of several pathologic changes including carcinogenesis. Evidence for this type of interaction between dermis and epidermis also starts to emerge [3]. Thus, keratinocytes cultured over dermal tissue organize in layers similar to those observed in the normal epithelium. In conclusion, fibroblastic cells appear to be very active cells, exerting several functions, which may vary according to age, location, and physiological or pathologic situations.

Fibroblasts in Culture

Fibroblastic cells are easily placed in culture and have therefore been intensely studied in vitro. When placed in a culture dish, fibroblasts reveal a certain number of features that are not always easy to appreciate in the whole tissue under normal conditions [2]. In culture, they are characterized by their polarity. Moreover, they are connected frequently by gap junctions or nexuses. Gap junctions are considered to be low-resistance pathways for intercellular communication; their presence between cultured fibroblasts suggests that unlike normal tissue fibroblasts, these cells are metabolically coupled. When examined by phase contrast or Nomarsky optics, cultured fibroblasts show several straight fibers (stress fibers), which usually run parallel to each other, and sometimes extend over long distances of the cell body. Stress fibers are characteristic features of cultured cells [2], but several recent observations have shown that they may exist in vivo in several cell types, and indeed be present in granulation tissue fibroblasts or myofibroblasts (see below) [4]. Stress fibers are mainly composed of contractile

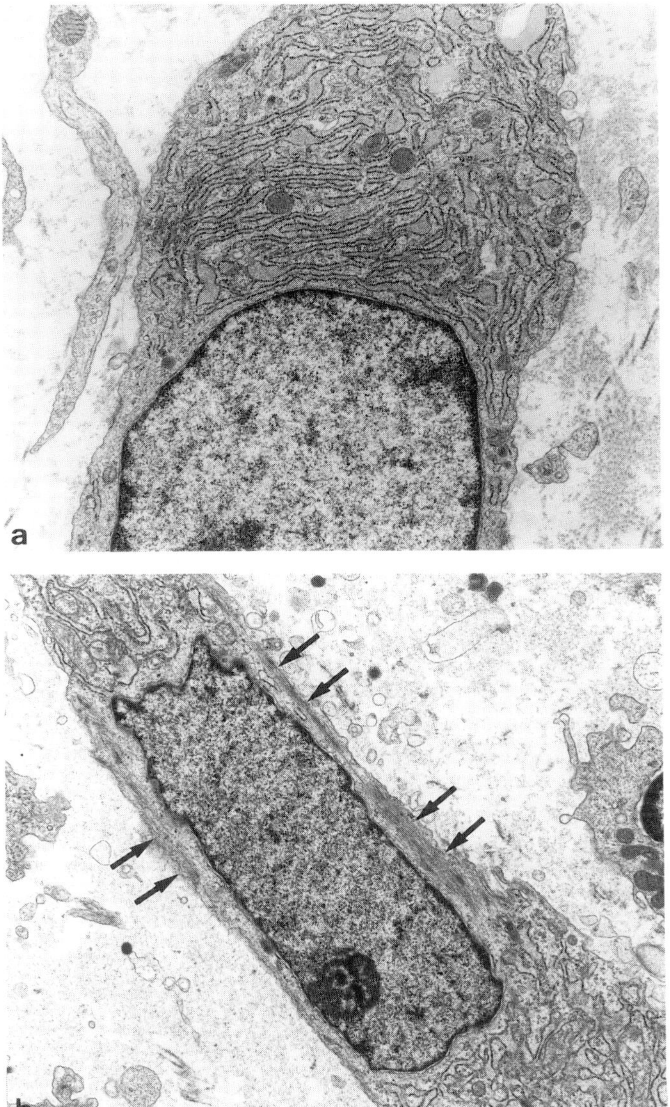

Figure 9.1 Electron micrographs of a rat dermis fibroblast (a) and of a myofibroblast from rat granulation tissue 10 days after production of an experimental wound (b). The fibroblast shows abundant rough endoplasmic reticulum while the myofibroblast also contains bundles of microfilaments (arrows) and scattered dense bodies (× 20,000; courtesy of Drs. L. Rubbia-Brandt and I. Darby, Department of Pathology, University of Geneva, Geneva, Switzerland).

proteins (such as actin and myosin) (Fig. 9.2) and probably reflect the capacity of these cells to develop a tensile strength. The presence of mitotic activity and of contractile and motile features, as well as the capacity of synthesizing collagen, collagenases, and proteoglycans, make cultured fibroblasts a good model of granulation tissue fibroblasts (see below). Cultured fibroblasts have been shown to possess the capacity of differentiating into several morphologic and biochemical types, which may correspond to modulations observed in vivo, in different organs, or after physiological and pathologic changes [5].

Features of Fibroblasts from Different Tissues

Fibroblastic cells have usually been conceived of as a uniform population from the morphologic, biochemical, and functional point of view. However, more and more evidence is accumulating to suggest that fibroblastic cells may be heterogeneous in different organs or may modulate their features according to functional and pathologic stimuli. As previously said, it has been reported that fibroblasts in vitro, may differentiate in different populations that can allegedly express different morphologic features [5]. The development of differentiation markers, particularly those connected to cytoskeletal elements, has allowed the distinction of several fibroblastic populations in different normal organs. Ultrastructural features, such as the presence of stress fibers, which are commonly present in culture, may be a discriminating criterion among different fibroblastic populations. Thus, fibroblasts with several degrees of smooth muscle differentiation have been described in the external theca of the ovary, in murine adrenal gland capsule, in the intestinal mucosa of humans and rabbits, in the periondotal ligament of several species, in the stroma of uterine mucosa, in lymphatic organs,

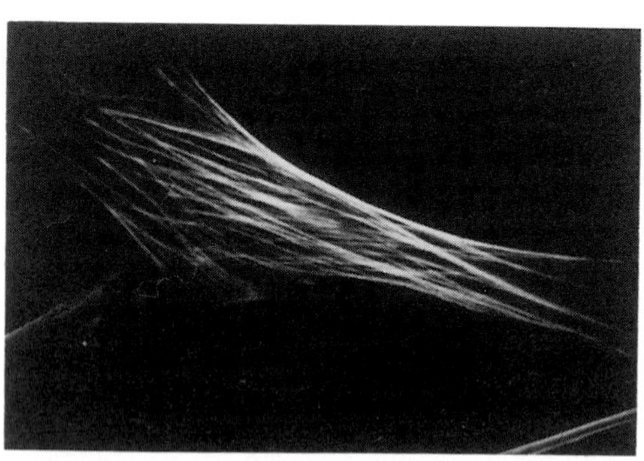

Figure 9.2 Immunofluorescence staining of a cultured rat fibroblast with general antiactin antibodies. Actin-positive stress fibers running parallel to the long axis of the cell are clearly visible in the flat preparation (× 400; from [4], with permission of the publisher).

including the spleen, of humans and rodents, and in the pulmonary septa of many mammalian species [4]. These differences in morphologic and biochemical features do not always correspond to known functional modulations. However, in some cases, it has been possible to find a correlation between morphologic modulation and functional activity. Thus, it has been suggested that through their contractile activity fibroblastic interstitial cells of the pulmonary alveolus regulate the tension of the alveoli, the amount of blood flow, and the organization of epithelial tissues [6]. It has been shown that these fibroblasts can contract and relax under the influence of several substances that contract and relax smooth muscle cells and in this way exert regulatory activities. All these morphologic and functional observations indicate that fibroblasts dispose of varying differentiation programs that may be function- and tissue-specific.

FIBROBLAST DURING WOUND HEALING: MYOFIBROBLAST

Morphology and Biochemical Features

Healing of an open wound is characterized by two phenomena: formation and contraction of granulation tissue and epithelialization. Granulation tissue consists of a temporary accumulation of small vessels and fibroblastic cells capable of retracting the wound space and finally resulting in scar formation. The cells responsible for these phenomena are a special kind of fibroblast that has modified its morphologic and biochemical features and acquired motile and contractile activities. These granulation tissue fibroblasts have been called myofibroblasts [7].

Myofibroblasts have ultrastructural and biologial properties close to smooth muscle cells, on one hand, and cultured fibroblasts, on the other hand [2]. They contain abundant actin microfilaments organized in stress fibers [7, 8] which probably play a role in their contractile activity (Fig. 9.1b). Immunofluorescence with antiactin and antimyosin antibodies shows a colocalization of these antigens in stress fibers [2]. The interaction between actin and myosin is known to be involved in the contracting process. Electron-opaque areas, called dense bodies, are scattered among the bundles of microfilaments or located beneath the plasmalemma similar to the attachment sites in smooth muscle cells or cultured fibroblasts. The remaining cytoplasm is occupied by packed cisternae of rough endoplasmic reticulum. Nuclei present multiple indentations or deep folds, an appearance quite unlike that of normal fibroblasts. Nuclear folds can be correlated with cellular contraction in several systems, such as smooth muscle cells [7]. As in cultured fibroblasts, gap junctions interconnect myofibroblasts [8]. Part of the myofibroblast surface is often covered by a basal lamina-like material, and dense zones in the fibrillar bundles immediately beneath the cell membrane are seen in areas facing this basement membrane. These structures, called hemidesmosomes, are also found in vivo to bind smooth muscle cells, endothelial cells, or pericytes, to their basal lamina [7]. Another transmembrane complex, the fibronexus, associates intracellular microfilaments of myofibroblasts and extracellular fibronectin fibers [9]. This complex is thought to fix myofibroblasts to extracellular matrix, thereby allowing to the cell to exert a tensile activity.

Myofibroblasts in Pathologic Wound Healing and Fibrocontractive Diseases

Myofibroblasts have been described not only in normal wound healing but also in several more chronic conditions that have been classified as follows: 1) situations related to inflammation, wound healing, and tissue remodeling, such as hypertrophic scars and burn contractures, retraction capsules on mammary implants, scleroderma, liver cirrhosis, pulmonary and kidney fibrosis, granulomas, and hepatic schistosomial fibrosis; 2) fibromatoses, which are proliferative fibroblastic lesions without prominent inflammatory components; these include Dupuytren's contracture, La Peronie's nodule, and plantar fibromatoses, as well as abdominal fibromatoses and nodular fasciitis; and 3) stromal response to neoplasia, particularly carcinomas, which are often inflammatory but sometimes consist of a vigorous proliferative reaction of myofibroblasts (for review see [10]).

Myofibroblasts Compared with Fibroblasts and Smooth Muscle Cells

It is accepted that myofibroblasts do not derive from circulating cells [1]; however, it is not sure from which local cell they do arise. The most likely candidates are fibroblasts, pericytes, and smooth muscle cells.

Pericytes have ultrastructural and immunohistochemical features similar to those of myofibroblasts; during early arterial development [11]), experimental arterial intimal thickening induced by endothelial injury, and when placed in culture [4], vascular smooth muscle cells also acquire a phenotype similar to that of myofibroblasts [12]. Thus, it seems that fibroblasts, as well as smooth muscle cells and pericytes, possess the potential capacity of modulating toward a myofibroblastic phenotype.

The availability of immunologic probes recognizing smooth muscle cell differentiation markers has been useful in the definition of the myofibroblastic phenotype. These antigens are intermediate filament proteins and actin isoforms. At least five distinct classes of intermediate filament proteins have been described (for review see [13]), including vimentin in cells of mesenchymal derivation, desmin in muscular cells, cytokeratins in epithelial cells, neurofilament proteins in neuronal cells, and glial fibrillary acidic proteins in glial cells (see [14]).

In mammals and birds, six actin isoforms have been identified, which migrate in three spots with different isoelectric points on two-dimensional gel electrophoresis. These have been called α, β, and γ [15]. Sequence analysis has allowed the determination of three actin isoforms with an α-electrophoretic motility: one specific for skeletal muscle, one specific for cardiac muscle, and one specific for smooth muscle, particularly vascular smooth muscle. β-Actin corresponds to a single isoform found in every cell and called cytoplasmic. Of the two isoforms that migrate with a γ mobility, one is cytoplasmic and the other is typical of smooth muscle, particularly parenchymal smooth muscle [16]. Two-dimensional gel electrophoresis, has shown that all smooth muscle tissues express α-, β-, and γ-actin isoforms, while fibroblasts express only β-and γ-isoforms [4]. Consequently, the expression of α-actin indicates the smooth muscle origin of a connective tissue or cell population.

Using these markers it has been possible to show that during normal wound healing in the rat, myofibroblasts not only show new ultrastructural features compared to in situ fibroblasts (see above) but also develop transiently smooth muscle differentiation features such as the appearance of α-smooth muscle actin ([17]; Fig. 9.3). This protein disappears after the wound is epithelialized. Because

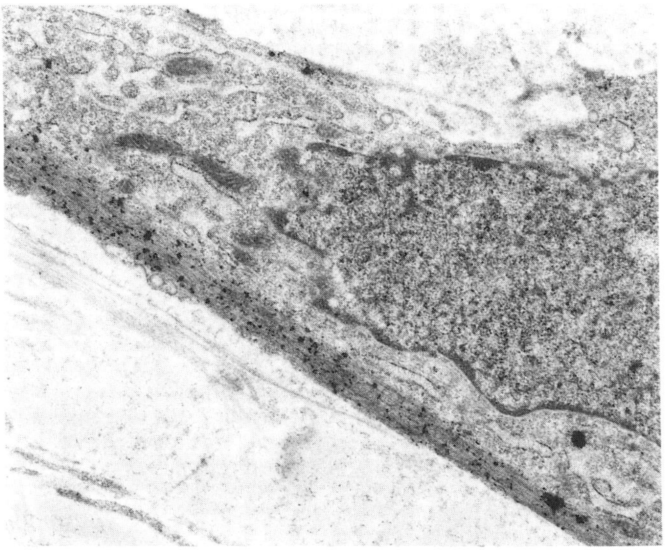

Figure 9.3 Immunogold staining with α-smooth muscle actin antibody of a myofibroblast in a rat granulation tissue 14 days after removal of a 4 cm^2 skin fragment. At this time, the bundles of microfilaments localized close to the plasmalemma are selectively marked with gold particles indicating that they contain α-smooth muscle actin (× 20,000; courtesy of Dr. I. Darby, Department of Pathology, University of Geneva, Geneva, Switzerland).

of the transient expression, it is not always possible to localize α-smooth muscle actin in normally healing wounds in humans. In contrast, in hypertrophic scars, fibromatoses, and stromal reaction to tumors, such muscle-differentiation antigens persist in myofibroblastic cells, suggesting that a perturbed expression of these proteins plays a role in the development of pathologic changes [18]. Thus in these situations, one can observe a heterogeneous myofibroblast population that comprises cells containing vimentin; vimentin and α-smooth muscle actin; vimentin, α-smooth muscle actin, and desmin; or, finally, vimentin and desmin (Figs. 9.4 and 9.5). The two last cell categories are never observed in myofibroblasts during normal wound healing.

These results represent a further indication that fibroblasts can modulate into several phenotypes that exert possibly different biological activities. The correlation between these phenotypes and their functional modulation is not known, but clearly the presence of certain phenotypes coincides with some pathologic situations. As an alternative, during these pathologic conditions a differential proliferation of fibroblasts, pericytes, and smooth muscle cells can result in the presence of a heterogeneous myofibroblastic population.

MODULATION OF THE PHENOTYPE

It is more and more clear that the fibroblastic stromal cell family is composed of several members, not only expressing different morphologic and biochemical features but also endowed with varied biological properties [19]. These fibroblastic cells modulate from one type to the other and vice versa during physiological and pathologic situations. This implies that local and systemic factors influence such modulations, and thus play a role in the evolution of several physiological and pathologic changes. Approaches other than the study of cytoskeletal elements and/or correlation of cytoskeletal changes with changes in the synthesis of extracellular components will probably be useful for the definition of fibroblastic modulations. The identification of new modulation markers will be instrumental in the understanding of fibroblastic physiology.

It is known that local factors liberated by cells such as macrophages and lymphocytes, or by fibroblasts themselves, called collectively cytokines, can modulate the activity of fibroblasts in physiological and pathologic conditions. Some of the factors have been shown to influence fibroblastic activities such as collagen production, wound healing, and even expression of α-smooth muscle actin [20]. Further studies along these lines may bring new data on the plasticity of fibroblastic activities. It has likewise been shown that the composition of extracellular matrix has profound influences on fibroblast morphology and behavior during development, culture conditions, and several in vivo situations. Again, studies along these lines may bring new information on the adaptation capacities of fibroblastic cells.

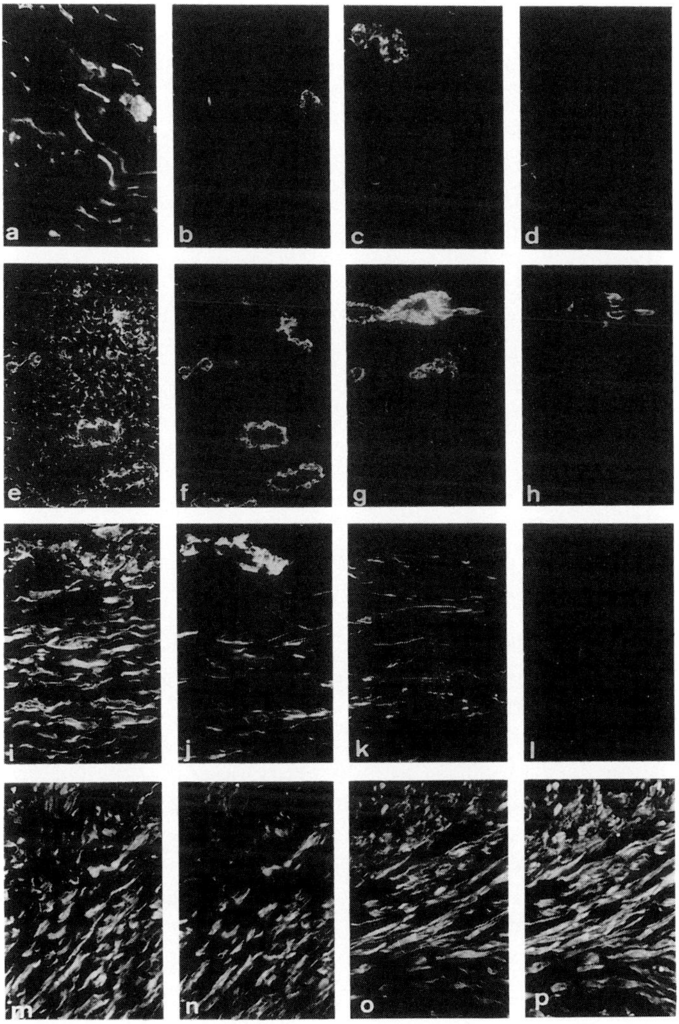

Figure 9.4 Double immunofluorescence staining of scar (a–d), eschar granulation tissue (e, f), normally healing granulation tissue (g, h), and two cases of hypertrophic scars (i–l, m–p), with antivimentin (a, e, i, m) and anti-α-smooth muscle actin (b, f, j, n) and with anti-α-smooth muscle actin (c, g, k, o) and antidesmin (d, h, i, p). Normal scar (a–d), eschar granulation tissue (e, f), and normally healing granulation tissue (g, h) are only positive for vimentin, whereas one case of hypertrophic scar (i–l) is positive for vimentin and α-smooth muscle actin, and the other (m–p) contains cells positive for vimentin, desmin, and α-smooth muscle actin (× 400; from [17], with permission of the publisher).

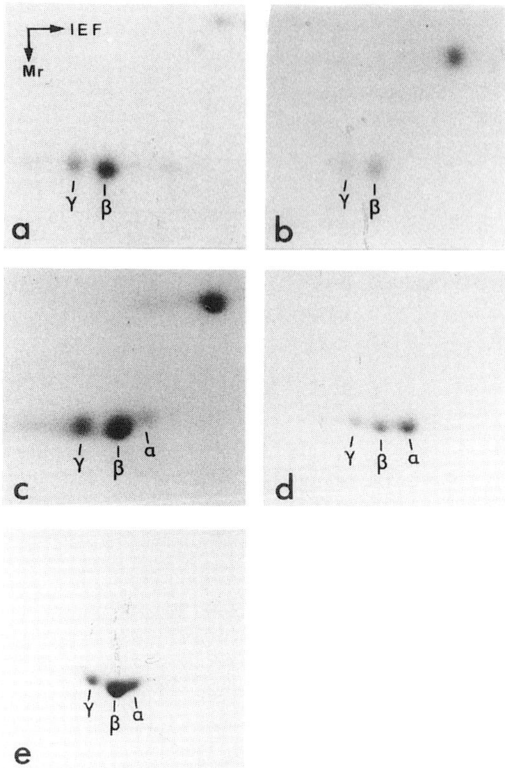

Figure 9.5 Two-dimensional gel pattern of actin isoforms in dermis (a), normal scar (b), hypertrophic scars (c, d), and palmar fibromatosis (e). Dermis and normal scar contain ß- and γ-actins whereas hypertrophic scars and palmar fibromatosis contain α-, ß- and γ-actins. V, vimentin; IEF, Mr, and the corresponding arrows indicate the direction of isoelectric focusing and second dimension, respectively (from [17], with permission of the publisher).

In conclusion, it appears that the fibroblastic stromal cells make up a family with several common features, but also with differing heterogeneous features and activities; these vary according to the location of the cell and to the external stimuli. Fibroblastic features can also modulate, both morphologically and functionally. Such considerations open the possibility of further understanding fibroblast biology, on one hand, and connective tissue physiology and pathology, on the other.

ACKNOWLEDGMENTS

This work has been supported in part by the Swiss National Science Foundation, grant 31-30796.91. We thank Mrs. M.-M. Rossire for typing the manuscript.

REFERENCES

1. Ross R, Everett NB, Tyler R. Wound healing and collagen formation. VI. The origin of the wound fibroblast studied in parabiosis J Cell Biol 1970; 44: 645–54.
2. Gabbiani G, Rungger-Brändle E. The fibroblast. In: Glynn LE, ed. Handbook of inflammation: tissue repair and regeneration, vol 3. Amsterdam: Elsevier/North-Holland Biomedical Press, 1981: 1–50.
3. Fusenig NE, Breitkreutz D, Boukamp P, et al. Epithelial–mesenchymal interactions in tissue homeostasis and malignant transformation. In: Johnson NW, ed. Markers of oral disease: oral cancer, vol 2. New York: Cambridge University Press, 1991:218–256.
4. Skalli O, Gabbiani G. The biology of the myofibroblast: relationship to wound contraction and fibrocontractive diseases. In: Clark RAF, Henson PM, eds. The molecular and cellular biology of wound repair. New York: Plenum Publishing, 1988: 373–402.
5. Bayreuther K, Rodemann HP, Hommel R, et al. Human skin fibroblasts in vitro differentiate along a terminal cell lineage. Proc Natl Acad Sci USA 1988; 85: 5112–6.
6. Adler KB, Low RB, Leslie KO, et al. Contractile cells in normal and fibrotic lung. Lab Invest 1989; 60: 473–85.
7. Gabbiani G, Hirschel BJ, Ryan GB, et al. Granulation tissue as a contractile organ. A study of structure and function. J Exp Med 1972; 135: 719–34.
8. Gabbiani G, Chaponnier C, Hüttner I. Cytoplasmic filaments and gap junctions in epithelial cells and myofibroblasts during wound healing. J Cell Biol 1978; 76: 561–8.
9. Singer II, Kawka DW, Kazazis DM, Clark RAF. In vivo codistribution of fibronectin and actin fibers in granulation tissue: immunofluorescence and electron microscope studies of the fibronexus at the myofibroblast surface. J Cell Biol 1984; 98: 2091–106.
10. Seemayer TA, Schürch W, Lagace R. Myofibroblasts in human pathology. Hum Pathol 1981; 12: 491 –2.
11. Kocher O, Skalli O, Cerutti D, et al. Cytoskeletal features of rat aortic cells during development: an electron microscopic, immunohistochemical and biochemical study. Circ Res 1985; 56: 829–36.
12. Chamley-Campbell J, Campbell GR, Ross R. The smooth muscle cell in culture. Physiol Rev 1979; 59: 1–61.
13. Steinert PM, Jones JCR, Goldman RD. Intermediate filaments. J Cell Biol 1984; 99: 22–7.
14. Rungger-Brändle E, Gabbiani G. The role of cytoskeletal and cytocontractile elements in pathologic processes. Am J Pathol 1983; 110: 359–92.

15. Garrels JI, Gibson W. Identification and characterization of multiple forms of actin. Cell 1976; 9: 793–805.
16. Vandekerckhove J, Weber K. At least six different actins are expressed in higher mammals: an analysis based on the amino acid sequence of the amino terminal tryptic peptide. J Mol Biol 1978; 126: 783–802.
17. Darby I, Skalli O, Gabbiani G. α-Smooth muscle actin is transiently expressed by myofibroblasts during experimental wound healing. Lab Invest 1990; *63*: 21–9.
18. Skalli O, Schürch W, Seemayer T, et al. Myofibroblasts from diverse pathologic settings are heterogeneous in their content of actin isoforms and intermediate filament proteins. Lab Invest 1989; 60: 275–85.
19. Sappino AD, Schürch W, Gabbiani G. Biology of disease. Differentiation repertoire of fibroblastic cells: expression of cytoskeletal proteins as marker of phenotypic modulations. Lab Invest 1990; 63: 144–61.
20. Hansson GK, Hellstrand M, Rymo L, et al. γ Interferon inhibits both proliferation and expression of differentiation-specific α-smooth muscle actin in arterial smooth muscle cells. J Exp Med 1989; 170: 1595–608.

10

Chemotaxis and Invasiveness

Adriana Albini, Antonella Melchiori, and Silvio Parodi
Istituto Nazionale per la Ricerca sul Cancro, Genoa, Italy

Hynda K. Kleinman
National Institutes of Health, Bethesda, Maryland

The ability of somatic cells to translocate inside the organism is a property vital to phenomena such as embryogenesis, development, differentiation, wound healing, and inflammation (for reviews, see [1–5]). Pathologic situations such as fibrosis and tumor cell metastasis also involve cell migration (for reviews, see [3, 6]). Chemotaxis is cell migration in response to a soluble gradient of a stimulatory substance (chemoattractant). Haptotaxis, a related phenomenon, is a directional migration on a gradient of a substrate-bound chemoattractant. Many cells are able to migrate, including leukocytes, smooth muscle cells, neurons, endothelial cells, fibroblasts, and tumor cells. During the processes of inflammation and metastasis, migratory cells acquire the capability to penetrate the dense extracellular matrix of the basement membrane. This process requires proteolytic degradation and is referred to as basement membrane invasion [7]. Although different chemoattractants as well as different physiological and pathologic situations are involved in cell migration and invasion, it is probable that similar, if not identical, mechanisms are at the basis of these phenomena. This hypothesis is supported by the fact that polymorphonuclear leukocytes and the slime mold *Dictyostelium discoideum* have closely related chemotaxis mechanisms [8]. The target cells most relevant to dermatology are leukocytes (inflammation) and fibroblasts (wound healing). Leukocyte chemotaxis has been extensively reviewed [8]. We will therefore focus on fibroblast chemotaxis. During wound healing, fibroblasts are stimulated to migrate by chemoattractants of diverse origin, produced at the site of the wound. Mitoattractants, or growth factors with chemotactic capabilities, will first stimulate the migration, then the growth of the recruited fibroblasts and their matrix production (Fig. 10.1). Furthermore, for the interest of the dermatologist–oncologist, we will review some tumor cell chemotactic and invasive properties. During the process of invasion, tumor cells must escape the bulk of the tumor, cross compartments of extracellular matrix, and reach capillary beds. Here the cells interact first with blood components and blood cells, then with endothelial cells through low-affinity interactions (via, for instance, selectins). After inducing retraction of endothelium, tumor cells strongly adhere to the underlying basement membrane through integrins or other cell-matrix receptors. This interaction triggers the production of proteolytic enzymes necessary for matrix digestion. Metastatic cells cross the degraded basement membrane and penetrate into the target organ, where autocrine and paracrine

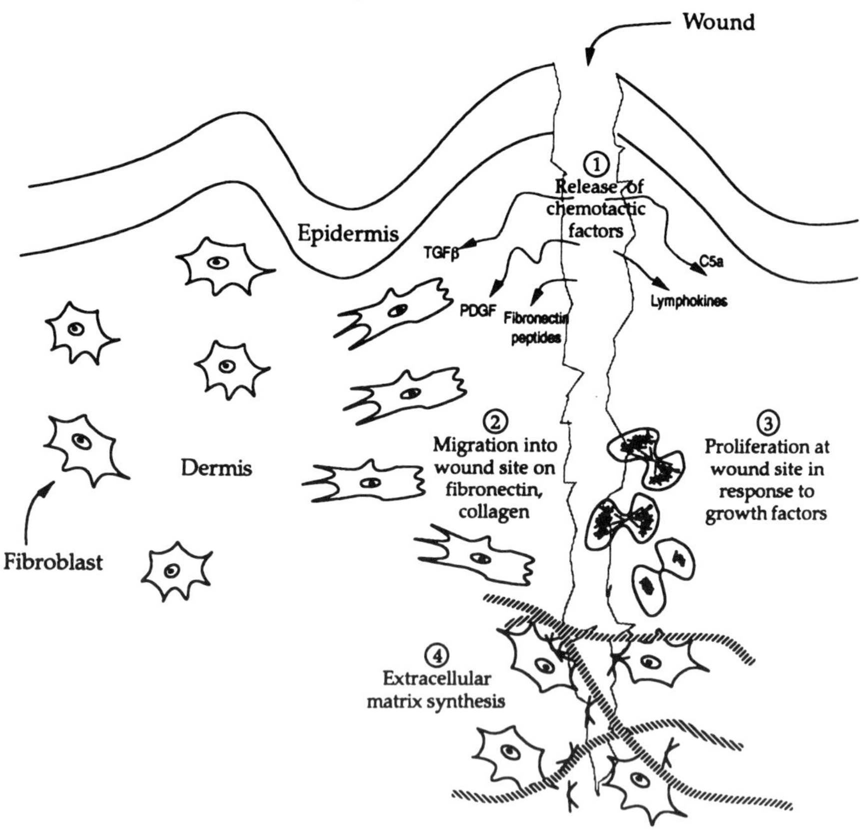

Figure 10.1 Fibroblast chemotaxis in wound healing.

growth factors stimulate their growth. Induction of neoangiogenesis and vascularization also supports the growth of a successful metastasis (Fig. 10.2).

EXPERIMENTAL SYSTEMS

Various experimental systems have been used for the study of cell migration [4]. The most widely used method for investigations on fibroblast and tumor cell chemotaxis employs blind well or Boyden chambers [9], in which chemoattractant and cells are separated by a microporous filter, often coated with attachment

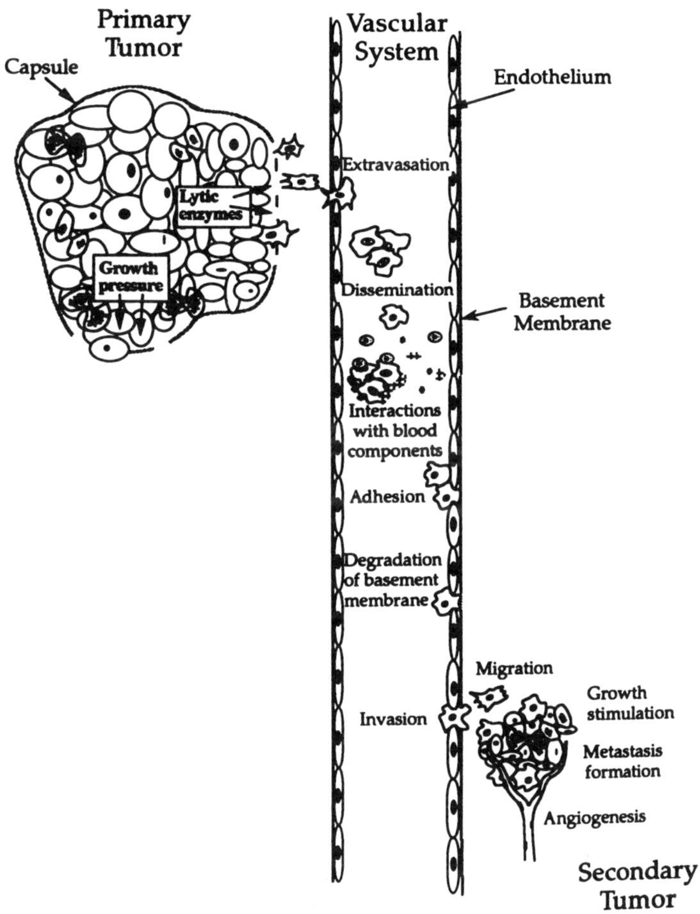

Figure 10.2 Steps in tumor cell invasion.

substrates. This chamber permits the formation of the steep gradients necessary for chemotactic stimulation. For assessment of invasion, physiological basement membranes (amnion, bladder walls, lens capsule, chicken chorioallantoic membrane, etc.), basement membranes synthesized in vitro (for example, by endothelial cell layers), and artificial or reconstituted basement membranes have been employed (for reviews, see [10, 11]). These membranes are often placed on top of the chemotaxis filters inside Boyden chambers, which allows their use in combination with factors eliciting the cell directional migration. Both motility and degradative activity are necessary for the cells to invade in this assay, closely reflecting the situation *in vivo*. We established the first assay [12], which uses Matrigel, a reconstituted basement membrane [13], in blind well chemotaxis chambers. Matrigel is extracted from the Engelbreth-Holm-Swaim (EHS) murine sarcoma, which produces authentic basement membranes, and is coated onto polycarbonate filters for use in the chambers. We refer to this assay as to the "chemoinvasion" assay. Variations and modifications of this assay have also been proposed [14–16]. An extensive comparison between invasion of the amnion and reconstituted basement membranes has been reported by Hendrix et al. [15]. Matrigel has also been successfully used for the study of tumor cell invasion directly in the tissue culture dish, especially for morphologic evaluations [12, 17]. When plated on a three-dimensional basement membrane gel (matrigel), fibroblasts are not able to grow and invade and develop only small, tight cellular clusters at the surface of the matrix. Transformed fibroblasts or sarcoma cells are capable of forming invasive, branching colonies, with the typical morphology shown in the lower panel of Figure 10.3.

CHEMOTAXIS

Fibroblasts respond to a large number of chemoattractants. Most of them are part of one of three major classes of molecules: extracellular matrix proteins, growth factors, and molecules involved in inflammation or blood clotting (see [4] for review). Tumor cells also respond to these chemoattractants. In addition, autocrine motility factor(s) are very powerful inducers of tumor cell migration [18].

Extracellular Matrix Molecules as Chemoattractants

Fibronectin [19] has been extensively investigated as a fibroblast chemoattractant. Not only intact fibronectin but also proteolytic fragments and synthetic peptides can also elicit chemotaxis (see [4, 20] for review). It is likely that proteolytic fragments, rather than the whole protein, form a gradient in situations where chemotaxis occurs. A major site in fibronectin involved in both cell attachment and migration is located 65–75 kD from the C-end of the molecule [21, 22]. The

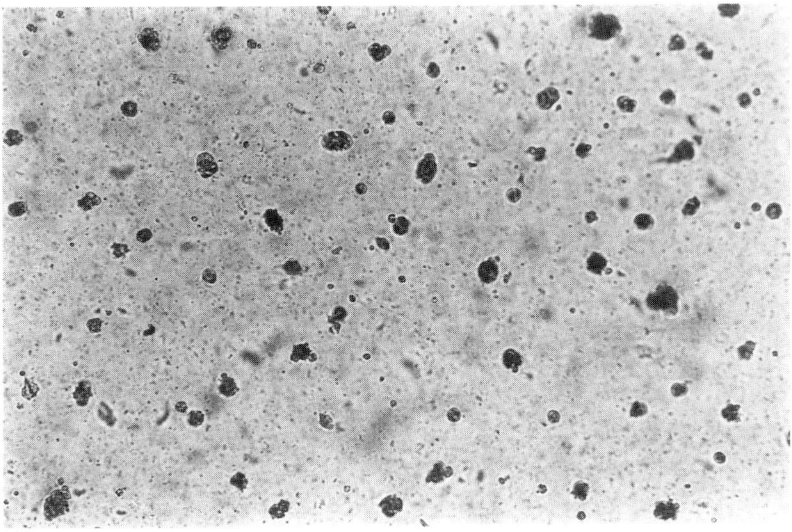

(A)

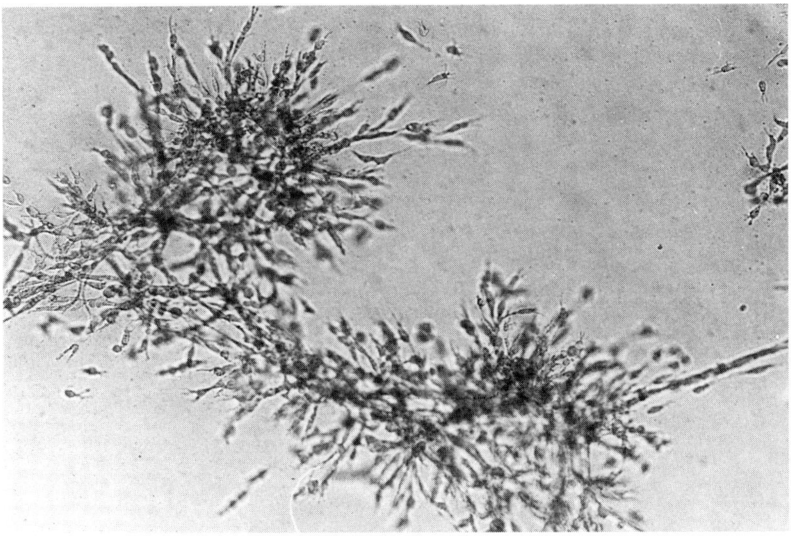

(B)

Figure 10.3 Growth of tumor cells in a reconstituted basement membrane. (A) Nonmetastatic cells. (B) Metastatic cells.

sequence responsible for both activities has been identified as RGDS [23, 24]. RGD is present in many adhesive proteins including thrombospondin, fibrinogen, tenascin, and laminin. RGD-containing peptides are able to mediate both chemotaxis and adhesion, although they are far less potent than the entire fibronectin molecule. The fibronectin receptor has been demonstrated to be involved in cell migration [24, 25]. The fibronectin receptor (and the many other matrix receptors of the integrin superfamily) is composed of two units, one α and one β (for a review, see [26]. The β-subunit contains the region that binds to RGD-containing sequences, but probably secondary interactions of the intact molecule (or of large fragments) with the α-subunits confer a stronger binding and a higher specificity. Other sites on fibronectin also seem to be involved in fibroblast cell adhesion [27], as well as fibroblast and tumor cell chemotaxis [28–30], possibly through different receptors. Integrin binding can also be RGD independent.

Laminin, a major glycoprotein of basement membranes [31], is a powerful stimulator of adhesion and migration for tumor derived and transformed cells (see [32] for review). Cells have high-affinity laminin receptors with an affinity of about 1 nM, which is 100–1000-fold higher than integrin-mediated binding [33–35]. The peptide sequence YIGSR that occurs within laminin appears to mediate high-affinity laminin binding to cells [36]. YIGSR can block cell adhesion to laminin and chemotaxis to laminin in some cell systems. Both RGD and YIGSR peptides inhibit experimental metastasis when injected in mice at the same time as tumor cells [37, 38], as well as inhibiting invasion in vitro (38, 39). YIGSR is likely to inhibit the binding of the injected cells to the laminin in basement membrane, while the RGD could be involved in blocking the interactions to stromal compartments (both of which the cell must cross in order to metastasize). Laminin also contains an RGD sequence in the murine A chain [40], which may function as an adhesive site for some cells. In the chick the CSAT antigen was shown to be a receptor for both fibronectin and laminin [41]. Integrin receptors for laminin are involved in cell adhesion to laminin of some tumor cells [42]. Highly metastatic melanoma cells have low-affinity receptors for laminin [43], and other receptors are likely to exist since laminin has multiple active sites. Both types of receptors, high-affinity and integrins, may exist on the same cells (for reviews of matrix receptors, see [44, 45]).

It has been observed previously that locomotion is optimal when the chemoattractant concentration is similar to the Kd of the receptor binding in diverse systems (for instance, in polymorphonuclear leukocytes) [8]. This also seems to be true for fibroblast migration to fibronectin, which is optimal at about 0.1 μM [4] and the Kd of fibronectin receptor binding is in the μM range [44]. Optimal melanoma cell migration to IGF-I (insulin-like growth factor I, see later) occurs at nM concentrations, which is within an order of magnitude of the Kd (= 0.3 nM) [46]. Since the optimal chemotactic concentration for laminin is very close to that of fibronectin [47], and similar to the integrin receptor Kd, it is possible that integrin laminin receptors are the main mediators of cell migration to laminin rather than the high-affinity receptors.

An RGDS-independent cell adhesion fragment from the heparin-binding region of fibronectin also inhibits metastasis in vivo as well as do large (440 and 330 Kd) chymotrypsin and thermolysin laminin fragments [48]. A 20 mer heparin-binding peptide from the B1 chain of laminin (position 641-660) not containing YIGSR is involved in adhesion and spreading on laminin [48–50].

Thrombospondin, a multifunctional glycoprotein secreted by stimulated platelets (for review, see [51]), is also a component of various extracellular matrices. Found in basement membranes and in the interstitium, it is produced by a variety of cells, including fibroblasts. Besides mediating cell attachment, thrombospondin is also able to induce tumor cell chemotaxis and haptotaxis [52]. The C-terminal region of thrombospondin is involved in melanoma cell haptotaxis, while chemotaxis seems to be mediated by the N-terminal heparin-binding domain of the molecule [52]. Although thrombospondin contains an RGD sequence, none of these interactions seem to be RGD mediated. RGD peptides also fail to inhibit tumor cell attachment or spreading on thrombospondin. Thrombospondin modulates endothelial cell adhesion and motility [53]. As for laminin, thrombospondin binds specifically to sulfated glycolipids and proteoglycans and these molecules probably mediate melanoma cell spreading and chemotactic response to thrombospondin [54, 55]. The polysulfonated compound suramine is, in fact, able to inhibit laminin and thrombospondin-mediated melanoma cell adhesion and migration [55].

Tenascin is a glycoprotein associated with mesenchymal–epithelial interactions in development and expressed by a variety of solid tumors (see [56] for review). It contains an RGD sequence recognized by various tumor cell lines and endothelial cells [57]. It is involved in neural crest cell migration [58]. Vitronectin, another RGD-containing attachment factor, also affects cell motility [59, 60]. The structural matrix proteins collagens and elastin are also chemotactic, these have been reviewed elsewhere [4].

Growth Factors as Chemoattractants

Various growth factors have been shown to promote chemotaxis at concentrations below that required for growth [3]. For example, the "mitoattractant" platelet-derived growth factor (PDGF) was found to be chemotactic for fibroblasts at concentrations one-tenth of that required for growth stimulation. It has been proposed that during wound healing the PDGF released by platelets initially recruits inflammatory cells and the fibroblasts into the site of injury. Higher quantities of the factor located at the wound site would then induce the migrated fibroblasts to replicate [3].

Many other growth factors have been reported to induce chemotaxis of cells for which they are mitogenic, such as endothelial cell growth factor (ECGF or acidic FGF) [61], basic FGF, and EGF [62]. Collagenase production by fibroblasts of different origins is stimulated differentially by chemotactically active bFGF and EGF [63]. Scatter factor, a fibroblast-derived cytokine very similar to hepatocyte growth factor, stimulates motility of various cells, among which epithelial and vascular endothelial cells [64]. TGFβ, which is able to stimulate the production of fibronectin, collagen, and proteoglycans by dermal fibroblasts, is a potent chemoattractant for fibroblasts [65]. Release of TGFβ from blood cells at sites of tissue injury may play a role in eliciting migration and matrix synthesis of neighboring connective tissue fibroblasts. The fibrotic reaction characteristic of certain tumors could be due to TGFβ production by the tumor cells [65]. On the other hand, TGFβ inhibits endothelial cell growth and also prevents endothelial cell migration [66]. TGFβ also has bifunctional effects on the migration of rat aorta smooth muscle cells [67]. It seems, therefore, that there is a correlation between growth promotion/induction of migration and growth inhibition/decreased migration. Probably there is a common cell specificity for induction of growth and migration by a "mitoattractant."

We have studied the responses to various growth factors (EGF, ECGF, PDGF, TGFα, TGFβ) of Kaposi's sarcoma cells and compared them to those of fibroblasts, smooth muscle, and endothelial cells [68]. It appeared that every cell had a very specific pattern of response and Kaposi's-derived cells resembled (but were not identical to) vascular smooth muscle cells. Thus, the responsiveness of a cell to a mitoattractant may, in some cases, be used to characterize cell type.

Tumor cells also respond chemotactically to growth factors [4]. Nerve growth factor (NGF) stimulates migration of mouse embryonal carcinoma cells. Insulin-like growth factor IGF-I, which stimulates migration and plasminogen activator release in human retinal pigment epithelial cells [69], has been shown to stimulate human melanoma cell migration [46]. In addition to their mitogenic properties, certain growth factors may enhance tumor cell metastasis by acting on cell motility.

The migration of dermal fibroblasts to one growth factor can be modulated by other growth factors [70]. This suggests that in vivo there might be a "network" of growth factors rather than a single one to regulate chemotactic migration.

Blood-Derived Chemoattractants and Other Molecules

"Blood"-derived factors, such as lymphokines, as well as complement-derived factors and products involved in the blood clotting cascade, are stimulators of fibroblast and tumor cell chemotaxis (for reviews, see [2, 4, 6]. Interleukin 1 is a potent stimulator of human neutrophil and T-lymphocyte migration and is also able to elicit chemotactic migratory responses in human tumor cell lines [71]. Interleukin 1 is released from the endothelium following stimulation and could be involved in metastatic cell trafficking through the endothelium [72].

INVASIVENESS

Malignant tumor cells have to cross extracellular matrix compartments in order to metastasize (for reviews, see [73, 74]. Since most cells metastasize via the vascular system, they must cross vascular basement membranes (Fig. 10.2), which are generally impermeable to normal cells. Trophoblasts of normal first-trimester human placenta are able to invade basement membranes in situ [75]. Also, supernatants of Kaposi's sarcoma (KS) cells, a tumor that has been postulated to recruit host vascular cells, are able to make endothelial and smooth muscle cells invasive ''in vitro'' [76]. This could be due to the presence in the conditioned media of high concentrations of certain growth factors able to stimulate invasion, such as FGF [77] or even PDGF [78], which induce collagenase secretion.

In order for invasion to occur a cell needs not only to be capable of migrating directionally but also to be able to degrade basement membranes through proteolytic activities [7]. Metastatic tumor cells produce high amounts of type IV collagenase and other metalloproteases able to digest basement membrane collagen [73]. Plasmin-mediated tissue degradation is also involved in basement membrane digestion and tumor cell invasion [79-81]; plasmin activates collagenase type IV as well [80]. Metastatic cell lines produce plasminogen activator, which converts the plasminogen to plasmin. Plasminogen activator levels are enhanced by laminin in breast carcinoma cells, and estrogen-sensitive MCF-7 cell production of urokinase-type plasminogen activator is stimulated by estradiol [82].

Invasive cells also show a decreased production of tissue-specific metalloprotease inhibitors (TIMPs). Human recombinant TIMP-1 is able to inhibit invasion in the amnion assay and experimental metastasis ''in vivo'' of B16-F10 mouse melanoma cells [83]. TIMP-2, a specific inhibitor of type IV collagenase, can also inhibit tumor cell invasion of basement membranes [84] and smooth muscle cell layers [85] when added exogenously.

Laminin is the major biologically active component of basement membranes [31, 32]. Metastatic and invasive cells preferentially adhere to laminin [86]. Exposure of tumor cells to laminin enhances their ability to form experimental metastasis [87] and also to attach to basement membranes [88]. Adhesion to laminin triggers the production of type IV collagenase [89] and of plasminogen activator. Laminin therefore has both direct and indirect effects related to tumor cell invasion.

MECHANISMS OF CHEMOTAXIS AND INVASIVENESS

In the first phase of directional migration, defined as the "sensory phase," the chemoattractant binds to the cell. Attractant binding stimulates shape changes and migration. Studies with antibodies to cell surface receptors and peptides from active domains of ligand protein have demonstrated that chemotaxis and invasion are indeed mediated through cell receptors [4, 20, 73].

Best investigated are the interactions between fibronectin and receptors of the integrin family. Antibodies to fibronectin receptors inhibit fibroblast chemotaxis [24]. The two subunits of the integrin receptor family molecules have a large extracellular domain, a transmembrane segment, and a short intracellular peptide [26], with the exception of the β4 subunit, which has a large cytoplasmic domain. Activity is Ca/Mg-dependent. The cytoplasmic part is in contact with the cytoskeleton. This interaction is important in the "intermediate phase" of chemotaxis, when microfilaments and microtubules are rearranged following binding of the chemoattractant to the cell surface, making the cell able to migrate [8]. The receptors are probably oriented in the direction of the source of chemoattractant, to make migration directional.

During the intermediate phase a cascade of events takes place, including protein phosphorylation, protein and phospholipid methylation, ionic fluxes, and changes in cyclic nucleotide levels. Phosphorylation of the receptor plays a major role in its function for *Dictyostelium* migration [8]. This could be true for fibroblast chemotaxis as well. In endothelial cells the B type receptor for PDGF mediates chemotactic response via activation of the receptor protein–tyrosine kinase [90]. In *Dictyostelium* the chemotactic signals are tranduced via G proteins. Pertussis toxin, a G protein inhibitor, completely blocks leukocyte chemotaxis. Guanidine nucleotides regulate the affinity of the chemoattractant binding site on leukocytes, macrophage membranes, and in *Dictyostelium*. A target of the receptor-activated G protein is phospholipase C, which is hydrolyzed upon activation and liberates inositol triphosphate. Inositol triphosphate is involved in calcium release and diacylglycerol, another product of phospholipase C hydrolysis, activates protein kinase C. Protein kinase C is involved in fibroblast chemotaxis to PDGF and fibronectin fragments [91]. Elevated cytoplasmic calcium also activates protein kinases, phospholipase A2, and actin-binding proteins. Activation of phospholipase A2 by elevated calcium or phorbol ester levels releases arachidonic acid. The invasive and metastatic activity of cancer cells is dependent on certain metabolites of arachidonic acid formed via the cyclooxygenase and lipoxiygenase pathways [92]. Inhibition of the lipoxygenase pathway blocks metastasis in vivo and invasiveness of tumor cells. One of the conversion products of arachidonic acid is leukotriene B4, which is a chemoattractant itself [93].

Some chemoattractants act by increasing cyclic AMP concentration via cell membrane adenyl cyclase [8]. Cyclic AMP and agents that increase cAMP levels also inhibit macrophage locomotion, while cGMP enhances this function. Directional migration requires orientation and shape changes [94]. Actin polymerization is observed during chemotaxis. It is not known which second messenger mediates changes in actin. Tubulin polymerization also is induced by chemoattractants and microtubules inhibitors inhibit cell polarity and reduce chemotaxis [8].

Most studies on the mechanisms of eukaryote chemotaxis have been done on leukocytes or *Dictyostelium*. When investigations on fibroblast chemotaxis have been done, similar mechanisms have proven to be in effect [4]. Less is known about the signals that play a role in tumor cell invasiveness. With the aim of understanding some of the mechanisms of invasion Welch et al. [95] tried several agents in a Matrigel invasion assay. Drugs that cause microtubule disruption (such as vincristine, vinblastine, colchicine, colcemid) inhibited invasion, as previously shown for fibroblastic cell chemotaxis [96]. Dibutyril cAMP, a cAMP agonist, was inhibitory (while, in contrast, 8-Br-cAMP stimulated invasion). Cholera toxin and forskolin, stimulators of adenyl cyclase, inhibited invasion; in contrast, pertussis toxin, a G protein inhibitor, had no effect. Pertussis toxin is also ineffective on insulin peptide-mediated melanoma cell chemotaxis [46]; however, it affects autocrine motility factor-induced migration [73].

It is not known which mechanisms of signal transduction are essential to fibroblast and tumor cell chemotaxis and tumor cell invasion. There are indications that different pathways of signal transduction are activated in tumor cell chemotaxis to different agents. It is possible that, as for other eukaryotic systems, there are redundant mechanisms for achieving a response.

ACKNOWLEDGMENTS

We are grateful to Dr. Douglas Noonan for revision of the manuscript and for the illustration.

The work in our laboratory has been made possible by grants from CNR, AIRC and MINISTERO DELLA SANITÁ; and a CNR bilateral grant to A. Albini.

REFERENCES

1. Le Douarin NM. Cell migrations in embryos. Cell 1984; 38: 353–60.
2. Varani J, Orr FW. Chemotaxis in non-leukocytic cells. In: Ward, P. ed. Handbook of inflammation. Amsterdam: Elsevier, 1983: 211–244.
3. Grotendorst GR, Martin GR. Cell movement in wound healing and fibrosis. In: K. Kühn and T. Krieg, eds. Connective tissue: biological and clinical aspects. Basel: Karger, 1986: 385–403.
4. Albini A, Adelmann-Grill B, Muller PK. Fibroblast chemotaxis. Collagen Rel Res 1985; 5: 283–96.

5. Mensing H. Importance of fibroblast chemotaxis in wound healing and tumor cell evasion. Klin. Wochenschr 1985; 63: 1–45.
6. Varani J, Ward PA. Tumor cell chemotaxis. In: I Hart, LA Liotta, eds. The biological basis of metastasis. The Hague: Martinus Nijhoff. 1982: 99–112.
7. Liotta LA. Tumor invasion and metastases: the role of basement membrane. Am J Pathol 1984; 117: 339–48.
8. Devreotes PN, Zigmond SH. Chemotaxis in eukaryotic cells: a focus on leukocytes and *Dictyostelium*. Ann Rev Cell Biol 1988; 4: 649–86.
9. Boyden S. The chemotactic effect of mixtures of antibody and antigen on polymorphonuclear leukocytes. J Exp Med 1962; 115: 453–66.
10. Terranova P, Hujanen ES, Martin GR. Basement membranes and the invasive activity of metastatic tumor cells. J Natl Cancer Inst 1986; 77: 311–6.
11. Albini A, Auckerman SL, Thompson EW, Melchiori A, Reich R, Shima TB, Martin GR, Iwamoto Y. Basement membranes, reconstituted to assess the invasiveness of tumor cells. In: GL Nicolson, IJ Fidler, eds. Tumor progression and metastasis. New York: Alan R. Liss, 1988: 261–69.
12. Albini A, Iwamoto Y, Kleinman HK, Martin GR, Aaronson SA, Kozlowski JM, McEwan RN. A rapid *in vitro* assay for quantitating the invasive potential of tumor cells. Cancer Res 1987; 47: 3239–45.
13. Kleinman HK, McGarvey ML, Hassell JR, Star VL, Cannon F, Laurie GW, Martin GR. Basement membranes complexes with biological activity. Biochemistry 1986; 25: 312–8
14. Erkell LJ, Schirrmacher V. Quantitative in-vitro assay for tumor cell invasion through extracellular matrix or into protein gels. Cancer Res 1988; 48: 6933–7.
15. Hendrix M, Seftor E, Misiorowski R, Saba P, Sundareshan, Welch D. Comparison of tumor cell invasion assays: human amnion versus reconstituted basement membrane barriers. Invasion-Metastasis 1989; 9: 278–97.
16. Repesh L. A new in vitro assay for quantitating tumor cell invasion. Invasion-Metastasis 1989; 9: 192–208.
17. Kramer RH, Bensch, KG, Wong J. Invasion of reconstituted basement membrane matrix by metastatic human tumor cells. Cancer Res 1986; 46: 1980–9.
18. Liotta LA, Mandler R, Murano G, Katz DA, Gordon RK, Chiang PK, Schiffman E. Tumor cell autocrine motility factor. Proc Natl Acad Sci 1986; 83: 3302–6.
19. Hynes RO. Fibronectins. Sci Am 1986; 254: 42–51.
20. Allavena G, Melchiori A, Aresu O, Ferreri-Santi L, McEwan R, Kitten G, Parodi S, Albini A. In vitro models for studying the malignant phenotype: chemotaxis and chemoinvasion. In G Prodi, LA Liotta, PL Lollini, S Garbisa, S Gorini, K Hellman, eds. Cancer metastasis. Biological and biochemical mechanisms and clinical aspects. New York: Plenum Press, 1988: 215–26.
21. Pierschbacher MD, Hayman EG, Ruoslahti E. Localization of the cell attachment site in fibronectin with monoclonal antibodies and proteolytic fragments of the molecule. Cell 1981; 26: 259–67.
22. Albini A, Richter H, Pontz BF. Localization of the chemotactic domain in fibronectin. FEBS Lett 1983; 156: 222–6.
23. Pierschbacher MD, Ruoslahti E. Cell attachment activity of fibronectin can be duplicated by small synthetic fragments of the molecule. Nature 1984; 309: 30–33.

24. Albini A, Allavena G, Melchiori A, Giancotti F, Richter H, Martin GR, Tarone G. Chemotaxis of 3T3 and SV3T3 cells to fibronectin is mediated through the cell attachment site in fibronectin and a fibronectin cell surface receptor. J Cell Biol 1987; 105: 1867–72.
25. Akiyama SK, Yamada SS, Chen WT, Yamada KM. Analysis of fibronectin receptor function with monoclonal antibodies: roles in cell adhesion, migration, matrix assembly, and cytoskeletal organization. J Cell Biol 1989; 109: 863–75.
26. Ruoslathti E, Pierschbacher MD. New perspectives in cell adhesion: RGD and integrins. Science 1987; 238: 491–7.
27. Humphries M, Yasuda Y, Olden K, Yamada K. The cell interaction sites of fibronectin in tumour metastasis. Ciba Found Symp 1988; 141: 75–93.
28. McCarthy JB, Hagen ST, Furcht LT. Human fibronectin contains distinct adhesion and motility-promoting domains for metastatic melanoma cells. J Cell Biol 1986; 102: 179–88.
29. Nagai T, Yamakawa N, Aota S, Yamada SS, Akiyama SK, Olden K, Yamada KM. Monoclonal antibody characterization of two distinct sites required for function of the central cell-binding domain of fibronectin in cell adhesion, cell migration, and matrix assembly. J Cell Biol 1991; 114: 1295–305.
30. Fukai F, Suzuki H, Suzuki K, Tsugita A, Katayama T. Rat plasma fibronectin contains two distinct chemotactic domains for fibroblastic cells. J Biol Chem 1991; 266: 8807–13
31. Martin GR, Timpl R. Laminin and other basement membrane components. Ann Rev Cell Biol 1987; 3: 57–85.
32. Kleinman HK, Cannon FB, Laurie GW, Hassel JR, Aumailley M, Terranova VP, Martin GR, Dubois-Dalcq M. Biological activities of laminin. J Cell Biochem 1985; 27: 317–325.
33. Lesot H, Kuhl U, von der Mark K. Isolation of a laminin binding protein from muscle cell membranes. EMBO J 1983; 2:861–5.
34. Malinoff HL, Wicha MS. Isolation of a cell surface receptor protein for laminin from murine fibrosarcoma cells. J Cell Biol 1983; 96: 1475–9.
35. Terranova VP, Rao CN, Kalebic T, Margulies IM, Liotta LA. Laminin receptors on human breast carcinoma cells. Proc Natl Acad Sci USA 1983; 80: 444–8.
36. Graf J, Ogle RC, Robey FA, Sasaki M, Martin GR, Yamada Y, Kleinman HK. A pentapetide from the laminin B1 chain mediates cell adhesion and binds the 67 000 laminin receptor. Biochemistry 1987; 26: 6896–900.
37. Humphries MJ, Olden K, Yamada KM. A synthetic peptide from fibronectin inhibits experimental metastasis of murine melanoma cells. Science 1986; 233: 467–70.
38. Iwamoto Y, Robey FA, Graf J, Sasaki M, Kleinman HK, Yamada Y, Martin GR. YIGSR, a synthetic laminin pentapeptide, inhibits experimental metastasis formation. Science 1987; 238: 1132–4.
39. Gehlsen KR, Argraves WS, Pierschbacher MD, Ruoslahti E. Inhibition of in vitro tumor cell invasion by Arg-Gly-Asp-containing synthetic peptides. J Cell Biol 1988; 106: 925–30.
40. Sasaki M, Kleinman HK, Huber H, Deutzmann R, Yamada Y. Laminin, a multidomain protein. The A chain has a unique globular domain and homology with the

basement membrane proteoglycan and the laminin B chains. J Biol Chem 1988; 263: 16536–44.

41. Horwitz A, Duggan K, Greggs R, Decker C, Buck C. The cell substrate attachment (CSAT) antigen has properties of a receptor for laminin and fibronectin. J Cell Biol 1985; 101: 2134–44.
42. Kramer RH, McDonald KA, Crowley E, Ramos DM, Damsky C. Melanoma cell adhesion to basement membrane mediated by integrin-related complexes. Cancer Res 1989; 49: 393–402.
43. Albini A, Aukerman SL, Noonan DM, Ogle RC, Fridman R, Martin GR, Fidler IJ. The in vitro invasiveness and interactions with laminin of K-1735 melanoma cells. J Clin Exp Metast 1989; 7: 437–451.
44. Buck A, Horwitz AF. Cell surface receptors for extracellular matrix molecules. Ann Rev Cell Biol 1987; 3: 179–205.
45. Mecham RP. Receptors for laminin on mammalian cells. FASEB J 1991; 5: 2538–46.
46. Stracke ML, Kohn E, Aznavoorian S, Wilson L, Salomon D, Krutzsch H, Liotta LA, Schiffmann E. Insulin-like growth factors stimulate chemotaxis in human melanoma cells. Biochem Biophys Res Commun 1988; 153: 1076–83.
47. Furcht LT, McCarthy JB, Palm SL, Basara ML, and Enenstein J. Peptide fragments of laminin and fibronectin promote migration (haptotaxis and chemotaxis) of metastatic cells. In Basement membranes and cell movement. CIBA Foundation Symposium. London: Pitman, 1984: 130–45.
48. McCarthy JB, Skubitz AP, Palm SL, Furcht LT. Metastasis inhibition of different tumor types by purified laminin fragments and a heparin-binding fragment of fibronectin. J Natl Cancer Inst 1988; 80: 108–16.
49. Charonis AS, Skubitiz APN, Koliakos GC, Reger LA, Dege J, Vogel AM, Wohlhueter R, Furcht LT. A novel synthetic peptide from the B1 chain of laminin with heparin-binding and cell adhesion-promoting activities. J Cell Biol 1988; 107: 1253–60.
50. Skubitz APN, McCarthy JB, Charonis AS, Furcht LT. Novel synthetic heparin binding peptides of laminin and fibronectin which promote the adhesion of melanoma cells. Invasion Metastasis 1989; 9: 89–101.
51. Lawler J. The structural and functional properties of thrombospondin. Blood 1986; 67: 1197–209.
52. Taraboletti G, Roberts DD, Liotta LA. Thrombospondin-induced tumor cell migration: haptotaxis and chemotaxis are mediated by different molecular domains. J Cell Biol 1987; 105: 2409–415.
53. Taraboletti G, Roberts D, Liotta LA, Giavazzi R. Platelet thrombospondin modulates endothelial cell adhesion, motility and growth: a potential angiogenesis regulatory factor. J Cell Biol 1990; 111: 765–72.
54. Roberts DD. Interactions of thrombospondin with sulfated glycolipids and proteoglycans of human melanoma cells. Cancer Res 1988; 48: 6785–93.
55. Zabrenetzky VS, Kohn EC, Roberts DD. Suramin inhibits laminin-and thrombospondin-mediated melanoma cell adhesion and migration and binding of these adhesive proteins to sulfatides. Cancer Res 1990; 50: 5937–42.
56. Chiquet-Ehrismann R, Mackie EJ, Pearson CA, Sakakura T. Tenascin: an extracel-

lular matrix protein involved in tissue interactions during fetal development and oncogenesis. Cell 1986; 47: 131–9.
57. Bourdon MA, Ruoslahti E. Tenascin mediates cell attachment through an RGD-dependent receptor. J Cell Biol 1989; 108: 1149–56.
58. Halfter W, Chiquet-Ehrismann R, Tucker RP. The effect of tenascin and embryonic basal lamina on the behaviour and morphology of neural crest cells in vitro. Dev Biol 1989; 132: 14–25.
59. Naito M, Hayashi T, Funaki C, Kuzuya M, Asai K, Yamada K, Kuzuya F. Vitronectin-induced haptotaxis of vascular smooth muscle cells in vitro. Exp Cell Res 1991; 194: 154–6.
60. Brown C, Stenn KS, Falk RJ, Woodley DT, O'Keefe EJ. Vitronectin: effects on keratinocyte motility and inhibition of collagen induced motility. J Invest Dermatol 1991; 96: 724–8.
61. Terranova VP, Florio RD, Lyall RM, Hic S, Friesel R, Maciag T. Human endothelial cells are chemotactic to endothelial cell growth factor and heparin. J Cell Biol 1985; 101: 2330–4.
62. Bade EG, Nitzgen B. Extracellular matrix (ECM) modulates the EGF-induced migration of liver epithelial cells in serum-free, hormone-supplemented medium. In Vitro Cell Dev Biol 1985; 21: 245–8.
63. Buckley-Sturrock A, Woodward SC, Senior RM, Griffin GL, Klagsbrun M, Davidson JM. Differential stimulation of collagenase and chemotactic activity in fibroblasts derived from rat wound repair tissue and human skin by growth factors. J Cell Physiol 1989; 138: 70–78.
64. Rosen EM, Jaken S, Carley W, Luckett PM, Setter E, Bhargava M, Goldberg ID. Regulation of motility in bovine brain endothelial cells. J Cell Physiol 1991; 146: 325–35.
65. Postlethwaite AE, Keski-Oja J, Moses HL, Kang AH. Stimulation of the chemotactic migration of human fibroblasts by transforming growth factor β. J Exp Med 1987; 165: 251–6.
66. Müller G, Behrens J, Nussbaumer U, Böhlen P, Birchmeier W. Inhibitory action of transforming growth factor β on endothelial cells. Proc Natl Acad Sci USA 1987; 84: 5600–4.
67. Koyama, N, Koshikawa T, Morisaki N, Saito Y, Yoshida S. Bifunctional effects of transforming growth factor-beta on migration of cultured rat aortic smooth muscle cells. Biochem Biophys Res Commun 1990; 169: 725–9.
68. Albini A, Mitchell CD, Thompson EW, Seeman R, Martin GR, Wittek AE, Quinnan GV. Invasive activity and chemotactic response to growth factors by Kaposi's sarcoma cells. J Cell Biochem 1988; 36: 369–76.
69. Grant MB, Guay C, Marsh R. Insulin-like growth factor I stimulates proliferation, migration and plasminogen activator release by human retinal pigment epithelial cells. Curr Eye Res 1990; 9: 323–35.
70. Adelmann-Grill BC, Wach F, Cully Z, Hein R, Krieg T. Chemotactic migration of normal dermal fibroblasts towards epidermal growth factor and its modulation by platelet-derived growth factor and transforming growth factor beta. Eur J Cell Biol 1990; 51: 322–36.
71. Orr FW, Buchanan MR, Tron VA, Guy D, Lauri D, Sauder DN. Chemotactic

activity of endothelial cell-derived interleukin 1 for human tumor cells. Cancer Res 1988; 48: 6758–63.

72. Dejana E, Bertocchi F, Bortolami ME, Regonesi A, Tonta A, Breviario F, Giavatei R. Interleukin 1 promotes tumor cell adhesion to cultured endothelial cells. J Clin Invest 1988; 82: 1466–70.
73. Liotta L, Wewer U, Rao N, Schiffmann E, Stracke M, Guirguis R, Thorgeirsson U, Muschel R, Sobel M. Biochemical mechanisms of tumor invasion and metastases. Prog Clin Biol Res 1988; 256: 3–16.
74. Thompson E, Reich R, Martin GR, Albini A. Factors regulating basement membrane invasion by tumor cells. In: ME Lippman, RB Dickson, eds. Breast cancer: cellular and molecular biolog. Boston: Kluwer Academic Publishers, 1988: 239–49.
75. Yagel S, Parher RS, Jeffrey JJ, Lala PK. Normal nonmetastatic human trophoblast cells share in vitro invasive properties of malignant cells. J Cell Physiol 1988; 136: 455–62.
76. Thompson EW, Nakamura S, Shima T, Melchiori A, Martin G, Salahuddin SZ, Gallo RC, Albini A. Supernatants of acquired immunodeficiency syndrome-related Kaposi's sarcoma cells induce endothelial cell chemotaxis and invasiveness. Cancer Res 1991; 51: 2670–1.
77. Mignatti P, Tsuboi R, Robbins E, Rifkin DB. In vitro angiogenesis on the human amniotic membrane: requirement for basic fibroblast growth factor-induced proteinases. J Cell Biol 1989; 108: 671–82.
78. Maslow DE, and Terranova VP. Modulation of cancer cell motility and invasiveness by epidermal and platelet-derived growth factors. Proc Am Assoc Cancer Res Annu Meet 1988; 29: 67.
79. Liotta LA, Goldfarb RH, Brundage R, Siegal R, Terranova V, Garbisa S. Effect of plasminogen activator (urokinase), plasmin, and thrombin on glycoprotein and collagenous components of basement membrane. Cancer Res 1981; 41: 4629–36.
80. Reich R, Thompson EW, Iwamoto Y, Martin GM, Deason JR, Fuller GC, Miskin R. Effects of inhibitors of plasminogen activator, serine proteinases, and collagenase IV on the invasion of basement membranes by metastatic cells. Cancer Res 1988; 48: 3307–12.
81. Meissauer A, Kramer M, Hofmann M, Erkell L, Jacob E, Schirrmacher V, Brunner G. Urokinase-type and tissue-type plasminogen activators are essential for in vitro invasion of human melanoma cells. Exp Cell Res 1991; 192: 453–9.
82. Pourreau-Schneider, N, Delori P, Boutiere B, Arnoux D, George F. Sampol J, Martin PM. Modulation of plasminogen activator systems by matrix components in two breast cancer cell lines MCF-7 and MDA-MB-231. J Natl Cancer Inst 1989; 81: 259–66.
83. Schultz RM, Silberman S, Persky B, Bajowski AS, Carmichael DF. Inhibition of human recombinant tissue inhibitor of metalloproteinases of human amnion invasion and lung colonization by murine B16-F10 melanoma cells. Cancer Res 1988; 48: 5539–45.
84. Albini A, Melchiori A, Santi L, Liotta L, Brown P, and Stetler-Stevenson WG. Tumor cell invasion inhibited by TIMP-2 J Natl Cancer Inst 1991; 83: 775–9.
85. DeClerk YA, Yean TD, Chan D, Shimada H, Langley KE. Inhibition of tumor

invasion of smooth muscle cell layers by recombinant human metalloproteinase inhibitor. Cancer Res 1991; 51: 2151–7.

86. Terranova VP, Liotta LA, Russo RG, Martin GR. Role of laminin in the attachment and metastasis of murine tumor cells. Cancer Res 1982; 42: 2265–9.
87. Terranova VP, Williams JE, Liotta LA, Martin GR. Modulation of the metastatic activity of melanoma cells by laminin and fibronectin. Science 1984; 226: 982–4.
88. Chakrabarty S, Brattain MG, Ochs RL, Varani J. Modulation of fibronectin, laminin, and cellular adhesion in the transformation and differentiation of murine AKR fibroblasts. J Cell Physiol 1987; 133: 415–25.
89. Turpeenniemi-Hujianen T, Thorgeirrson UP, Rao CN, Liotta LA. Laminin increases the release of type IV collagenase from malignant cells. J Biol Chem 1986; 261: 1883–9.
90. Westermark B, Siegbahn A, Heldin CH, Claesson-Welsh L. B-type receptor for platelet-derived growth factor mediates a chemotactic response by means of ligand-induced activation of the receptor protein-tyrosine kinase. Proc Natl Acad Sci USA 1990; 87: 128–32.
91. Adelmann-Grill BC, Wach F, Behr J, Krieg T. Involvement of protein kinase C in signal transduction during fibroblast chemotaxis to platelet-derived growth factor and a fragment of fibronectin. Eur J Cell Biol 1989; 50: 128–31.
92. Reich R, Segui-Real B, Royce L, Martin G, Goldberg G. Reduction of the malignant behaviour of tumor cells by polyunsaturated fatty acids. J Cell Biol 1988; 107: 45A.
93. Mensing H, Czarnetzky BM. Leukotriene B4 induces in vitro fibroblast chemotaxis. J Invest Dermatol 1984: 9–12.
94. Raz A, and Ben-Ze'ev A. Cell-contact and -architecture of malignant cells and their relationship to metastasis. Cancer and Metast Rev 1987; 6: 3–21.
95. Welch DA, Lobl TJ, Seftor EA, Wack PJ, Aeed PA, Yohem KH, Seftor REB, Hendrix MJC. Use of the membrane invasion culture system (MICS) as a screen for anti-invasive agents. Int J Cancer 1989; 43: 449–57.
96. Gauss-Muller V, Kleinman HK, Martin GR, Schiffmann E. Role of attachment factors and attractants in fibroblast chemotaxis. J Lab Clin Med 1980; 96: 1071–80.

11

Cell–Cell and Cell–Matrix Interactions

Betty V. Nusgens
University of Liège, Sart Tilman, Belgium

In multicellular organisms, interactions of the cells with extracellular matrices (ECM), interstitial connective tissues, and basement membranes, as well as with other cells are decisive events in many developmental, biological, and pathologic processes. These include embryogenesis, growth, differentiation and repair, immunologic reaction, tumoral invasion, and metastasis. Two classes of operative molecules deliver information to the cells: soluble factors such as hormones, cytokines, and growth factors; and insoluble ECM components. Both classes of molecules interact with the cells through specific membrane recognition systems: the growth factor receptors and the integrins. The extracellular matrix, made of a network of multidomain molecules extensively linked to each other, not only provides a mechanical support to the cells but also contains cues that profoundly influence cell behavior, such as anchorage, shape, proliferation, migration, and differentiation. Under the effect of the diffusible factors, cells constantly influence the composition of the matrix, which in turn modulates their activity and responsiveness to growth factors. This concept of dynamic reciprocity adds to the complexity of the system. Moreover, the ECM can bind diffusible growth factors with a high affinity and, by its sequestering and releasing capacities, may operate a spatiotemporal control of their activity. During the last decade, in vitro experiments using simplified models have allowed us to progress in our understanding of the mechanisms underlying these complex interactions. The cell–matrix interaction will be specified by the chemical nature of the structure recognized by the cells and their membrane-binding properties. The set of integrins expressed by fibroblasts is not identical to that of endothelial cells, keratinocytes, or smooth muscle cells, and others. Cell–cell interactions will occur using two mechanisms. Each type of cell produces and releases cytokines acting in an autocrine or paracrine fashion. Enzymes are also secreted that can degrade the ECM and release diffusible fragments able to bind to cell membranes. Under these multiple influences, the biosynthetic program of the connective tissue cells is tuned up, resulting in variations in the polymeric structures of the ECM and in their interactive properties with the cells.

The skin is a representative example of this cell–matrix and cell–cell interaction, since it is made of a complex connective tissue supporting and interacting with specialized epithelial structures.

INFORMATIONAL MOLECULES OF THE ECM

The dermis is made of polymers of macromolecules and glycoproteins organized in a three-dimensional network of fibers embedded in a hydrated ground substance. The major dermal structural proteins are collagens type I and III which form hybrid fibrils by copolymerization, in association with the minor collagen type V, which forms the axial nucleus of the fibril. The relative proportion of type I and type III would regulate the size of the fibrils. Type VI collagen is present in the skin in the form of beaded microfilaments participating in the cohesion of the bundles of fibrils. Collagen type XIV covers the fibrils of interstitial collagens, having a function similar to the FACIT collagens, such as type IX in cartilage and type XII in tendons (for details, see Chapter 1 and [1]). The elastic fibers are composed of a microfibrillar meshwork of fibrillin, within which elastin progressively polymerizes (Chapter 3). The extrafibrillar space is composed of hydrated hyaluronan associated with proteoglycans. Some of these, as such as fibromodulin and decorin, are directly associated with the collagen fibrils and accentuate the 64 nm periodicity seen on electron microscopic examination (for details, see Chapter 2 and [2]). The main glycoprotein in the dermis is fibronectin, a widely recognized cell adhesion protein that is also able to interact with other macromolecules such as collagens, fibrin, heparin (see Chapter 5). Other glycoproteins, such as tenascin (mainly present in embryonic and neoplastic tissues) is also found in the papillary dermis and along the epithelial adnexae. It is considered a contra-adhesive protein [3].

The basement membrane at the dermoepidermal junction is the support for keratinocytes and separates the epidermis from the dermis. The structural element ensuring the mechanical stability of the basal lamina is collagen type IV. It assembles by association of amino and carboxy-terminal extremities and lateral aggregation to form a loose meshwork that will serve as a frame to which other basement membranes proteins can attach. The laminin–nidogen complex binds to type IV polymers through the amino-terminal domain of nidogen, while the BM-40 protein binds to the triple helix. Proteoheparan sulfates are linked to laminin and nidogen. A zone beneath the basal lamina contains collagen type VII, which forms the fibrils anchoring the basement membrane to the anchoring plaques in the papillary dermis. More recently described, the BM-600 (or Kalinin or niceine) is probably involved in the attachment of keratinocytes to the basal lamina, as suggested by its alteration in patients with lethal junctional bullous epidermolysis (see [4] and Chapter 4).

It is obvious from the above enumeration of the constituents of the dermis that the variety of macromolecules involved in its edification can explain the diversity of its functions. The fibrillar structures are made of a composite biomaterial that, depending upon their relative proportion, will modulate the structural organization of the tissues and the type of information delivered to the cells. Several isoforms of the structural glycoproteins have also been described arising either from different genes, as for laminin (merosin, form "S"), or from alternative splicing, as for fibronectin and tenascin. These glycoproteins are made of a succession of distinct functional domains, which can be expressed or deleted, allowing a further modulation of their activity. Three main types of domain can be defined in these informational macromolecules. Some of them allow macromolecules to self-assemble or to link to each other. Specific domains are the sites of interactions with the cells and have been extensively studied, such as the RGD sequence in fibronectin. Several different cells recognition sites have been described on the same protein, as in laminin. Some of them can be cryptic in the intact molecule. The third type of domain is the EGF-like repeats identified in several extracellular macromolecules including laminin, tenascin, and thrombospondin. They might function as signals for modulating cell activity [5]. It is worth noting that some extracellular macromolecules posses binding capacity for growth factors. This is the case for heparan sulfate proteoglycans, which fix the FGFs, while TGF-beta interacts primarily with the protein core of proteoglycans and fibronectin. This confers on the extracellular matrix a reservoir property allowing a further mechanism of regulation [6].

Cell recognition sequences have been localized by using enzymatic fragments of proteins and their involvement in the regulation of functions by competition and inhibition experiments in vitro. Homologous synthetic peptides and production of engineered peptides by directed mutagenesis are now largely developed. Laminin and fibronectin are the best characterized structural glycoproteins. Each of them possess several sites recognized by the cells and directing different functions.

In laminin, the fragment P_1 corresponding to the cross of the molecule induces cell adhesion and proliferation. It is also chemotactic. This activity could be assigned to a RGD sequence in the A chain of laminin. This site is only functional after proteolytic degradation of the protein, suggesting that the breakdown products could be also involved in cellular regulation. This consideration might be significant when the basement membranes are degraded during neoplastic invasion and metastases. Another major site of cell recognition is located on the long arm of the molecule (E8). It is responsible for cell adhesion, epithelial differentiation, and neuritic outgrowth [7].

The RGD sequence in fibronectin was the first recognized cell attachment and spreading site in proteins. RGD sequences are not the universal cell recognition sequences since in some proteins RGD sequences exist that are not involved in cell attachment, while many cells use attachment processes that are RGD-independent. Other cell adhesion sites have been identified in fibronectin, such as as the LDV-containing sequence that displays cell-type specificity and alternative splicing. Recent studies indicate that the conformation and other regions of the protein play a helper or synergistic role that can modulate the activity of such sequences.

A number of other proteins posses cell recognition sequences. Type I collagen, besides having two RGD sequences, interact via a DGEA site with a specific integrin alpha$_2$ beta$_1$, allowing the expression of retractile properties of fibroblasts. The biological relevance of these recognition sites in vivo remains to be established (for review, see [8]).

CELL MEMBRANE RECOGNITION MOLECULES

Among the cell surface molecules able to recognize the insoluble ECM macromolecules, the integrins are the most widely expressed. They appear to be the major cell surface adhesion receptors. They also mediate cell–cell contact and are involved in inflammatory and immune processes [9]. Integrins are transmembrane heterodimers made of one subunit alpha noncovalently associated to a beta subunit. Up to now, there have been eight described beta and fourteen known alpha subunits and their number is growing. The complexity of the family is still enhanced by the occurrence of alternative splicing. Conformational activation and deactivation depending on cell differentiation modulate their affinity and specificity. It gives these proteins versatile features that do not always appear in in vitro experiments and are probably most significant in vivo (see [10] and Chapter 7). There is increasing evidence that integrins, in their active state, receive information from matrix that they transfer to the cells. The link between the intracytoplasmic domain of the integrin beta subunit and the cytoskeleton occurs through talin, vinculin, alpha-actinin, and probably other proteins [11]. These structures are most significant in the transduction of the mechanical signals between the ECM and the cell. The occupation of integrin receptors by their ligand leads to a cascade of intracellular events that is still largely unknown.

Cell surface proteoglycans, such as the syndecan family, also behave as matrix receptors [12]. They bind selectively to ECM components (collagen I, III, V, fibronectin) and associate intracellularly with the cytoskeleton. They also bind growth factors as b-FGF. They are developmentally regulated and found mainly in mature epithelia. They share homologies with the fibroblastic matrix-type proteoheparan sulfate. In addition to these two main classes of receptors, a number of proteins binding to ECM macromolecules have been recognized as potential cell receptors, such as the 67 kD laminin binding protein, the anchorins, and others (see Chapter 7).

CELL–MATRIX INTERACTIONS REGULATE CELLULAR PHENOTYPE

The complexity of the three-dimensional network of the extracellular matrices and the diversity of the cellular receptors make difficult the analysis of the mechanisms operating in vivo in cell–matrix interactions. The basic mechanisms, mostly investigated in vitro, address all the functions of the cells triggered or regulated by ECM macromolecules. They are attachment and cell shape, mobility including haptotaxis and chemotaxis, contraction and retraction, and all secondary events such as cell division and expression of a differentiated phenotype. The ECM macromolecules under investigation can be layered on a suitable support or organized in a three-dimensional gel. Competition experiments can use proteolytic fragments, synthetic peptides, and other methods.

A good illustrative example is the migratory behavior of keratinocytes during wound healing. When freshly isolated from normal skin, keratinocytes do not express fibronectin receptors and do not attach to fibronectin-coated dishes. However, in long-term culture or when isolated from wound tissue, they express specific fibronectin integrins and attach to fibronectin. This function is probably operational during the closure of the wound, when keratinocytes attach to and migrate on the provisional fibronectin-containing wound matrix [13].

The reconstitution of a simplified three-dimensional network of macromolecules seems more appropriate to mimic the regulation operated by the ECM. A basement membrane can be reconstituted by polymerizing molecules extracted from the murine EHS tumor (Matrigel). This material has been widely used and was shown to allow a partial retention of the differentiated phenotype of several parenchymal or epithelial cells [14]. The Matrigel also rapidly promotes the organization into tubelike structures of endothelial cells cultured at its surface. A similar pattern of vasculogenesis is observed with type I or type III collagen gel, but only when the apical side of the cell is in contact with the collagen fibrils and only at a low cell density (C. Deroanne, personal communication). This suggests the existence of restricted localization of receptors and points to the importance of cell–cell contact and cell–matrix interaction to switch on and off programs of differentiation (see [15]).

MATRIX–CELLS INTERACTIONS AND MECHANICAL FORCES

A three-dimensional network of collagen polymers represents a subtitute for connective tissue in which mesenchymal cells isolated from their environment and cultured in vitro have been shown to recover their differentiated behavior. Fibroblasts, smooth muscle cells, and myofibroblasts assume in a collagen lattice an elongated bipolar shape and induce a progressive retraction of the gel. It has recently been demonstrated that the contraction is mediated by a non-RGD-dependent $alpha_2$ $beta_1$ integrin receptor expressed under the effect of PDGF. Cells defective in collagen adhesion, as are some tumoral cell lines and dermatosparactic fibroblasts lacking anchorins, are not able to retract the collagen lattice. Besides appropriate adhesive receptors and seric factors, an intact cytoskeleton as well as an active protein synthesis are required for retraction to occur. In retracting lattices, fibroblasts stop proliferating and their biosynthetic phenotype is profoundly modified. The mRNA level and the synthesis of the various types of intertitial collagen and fibronectin drop down, while those of collagenase and stromelysin (two enzymes involved in degradation) are strongly activated [16]. As discussed in details in a recent review by Ingber and Folkman [17], cells generate force within their intracellular cytoskeleton and exert an outward tension on their extracellular adhesions. When plated on malleable substrata that can be deformed in response to cell-generated forces, the tension dissipates. The model of freely retracting collagen gel is one typical example. If the cells are placed on a rigid substratum that both promotes anchoring of the cytoskeleton through integrins and physically resists, an inward tension is transmitted in return to the cell. This condition is fulfilled when the collagen lattice is immobilized. The mechanical tension developed by the cells and transmitted by the collagen polymers can be measured by a device using strain gauges [18]. It takes a few hours to attain its maximal value, which lies around 0.5–1 millinewton for 10^6 human skin fibroblasts and remains stable for several hours. It is higher in smooth muscle cells and intermediate in human granulation tissue myofibroblasts (P. Lefèbvre, personnal communication). It increases as a function of cell number and also with the collagen density of the lattice. If one stretches or relaxes the gel, the initial value of the mechanical tension is recovered within 2–3 hr, suggesting that cells can respond to mechanical disequilibrium by readjusting tension. As compared to a freely contracting lattice, the mRNA levels for collagen I, III, and VI, fibronectin as well as that of actin, is largely increased in the lattice under tension while that of collagenase is lower [16]. These data are further arguments for considering mechanical forces as biological regulators. How the mechanical signal is transduced into a biochemical signal begins to be clarified (for review, see [19].) The transmission of the forces across the integrins system plays a significant role in controling morphogenesis and tissue repair in vivo. They are probably also involved in various fibrotic processes, such as in vascular hypertension, burn retraction, and others.

Cell–matrix and matrix–cell interactions not only control the proliferative and biosynthetic activities of the cell through a direct regulation of genomic expression but can also modulate the activity of cytokines and growth factors. Some components of the ECM, including the heparan sulfate proteoglycans or the syndecans, can immobilize heparin-binding growth factors. The protein core of proteoglycans binds TGF-beta. Both might play a role in protecting the activity and/or a role of reservoir. EGF is a growth factor that has been shown to improve wound healing in vivo by increasing the tensile strength of the wound and its content in collagen. When examined in vitro, EGF inhibits collagen synthesis and activates collagenase of fibroblasts cultured in monolayer on plastic. An opposite effect similar to the in vivo situation is observed when fibroblasts are maintained in a collagen lattice, although the number and the affinity of the EGF receptors are not modified by the interaction with the collagen support [20].

Pathologic conditions related to defective cell–matrix interactions begin to emerge. Their involvement in platelet aggregation, in the immune response, and in tissue repair make them potential candidates for altered functions. Some diseases are already known to be caused by mutations in integrins genes, such as the leukocyte adhesion deficiency. The Ehlers-Danlos type X is linked to a lack of fibronectin function. The lack of regenerative capacities of the adult central nervous system might be related to a lack of expression of laminin able to promote the outgrowth of neurites. Laminin-containing implants in brain lesions could improve the restoration of nervous connections [21]. This opens potential therapeutic approaches using ECM macromolecules as demonstrated with fibronectin for facilitating the healing of corneal ulcers. Cell–matrix interactions are also of prime importance in cancer invasion and metastasis, since they control the cellular locomotory and anchoring properties. The growing knowledge of these interactions and the determination of the peptidic sequences involved are being exploited in the design of agents able to control tumoral cell behavior [22].

CELL–CELL INTERACTIONS

The dialog by exchange of information between cells depends upon the production of active soluble factors that can act at distance, such as the endocrine system of delivery of hormones or, as described for lymphokines and growth factors, in a paracrine fashion on neighboring cells or in an autocrine loop. Cytokines display a variety of activities to modulate the phenotype of the cells that express the specific membrane receptors (see Chapter 12). A few examples related to the skin will illustrate their participation in cell–cell interactions. The mutual influence of keratinocytes and dermal fibroblasts can be demonstrated by using in vitro reconstructed skin. In this system, the fibroblasts have been shown to promote keratinocyte proliferation [23] with variable competence, the hair papilla cells displaying the highest activity [24]. The reverse has also been reported: a stimulation of fibroblast proliferation under the influence of keratinocytes probably through the secretion of IL1 [25]. In a similar reconstituted skin, we observed that keratinocytes were able to stimulate collagenase production and inhibit collagen synthesis by modulating the level of expression of their respective mRNAs [26]. This exchange of information is negatively regulated by retinoids [27]. Several other cell–cell interactions through the paracrine secretion of growth factors and cytokines such as endothelial cells–leukocytes [28], smooth muscle cell–endothelial cells [29], mast cells–fibroblasts and others [30], have been thoroughly investigated.

Cooperation between cells also exists in the building of structures. Fibroblasts are able to induce the assembly of the macromolecules forming the basement membrane and secreted by epithelial cells [31]. Epithelial–mesenchymal cell interactions likewise enhance the expression of type VII collagen forming the anchoring fibrils [32]. Some breast adenocarcinoma cells are not able by themselves to produce the degradation enzymes necessary to invade the surrounding tissues, but they induce the host fibroblasts to synthesize and secrete metalloproteinases that will be captured by the tumoral cells, perhaps through a membrane receptor. MCF7 cells are likewise able by a paracrine or juxtacrine secretion to stimulate normal fibroblasts to produce instertitial macromolecules through a pretranslational regulation. This observation might be related to the desmoplastic reaction occurring in scirrhous breast carcinoma [33].

The large network of cell–matrix–cell interactions operating by the recognition of signals, diffusible or insoluble, is obviously involved in most developmental processes. Alterations in the mutual exchange of information might be responsible for those yet not understood congenital disorders.

REFERENCES

1. Burgeson RE. New collagens, new concepts. Annu Rev Cell Biol 1988; 4: 551–77.
2. Gallagher JT. The extended family of proteoglycans: social residents of the pericellular zone. Curr Opin Cell Biol 1989; 1: 1201–18.
3. Chiquet-Ehrismann R, Mackie EJ, Pearson CA, Sakakura T. Tenascin: an extracellular matrix protein involved in tissue interactions during fetal development and oncogenesis. Cell 1986; 47: 131–9.
4. Timpl R. Structure and biological activity of basement membrane proteins. Eur J Biochem 1989; 180: 487–502.
5. Engel J. Domains in proteins and proteoglycans of the extracellular matrix with functions in assembly and cellular activities. Int J Biol Macromol 1991; 13: 147–51.

6. Flaumenhaft R, Rifkin D. Extracellular matrix regulation of growth factor and protease activity. Curr Opin Cell Biol 1991; 3: 817–23.
7. Sonnenberg A, Linders CJT, Modderman PW, Damsky CH, Aumailley M, Timpl R. Integrin recognition of different cell-binding fragments of laminin (P1, E3, E8) and evidence that alpha-6-betal but not alpha-6-beta-4 functions as a major receptor for fragment E8. J Cell Biol 1990; 110: 2145–55.
8. Yamada KM. Adhesive recognition sequences. J Biol Chem 1991; 266: 12809–12.
9. Ryan US, Worthington RE. Cell–cell contact mechanisms. Curr Immunol 1992; 4: 33–7.
10. Hynes RO. Integrins: versatility, modulation and signaling in cell adhesion. Cell 1992; 69: 11–25.
11. Burridge K, Fath K, Kelly T, Nuckolls G, Turner, C. Focal adhesions: transmembrane junctions between the extracellular matrix and the cytoskeleton. Annu Rev Cell Biol 1988; 4: 487–525.
12. Bernfield M, Sanderson RD. Syndecan, a developmentally regulated cell surface proteoglycan that binds extracellular matrix and growth factors. Philos Trans R Soc Lond [Biol] 1990; 327: 171–86.
13. Clark RA. Fibronectin matrix deposition and fibronectin receptor expression in healing and normal skin. J Invest Dermatol 1990; 94: 128–34S.
14. Kleinman HK, McGarvey ML, Hassell JR, Star VL, Cannon FB, Laurie GW, Martin GR. Basement membrane complexes with biological activity. Biochemistry 1986; 25 312–8.
15. Carey DJ. Control of growth and differentiation of vascular cells by extracellular matrix proteins. Annu Rev Physiol 1991; 53: 161–77.
16. Lambert CA, Soudant EP, Nusgens B, Lapière CM. Pretranslational regulation of extracellular matrix macromolecules and collagenase expression in fibroblasts by mechanical forces. Lab Invest 1992; 66: 444–51.
17. Ingber DE, Folkman J. Tension and compression as basic determinants of cell form and function: utilization of a cellular tensegrity mechanism. In: Cell shape: determinants, regulation and regulatory role. Orlando, FL: Academic Press, 1991: 3–31.
18. Delvoye P, Wiliquet P, Leveque JL, Nusgens BV, Lapière CM. Measurement of mechanical forces generated by skin fibroblasts embedded in a three-dimensional collagen gel. J Invest Dermatol 1991; 97: 898–902.
19. Vandenburgh HH. Mechanical forces and their second messengers in stimulating cell growth in vitro. Am J Physiol 1992; 262: R350–5.
20. Colige A, Nusgens B, Lapière CM. Response to epidermal growth factor of skin fibroblasts from donors of varying age is modulated by the extracellular matrix. J Cell Physiol 1990; 145: 450–7.
21. Davis GE, Blaker SN, Engvall E, Varon S, Manthorpe M, Gage FH. Human amnion membrane serves as a substratum for growing axons in vitro and in vivo. Science 1987; 236: 1106–9.
22. Liotta LA. Tumor invasion and metastases—role of the extracellular matrix: Rhoads memorial award lecture. Cancer Res 1986; 46: 1–7.
23. Coulomb B, Lebreton C, Dubertret L. Influence of human dermal fibroblasts on epidermalization. J Invest Dermatol 1989; 92: 122–5.

24. Reynolds AJ, Oliver RF, Jahoda CA. Dermal cell populations show variable competence in epidermal cell support: stimulatory effects of hair papilla cells. J Cell Sci 1991; 98: 75–83.
25. Delaporte E, Croute F, Vincent C, Bonnefoy JY, Robert J, Thivolet J, Nicolas JF. Keratinocyte–fibroblast interactions: I. Production by the keratinocytes of soluble factors stimulating the proliferation of normal human skin fibroblasts. Pathol Biol 1989; 37: 875–80.
26. Lacroix M, Lapière CM. Keratinocytes modulate the steady-state level of matrix proteins mRNAs in dermal fibroblasts. J Invest Dermatol 1990; 95: 477.
27. Drèze S, Bailly C, Asselineau D, Nusgens B, Darmon M, Lapière C M. Synergism between human skin fibroblasts and keratinocytes to produce collagenase: negative regulation by retinoids. In: Reichert V, Schroot B, eds. Pharmacology of retinoids in the skin, vol 3. Karger, Basel, 1989: 92–93.
28. Mantovani A, Dejana E. Cytokines as communication signals between leukocytes and endothelial cells. Immunol Today 1989; 10: 370–5.
29. Campbell JH, Horrigan S, Merrilees M, Campbell GR. Endothelial–smooth-muscle interactions—possible role in the pathogenesis of atherosclerosis. In Endothelial cell function in diabetic microangiopathy: problems in methodology and clinical aspects,'' vol 9. 1990: 108–17.
30. Levis-Chaffer F, Segal V, Shalit M. Effects of interleukins on connective tissue type mast cells co-cultured with fibroblasts. Immunology 1991; 72: 174–80.
31. Delvoye P, Pierard D, Noël A, Nusgens B, Foidart JM, Lapière CM. Fibroblasts induce the assembly of the macromolecules of the basement membrane. J Invest Dermatol 1988; 90: 276–82.
32. Konig A, Bruckner-Tuderman L. Epithelial–mesenchymal interactions enhance expression of collagen VII in vitro. J Invest Dermatol 1991; 96: 803–8.
33. Noël A, Munaut C, Boulvain A, Calberg-Bacq CM, Nusgens B, Lapière CM, Foidart JM. Modulation of collagen and fibronectin synthesis by normal and malignant cells J Cell Biochem 1992; 48: 150–61.

12

Effect of Cytokines and Growth Factors on Fibroblast Activity

Konrad Herrmann and Hans-Joachim Böhme
University of Leipzig, Leipzig, Germany

The extracellular matrix (ECM) is a dynamic network of proteins and proteoglycans that not only provides structural support to the organism but also has a strong influence on a wide range of biological processes.

Fibroblasts are the most frequent cells in connective tissue producing and forming the ECM. Interstitial collagens are the primary structural proteins of all tissues and the major structural component of connective tissue. Their metabolic turnover (synthesis and degradation) is normally under tightly controlled physiological conditions. The regulation of fibroblast activity is achieved by its interaction with other cells and with the surrounding ECM, as well as by the influence of cytokines and growth factors. Several studies have demonstrated a close correlation between the biosynthetic activity of fibroblasts and the organization or reorganization of the ECM.

Most of the information on regulation of fibroblast activity, especially of the metabolism of structural proteins by cytokines and growth factors, has been obtained from in vitro studies of cultured cells, but there is little experimental evidence about their in vivo role. Up to now, it has been well accepted that these mediators are involved in physiological and pathologic processes, such as wound healing or development and maintainance of fibrosis. In these processes a variety of biological events including inflammation, activation of different connective tissue cells, and migration and proliferation of fibroblasts are involved. Besides cell–cell and cell–matrix interactions, cytokines and growth factors being released from activated cells play an important role in the regulation of fibroblast activity.

Our knowledge of the mediators involved in connective tissue activation increased in the last years when most of them became available as recombinant proteins. Qualitative and quantitative effects of recombinant mediators on the metabolism of matrix proteins have been studied by using in vitro cell culture techniques. The results of these in vitro investigations, however, cannot be directly extrapolated to the in vivo situation because there are also interactions between fibroblasts and inflammatory cells as well as degradation products of components of the ECM that might be involved. Cytokines and growth factors secreted by connective tissue cells (e.g., fibroblasts and endothelial cells) and by inflammatory cells can also interact and exert their biological effects in a concerted manner.

Because cytokines and growth factors have important functions in normal cellular processes, to explain their roles in pathologic processes we must assume an excessive production or an inadequate inhibition of them. Furthermore, some factors may even be able to antagonize or oppose the effects of others. In addition, specific inhibitor molecules appear to exist that block the biological effect of these factors.

This review outlines our current understanding of several major aspects of the cytokine-mediated regulation of fibroblast activity. In this context, the network of the synergistic and antagonistic action of cytokines and growth factors in the development of fibrosis will be discussed in more detail. One of the most consistent features of connective tissue fibrosis is the overproduction and accumulation of matrix proteins, especially of collagen, in the involved tissues. Reviewing the contradictory data about cytokines in ECM metabolism, we try to create a better understanding of the complicated network of the regulation of fibroblast activity.

TRANSFORMING GROWTH FACTOR-β

Transforming growth factor β (TGF-β) comprises a family (TGF-β1, -β2, -β3, and -β4) of highly conserved homodimeric polypeptides with a molecular mass of 25 kDa [1]. Most mammalian cells including fibroblasts synthesize and secrete this growth factor as a larger precursor that is processed by limited proteolysis to the mature polypeptide [2]. In vitro, the activation of the TGF-β precursor can be achieved by incubation at lower pH values or by treatment with proteases; the mechanism of its in vivo activation, however, is unknown. There is evidence that coculturing of fibroblasts with endothelial cells and pericytes leads to the activation of latent TGF-β. The same mechanism may also take place under physiological conditions [3].

The effect of TGF-β on its target cells seems to be mediated by binding to a specific membrane receptor(s), the existence of which has been detected in a wide variety of cell types. After the binding of TGF-β to the membrane receptor, the target cells respond via an unknown transmembrane signaling mechanism with an increased interaction of the nuclear factor 1 with the collagen promoter, leading to a stimulation of collagen mRNA expression [4].

With the use of immunohistologic staining and in situ hybridization techniques, TGF-β1 and its specific mRNA were also detected in mesenchymal derived tissues, including connective tissue. Therefore, we will focus the following discussion of the biological effects on the subspecies TGF-β1.

In general, TGF-β1 is a pleiotropic growth factor for fibroblasts acting by autocrine and paracrine mechanisms. Concerning the autocrine effect, there is good evidence that TGF-β stimulates the synthesis of platelet-derived growth factor (PDGF)-B-and/or A-chain by inducing the *c-sis* mRNA as well as the secretion of PDGF-like peptides, which in turn leads to cell proliferation via the PDGF-mediated pathway.

The regulatory effects of TGF-β1 on gene expression of various matrix components are by far the best studied biological phenomena of this compound. TGF-β1 is known to activate the transcription of collagen type I, type III, type VII, fibronectin, the β-subunit of the fibronectin receptor, β-actin, and several proteoglycans and glycosaminoglycans. It is worthwhile to note that in fibroblasts the steady state levels of collagen type I and fibronectin mRNAs are regulated coordinatively. TGF-β1 inhibits collagenase synthesis on the transcriptional level, and suppresses the synthesis of proteases inhibitors such as collagenase inhibitor TIMP and plasminogen-activator inhibitor. These data indicate that TGF-β1 enhances the formation of ECM both by suppressing matrix degradation and by stimulation of the de novo synthesis of ECM components [5]. Furthermore, TGF-β1 acts as a potent chemoattractant for fibroblasts and stimulates their total protein synthesis but does not directly affect diploid fibroblast proliferation.

There is also in vivo evidence for the potency of TGF-β1 to induce ECM production. Its injection into the dermis of mice gives rise to a marked formation of granulation tissue, while its application in wound healing models leads to an increase of connective tissue accompanied by an enhanced migration of fibroblasts into the wounded area and a significant deposition of collagen. In another experimental wound healing model, TGF-β1 exerts its regulatory effect at two different levels. Before matrix reorganization, it promotes matrix protein synthesis but has little effect on fibroblast proliferation. However later, during matrix reorganization, TGF-β1 causes decreased DNA and collagen synthesis [6].

In situ hybridization experiments using scleroderma skin biopsies showed a coexpression of TGF-β1 and collagen type I mRNA in a coordinative manner. The concept of an involvement of TGF-β1 in the induction and maintenance of fibrosis is further supported by the detection of high TGF-β1 mRNA concentrations in fibroblasts derived from patients with early stages of scleroderma [7].

The recent observation that the activation of collagen gene expression by TGF-β1 is counteracted by TNF-α and IFN-γ further emphasizes the idea that cytokines and growth factors may influence each other both synergistically and antagonistically [8].

Addition of low dosages of TGF-β1 to the medium of cultured fibroblasts resulted in an accelerated ECM reorganization consistent with its ability to promote these cells to contract collagen gels. [9]. This effect may be responsible for wound contraction during wound healing.

The most potent activator of collagen synthesis and of collagen mRNA expression in fibroblasts is TGF-β, which causes a severalfold increase of collagen production both under in vitro conditions and in in vivo wound healing models, as well as in fibrotic diseases such as scleroderma and keloids. This mediator, which is produced and released locally, augments and accelerates at first the inflammatory response and then upregulates the biosynthetic metabolism of fibroblasts in a concerted manner. Thus, TGF-β possesses the potential to exert both agonistic and antagonistic effects in the modulation of fibroblast activity.

PLATELET-DERIVED GROWTH FACTOR

PDGF and PDGF-like peptides are structurally closely related competence factors for cell growth. Originally identified as a platelet-derived factor this mediator was later detected also in other mammalian cells including fibroblasts. PDGF is a heterodimer of α and β chains linked by disulfide bridges; the two genes reside on separate chromosomes. Recently, homodimers of α or β chains have also been described.

Fibroblasts and other target cells possess two distinct PDGF receptors denoted type A and type B. The A-type receptors binds all three isoforms of PDGF, whereas the B-type receptor binds the PDGF ββ-homodimer with high affinity, the αβ-heterodimer with lower affinity, and does not appear to bind the αα-homodimer at all. These different receptor types are structurally and functionally related and belong to the tyrosine kinase family [10]. The B-type receptor is a transmembrane glycoprotein of approximately 180 kDa composed of an external cytokine-binding domain, a small transmembrane domain, and a cytosolic tyrosine kinase domain. The spacing of the 10 cysteine residues of the external part of the receptor predicts that it consists of 5 immunoglobulinlike domains. The A-type receptor is synthesized as a 140 kDa precursor that matures by N-linked glycosylation to a 170 kDa species.

Upon binding of PDGF to the extracellular domain of the receptor, the cytosolic tyrosine kinase becomes activated by a process that is presently not fully understood. A possible explanation of this activation of the B-type PDGF receptor was suggested by the observation that binding of ββ-PDGF dimer induces dimerization of the B-type PDGF receptor in a concentration-dependent manner. In connection with the dimeric structure of the growth factor, this finding indicates that each ββ-dimer binds two receptor molecules. Because it was found that dimerization of the receptor is closely associated with the activation of the tyrosine kinase activity, it is conceivable that the dimerization of the PDGF receptor gives rise to an interaction between the two tyrosine kinase domains, which in turn leads to their activation. A similar mechanism was also proposed [11] for activation of the EGF receptor.

An unusual autocrine activation could be demonstrated in the case of this growth factor by a careful investigation of the apparent paradox that although SV 40 induces neoplasia by expression of the *v-sis* oncogene, which codes for the β chain of PDGF, exogenous PDGF does not induce neoplasia even when added to cells bearing PDGF receptors. It was found that after a *v-sis* (or *c-sis*) induction, the newly synthesized PDGF β-chains can bind within the rough endoplasmic reticulum to their receptor. Thus, autocrine activation is achieved without secretion of the ligand or expression of the membrane receptor.

Apart from being stored in platelets, PDGF has been found to be synthesized by a number of cells such as smooth muscle cells, activated macrophages, endothelial cells, and mitogen-stimulated fibroblasts. Although the in vivo function of PDGF is still unclear, the sites of its synthesis, in combination with the fact that it stimulates proliferation of connective tissue, suggest that PDGF has a role in tissue repair. This postulation is strengthened by the fact that PDGF also stimulates chemotaxis of fibroblasts as well as of neutrophils and monocytes. Experimental support of this hypothesis came from the following observations: the PDGF levels are elevated during wound healing and in early stages of scleroderma; PDGF selectively stimulates the synthesis of type V collagen accompanied by a reciprocal decrease of type III collagen; PDGF causes a stimulation of type I collagen synthesis in some but not all fibroblast cultures; in synovial fibroblasts PDGF inhibits collagenase expression, but it shows only little, if any, effect on the transcription of this enzyme in dermal fibroblasts.

Like TGF-β, PDGF is involved in wound contraction. Using lattices, PDGF promotes fibroblast contraction of collagen gels. The promoting influence of recombinant PDGF on chemotaxis using a Boyden chamber is well accepted. This in vitro observation is further supported by the fact that in animal wound healing models the chemotaxis of fibroblast is abolished by the addition of antibodies against PDGF.

INTERFERON-γ

Interferon-γ (IFN-γ) is a 17 kDa protein that forms a homodimer exhibiting antiviral, antiproliferative, and immunoregulative properties in a variety of mammalian cells, including fibroblasts. This cytokine is mainly released by activated lymphocytes and encoded by a single gene. Its biological activity is mediated by binding to a high-affinity cell surface receptor. The signal transduction involves activation of both the membrane-bound and soluble protein kinase C.

Many studies reported that the ability of IFN-γ to express the class II major histocompatibility antigen (HLA-DR) [12] as well as intercellular adhesion molecule (ICAM-1) in various cells including fibroblasts may be important both for antigen presentation and for trafficking of lymphocytes into the dermis [13]. The biological significance of HLA-DR expression in fibroblasts in response to IFN-γ is speculative because of their inability to provide additional antigen presenting signals. The available experimental data suggest a model in which IFN-γ-stimulated fibroblasts are able to activate resting T lymphocytes, which in turn leads to their proliferation and to the liberation of several cytokines, especially interleukins.

The best-investigated effect in connective tissue of IFN-γ is its ability to suppress the collagen synthesis of fibroblasts on the protein as well as the mRNA level [14, 15]. It has recently also been reported that IFN-γ depressed markedly the enhanced collagen synthesis of cultured scleroderma fibroblasts and induces a collagen low-producer phenotype. This inhibition leads to a coordinate decrease in the synthesis of both type I and type III collagen in normal as well as scleroderma fibroblasts. The observation that the level of collagen mRNA is also decreased points to an involvement of IFN-γ in the regulation of gene expression [15]. The repression of collagen synthesis is further enhanced by an incubation of fibroblasts with IFN-γ and TNF-α, suggesting a coordinative transcriptional down regulation by these cytokines [16].

In a concentration-dependent manner, IFN-γ causes a strong elevation of fibronectin mRNA transcription whereas only a slight increase of protein level could be observed [14, 17]. The synthesis of glycosaminoglycans, another important component of the ECM, is also upregulated by IFN-γ whereas the activity of collagenase, the opponent of the accumulated collagen in fibrotic tissues, is markedly diminished [17]. Because in these experiments no evidence was found for an effect of IFN-γ on the activation of latent collagenase, a direct influence of this growth factor on collagenase synthesis was proposed. The exact mechanism of this effect, however, remains unclear.

The chemotactic response of human dermal fibroblasts using different chemoattractants is strongly inhibited by IFN-γ. Antibodies against this cytokine block this inhibition [18]. The attachment of skin fibroblast to components of the ECM is also modulated by this polypeptide [19] and it is assumed that both effects may be important in wound healing.

Recent studies showed that IFN-γ inhibits the collagen synthesis and decreases collagen accumulation also under in vivo conditions in animal models of fibrosis [20]. Several clinical trials to treat fibrotic diseases such as scleroderma, keloids, hypertrophic scars, and idiopathic pulmonary fibrosis, with IFN-γ are now in progress.

INTERLEUKIN-1

Interleukin-1 (IL-1) is synthesized as a 33 kDa precursor that is proteolytically activated to the 17 kDa mature protein. The exact mechanism of its secretion is poorly understood. IL-1 is mainly produced by monocytes and macrophages. Its main function in connective tissue seems to be the assembling and degradation of ECM by inducing synthesis of matrix proteins and proteases, including collagenase. Two forms of IL-1 (α and β) have been described that share 26% homology in their amino acid sequence. Although IL-1β is mainly found in the supernatant of activated monocytes, IL-1α acts primarily as a membrane-bound molecule. Both subtypes bind to the same receptor species but with different affinity. Human fibroblasts are able to synthesize IL-1β in response to incubation with both recombinant IL-1α and IL-1β. Furthermore, a synergistic upregulation of IL-1β mRNA could be shown after simultaneous addition of IL-1 and TNF-α to cultured human lung fibroblasts [21]. The IL-1β production of activated fibroblasts also seems to be under posttranscriptional control, since the IL-1β mRNA levels do not correlate with the release of the corresponding protein [21]. The pro-IL-1β, which will not be secreted extracellularly, may have important intracellular regulatory effects.

Cultured dermal fibroblasts respond to IL-1α with increased proliferation and modulation of their metabolism. IL-1 induces procollagen type I and type III expression in human fibroblasts. Type III procollagen mRNA is found in higher concentration than those of type I. The levels of α1(I) and α2(I) mRNAs are regulated coordinately at a pretranslational level in dermal fibroblast. Synovial fibroblasts, however, display decreased type I procollagen mRNA after incubation with IL-1. A reason for this observation may be its ability to increase prostaglandin E2 production in synovial fibroblasts, which act as a strong inhibitor for collagen type I gene expression [22]. IL-1 was also shown to be capable of inducing the production of fibronectin and proteoglycans in fibroblasts.

Recent studies have further shown that the effect of IL-1 on collagen synthesis is dose-dependent; low concentrations cause a stimulation but high dosages lead to an inhibition of the expression of type I and type III collagen [23, 24]. These concentration-dependent responses may be one of the reasons for the contradictory results in the literature concerning the influence of IL-1 on collagen metabolism.

In cultured fibroblasts, IL-1 and TNF-α were shown to cause an enhancement of *c-fos* and *c-myc* proto-oncogene mRNA steady-state levels. The corresponding proteins stimulate the secretion of interleukin-6 (IL-6). In human fibroblasts, both mediators cause a rapid accumulation of intracellular cAMP and an activation of cAMP-dependent protein kinase. This is the first evidence for the mechanism of the molecular action of these cytokines [25].

Both IL-1α and IL-1β may induce the synthesis of collagenase and of neutral proteases (e.g., elastase) in synovial as well as dermal fibroblasts, but also the synthesis of tissue inhibitor of metalloproteinases (TIMP) [26], which most likely plays a key role in modulating collagenase activity. A coincubation of fibroblast with IL-1 and PDGF increases the expression of stromelysin, an interstitial collagenase, up to 23-fold [27].

IL-1 can potentiate the chemoattractive potency of EGF and PDGF on dermal fibroblasts by increasing their migratory response. In addition, IL-1 may also contribute to fibroblast proliferation either directly or indirectly by stimulating the production of PDGF.

INTERLEUKIN-6

Interleukin-6 (IL-6) is a pleiotropic cytokine produced by fibroblasts and a wide range of other mammalian cells; it interacts with most cell types resulting in a variety of biological activities. IL-6 is a 21 kDa glycoprotein containing 184 amino acid residues and is synthesized as a precursor peptide with 212 amino acids. The human IL-6 gene is located on chromosome 7. The expression of the IL-6 gene was found to be under the control of a nuclear binding factor (NF-IL-6) that binds to IL-1-responsive elements in the IL-6 gene and also to similar regulatory regions identified in the genes of several other cytokines and acute-phase proteins.

The high-affinity IL-6 receptor is expressed in a variety of different mammalian cells. Molecular cloning of the receptor gene demonstrated that this receptor possesses one immunoglobulinlike domain in the N-terminal extracellular part of the molecule as other members of the cytokine receptor superfamily [28]. The mechanism of signal transduction is still unclear. IL-6 does not stimulate the prostaglandin E2 production of fibroblasts, suggesting that its biological effects are not mediated by such metabolites.

In cultured dermal fibroblasts, IL-6 stimulates the synthesis of collagen and glycosaminoglycans, especially of hyaluronic acid, chondroitin-4 sulfate, chondroitin-6 sulfate, and dermatan sulfate, whereas fibronectin metabolism and total protein synthesis were not affected [29]. Addition of specific antibodies directed against IL-6 could abolish these stimulatory effects. In a dose-dependent manner, IL-6 also induces the expression of the collagenase gene, giving rise to increase of collagenase activity [30]. In contradiction to these observations, IL-6 was identified as a potent inducer of the de novo synthesis of TIMP and as ineffective with respect to collagenase expression [31].

IL-6 has recently been reported also to stimulate the production of the complement components factor B and C3 in cultured human skin fibroblasts [32] and is known as one of the most potent agents for fibroblast proliferation.

Since cultured dermal fibroblasts synthesize and secrete IL-6 in basal amounts constitutively and in enhanced amounts after incubation with different cytokines such as IL-1, TNF-α, TNF-β, it is likely that fibroblasts are a main producer of this powerful cytokine in connective tissue.

Besides its influence on the synthesis of matrix proteins by fibroblasts, IL-6 is one of the most potent agents for fibroblast proliferation.

The results discussed above suggest that IL-6 could play an important role in the regulation of matrix formation and/or remodeling such as occurs in wound healing and pathologic fibrotic reactions.

EPIDERMAL GROWTH FACTOR

Epidermal growth factor (EGF) is a small polypeptide (52 amino acids) that directly stimulates growth and differentiation in a number of epithelial tissues, stimulates the growth of mesenchymal and endothelial cells, and has multifunctional effects such as ion secretion, muscle contraction, and cell movement. EGF is present in human platelets and is found in all body fluids, even sweat. TGF-α has overall but limited homology to EGF and is antigenically related and binds to the EGF receptor. All known effects of EGF are mediated by its receptor whose amino acid sequence was deduced using cDNA clones from placenta. A close similarity between the predicted sequence of the *v-erbB* mRNA oncogene product of the avian erythroblastosis and the EGF receptor transmembrane and cytoplasmic domain was noted.

The EGF receptor is a single-chain 170 kDa glycoprotein and belongs to the tyrosine kinase family. It is composed of at least three different domains: an external EGF-binding domain of about 100 kDa, a relatively small transmembrane portion, and a cytoplasmic domain of about 60 kDa. The cytoplasmic domain contains the endogenous EGF-dependent tyrosine kinase activity and a number of autophosphorylation sites. How extracellular EGF binding regulates the cytoplasmatically located tyrosine kinase activity is not clear but may involve a specific threonine and/or receptor dimerization. The first molecular event mediated by EGF after binding to its surface receptor is the stimulation of tyrosine phosphorylation of cellular substrates including rapid autophosphorylation. This intrinsic protein tyrosine kinase activity is essential for signal transduction [33].

Especially intriguing was the observation that binding of EGF at physiological concentrations (1 nM) to cells expressing the human EGF receptor stimulates a rapid tyrosine phosphorylation of a phospholipase C isozyme (PLC-II), as revealed by immunoblotting analysis with phosphotyrosine-specific antibodies [34]. Two other phospholipase C isozymes (PLC-I and PLC-III) were not significantly phosphorylated in response to this growth factor. It is interesting that antibodies specific for PLC-II were able to coprecipitate the EGF receptor and antibodies against the EGF receptor coprecipitate PLC-II. According to this study about 1% of EGF receptor molecules are associated with PLC-II molecules. The tyrosine kinase inhibitor tyrphostin, which blocks EGF-stimulated cell proliferation, blocks also EGF-dependent phosphorylation of PLC-II, its association with EGF receptor, as well as EGF-mediated calcium release. Hence, EGF-induced tyrosine phosphorylation of PLC-II may be a regulatory event linking the intrinsic tyrosine kinase activity of EGF receptor to the inositol trisphosphate signaling pathway. The association with PLC-II is not unique to the EGF receptor, because it was found that PLC-II is also phosphorylated in response to PDGF. However, neither insulin nor colony-stimulating factor is capable of promoting PLC-II phosphorylation, suggesting that not all tyrosine kinases are able to induce this phenomena.

As do most other types of cells, fibroblasts possess EGF receptors and respond to exogenous EGF in culture. After addition, human gingival fibroblasts cultured as monolayer synthesize a greater amount of DNA and of total protein, but collagen biosynthesis is not affected [35]. Although an increase in prolyl hydroxylase was observed in osteoblastic cells, a decrease in collagen synthesis was noted [36]. On the other hand, several recent reports have demonstrated that wound healing in vivo is accelerated by EGF both by accumulating mesenchymal cells in the granulation tissue and by stimulating collagen synthesis [37, 38]. Hence the proposal that EGF, together with other growth factors (e.g., fibroblast growth factor and PDGF, present in platelets), represents a physiological stimulus in the process of wound healing is most acceptable.

The reason for the discrepancy between the results obtained in experiments with fibroblasts cultured as monolayer and the observations in wound healing in in vivo models seems to be the interaction of fibroblasts with the extracellular matrix. It was demonstrated [39] that fibroblasts cultured in a three-dimensional collagen lattice respond to EGF with an increased production of both noncollagen protein and collagen synthesis, as observed in wound healing. It is obvious that the three-dimensional collagen lattice resembles the physiological environment better then a two-dimensional culture on plastic or plastic-coated petri dishes with various macromolecules of the extracellular matrix. Fibroblasts isolated from their physiological environment acquire properties different from those in situ because of the loss of some regulative signals arising from the extracellular matrix in which they normally reside.

INSULIN-LIKE GROWTH FACTORS

Two distinct insulin-like growth factors (IGF-I and IGF-II) exist in human plasma; both are quite similar chemically. IGF-I appears to be a primary regulator of the growth of an organism. It is produced mainly by the liver in the response to secretion of growth hormone by the pituitary gland. Its ability to stimulate growth is largely mediated by a membrane receptor that shares a number of properties, including molecular weight and tyrosine kinase activity, with the insulin receptor. The IGF-I receptor prefers IGF-I to IGF-II and interacts with high concentrations of insulin. The IGF-I receptor tyrosine kinase shares many properties with the tyrosine kinases associated with other receptors for growth factors, especially the insulin receptor. Nonetheless, subtle differences in the specificity of the receptor kinases for synthetic substrates suggest that natural substrates, even for these two closely related receptor kinases, differ. IGF-II is also mainly synthesized by the liver. Its receptor is identical with the mannose 6-phosphate receptor and does not recognize insulin.

A significant aspect of IGF-I physiology is that plasma and other biological fluids contain multiple proteins that specifically bind IGFs [40, 41]. Three different classes of IGF-binding proteins (IGFBPs) have been identified. IGFBP-1 was first identified in amniotic fluid and purified from this source. It is regulated by insulin and glucose. The second type of IGFBP, IGFBP-2, was originally purified from medium conditioned by the rat-liver-derived cell line BRL-3A. IGFBP-3, also known as BP-53, is growth-hormone-dependent and forms in the presence of a acid-labile 85 kDa protein and IGF-I or IGF-II, the high-molecular-weight complex in which most of the IGFs are found in the circulation. Target cells for IGFs, including bone, liver, and muscle cells, and fibroblasts have been shown to produce different IGFBPs in vitro [42].

IGF-I (and insulin) is able to stimulate cell multiplication in chick fibroblasts. In human skin fibroblasts, however, other factors in addition to IGF-I (or insulin) are required for triggering cell proliferation. Binding of a ligand (insulin or IGF-I) to the IGF-I receptor of human fibroblasts stimulates DNA synthesis.

TUMOR NECROSIS FACTOR-α

Tumor necrosis factor-α (TNF-α) is a macrophage-derived pleiotropic cytokine that occurs in a transmembrane form with a molecular mass of 26 kDa and in a soluble form with a molecular mass of 17 kDa.

TNF-α binds to a specific receptor with a molecular mass of approximately 90–100 kDa. IFN-γ increases the number of membrane receptors, whereas IL-1 and TNF-α itself down regulate the receptor expression [43]. Little is known about the mechanism of signal transduction. Two early events are the accumulation of cAMP and the increase in cAMP-dependent protein kinase activity observed within minutes after TNF exposure.

Upon binding to its receptor, TNF-α activates a number of genes, such as the proto-oncogenes *c-fos*, *c-myc*, and *c-jun*, transcription factors NF-kB and IRF-1 and others. Some of these mRNAs, which are only transiently (about 30–120 min) elevated in response to TNF-α (e.g., *c-fos*, *c-myc*, or the transcription factor IRF-1), may be important for the control of other genes.

In addition to its multiple biological activities on immune and tumor cells, TNF-α is also able to modulate fibroblast functions. In human fibroblasts and 3T3 cells cultured in the presence of different concentrations of fetal calf serum, this cytokine decreases the collagen type I and type III gene transcription and the synthesis of the corresponding proteins up to 50% [44, 45]. Because previous reports could clearly demonstrate that TNF-α significantly stimulates the secretion of the prostaglandin E2 by dermal fibroblasts in a dose-dependent manner, it seems to be possible that the stimulated prostaglandin liberation is responsible for the inhibition of the collagen synthesis. In contrast to this, for human lung fibroblasts growing in a serum-free medium, TNF-α stimulates type I collagen mRNA steady state levels. These data might suggest that the biological effect of TNF-α is modulated by serum factors. IFN-γ acts synergistically to TNF-α in this system. Since collagen type I and type III mRNA steady state levels are also reduced, this effect must occur at a pretranslational level.

Besides its influence on collagen production, TNF-α and β also enhance the synthesis of glycosaminoglycans, while fibronectin synthesis seems to be inhibited [44]. The collagenase activity is more than 10-fold elevated after incubation with TNF-α or TNF-β.

TNF also acts synergistically with IL-1 and increases the level of IL-1β mRNA in human lung fibroblasts, but this intracellular accumulation of IL-1β mRNA is not associated with the release of the IL-1β protein by these fibroblasts [21]. The finding that posttranscriptional mechanisms prevent cytokine-stimulated fibroblasts from secreting the cytokine might play an important role in terminating inflammatory processes.

Furthermore, TNF-α stimulates fibroblasts to produce IFN-β, which can modulate fibroblast metabolism and enhances IL-6 production in cultured human fibroblasts as well as in an in vivo mouse model [46].

TNF-α has been reported to stimulate the proliferation of human fibroblasts; this effect could be related to the enhanced expression of the EGF receptors [47]. The growth-stimulatory activity of this mediator was more marked in the presence of fetal calf serum and blocked by a monoclonal antibody neutralizing its cytotoxic activity [48].

FIBROBLAST GROWTH FACTORS

Fibroblast growth factors (FGFs) are a family of at least eight proteins with a great extent of structural homology that exert mainly mitogenic activity to fibroblasts. Up to now, interest has focused on two FGFs that differ in their isoelectric points: basic and acidic FGF (bFGF, aFGF) with a molecular mass of approximately 16 kDa. Fibroblasts express a specific receptor with a molecular mass of 140–160 kDa [49]. The binding of FGF on its receptor is accompanied by the formation of inositol phosphates, activation of protein kinase C, and a decrease in intracellular cAMP levels. At least two types of G-proteins may be involved in the intracellular signaling pathway of FGF.

Furthermore, FGF binds on glycosaminoglycans, especially heparin. This complex will be much more stable against denaturation and proteolytic degradation. Dermal fibroblasts are significantly stimulated by aFGF in the presence of heparin. It induces DNA synthesis and increases the cell number of fibroblasts, cultured in monolayer or in a three-dimensional collagen gel, in a dose-dependent manner. It is interesting that FGF-stimulated fibroblasts growing in such a gel do not contract this gel as untreated fibroblasts do [50]. Collagenase is also induced by a transcriptional regulation. In an animal wound-healing model, it could be shown that bFGF supports matrix formation and formation of granulation tissue. In those cells that secrete bFGF, this growth factor stimulates the expression of the oncogenes *c-fos*, *c-jun*, and *junB*.

INFLUENCE OF THE EXTRACELLULAR MATRIX ON CYTOKINE ACTION

The extracellular matrix contains a number of large multidomain macromolecules: various collagen types, fibronectin, elastin, laminin, and proteoglycans. A number of different cells including endothelial cells and fibroblasts have been demonstrated to interact with specialized domains of these proteins that control cellular attachment and differentiation. The interaction is achieved via specific receptors located on the cell surface and recognizing distinct sequences of the macromolecules (see Chapters 7 and 11).

In addition to this attachment, these macromolecules of the extracellular matrix contain domains with growth factor activity that may stimulate target cells in a much more selective way than diffusible growth factors. Such growth factor domains, with a close or more distant homology with EGF and TGF-α have been identified in matrix proteins such as laminin, tenascin, and thrombospondin [51].

The complex network of intracellular events is controlled by small diffusible growth factors and cytokines that lead to growth, proliferation, and reorganization of connective tissue. Little is known about the spatial organization of growth factors in tissues. Concentration gradients are important and for some growth factors interactions with proteoglycans may also be involved. Until recently it was believed that the functions of proteoglycans vary from the formation of an elastic pad in cartilage to prevention of premature association of antigenic peptides with class II histocompatibility antigens. However, many of the proteoglycans function as modulators of growth factors. It is well known that heparan sulfate binds the fibroblast growth factors [52] and protects them from degradation. More recently it has been shown that the binding of basic FGF to its receptor requires prior binding either to heparan sulfate side chains of a membrane heparan sulfate proteoglycan or to free heparan sulfate chains. The FGF receptor of cells lacking heparan sulfate does not bind basic FGF. The binding function can be restored by adding the growth factor as heparin–basic FGF complex [53].

The binding of growth factors by proteoglycans is not limited to the FGF–heparan sulfate interaction. Growth factors that bind to heparan sulfate include granulocyte–macrophage colony-stimulating factor, interleukin-3, and platelet factor 4 [54]. The latter binds also with high affinity to chondroitin sulfate proteoglycan serglycin [55].

While the above-mentioned growth factor proteoglycan interactions are mediated by the glycosaminoglycan chains of the proteoglycans, at least one growth factor, TGF-β-, binds to proteoglycans through the core protein. One of the three receptors for TGF-β is a proteoglycan named betaglycan. Betaglycan apparently does not act in signal transduction but in binding TGF-β and delivering the growth factor to the signal-transducing receptor.

TGF-β binds also to decorin, a proteoglycan of extracellular matrix [56]. Decorin is a member of a family of leucine-rich proteins and is associated with type I collagen fibrils. Decorin not only binds TGF-β but also neutralizes the activity of the growth factor. This observation, together with the fact that the synthesis of decorin in a variety of cells is stimulated by TGF-β, suggests that decorin may be an effector molecule in a negative feedback loop that regulates TGF-β activity.

Because proteoglycans are abundant and ubiquitous molecules, it is likely that they are able to bind most of the growth factors and cytokines. The result is that these factors can only act over short distances in the tissue due to their immobilization by cell surface or extracellular matrix proteoglycans.

CYTOKINES AND GROWTH FACTORS IN VIVO

Cytokines and growth factors are soluble, low-molecular-weight polypeptides that modulate the biological activity of their target cells via specific cell surface receptors (Tables 12.1 and 12.2). Most of them act by autocrine or paracrine mechanism but endocrine effects must also be taken into consideration. The mechanism of signal transduction is in most cases not completely understood. Many of the receptor molecules are protein tyrosine kinases that phosphorylate intracellular target proteins in response to the binding of the corresponding ligand. However, the discussed mediators may also influence other signal transduction systems, such as the activation of the phospholipase C-II by the EGF receptor kinase. In some cases G-proteins may also be involved in the transmembrane signaling mechanism.

The biological function of the fibroblast is related to and influenced by the other components of the connective tissue (endothelial, smooth muscle, immune, mast cells, and the macromolecules of the ECM). The specific interactions with these cells and macromolecules to a great extent determine the specific reaction of the fibroblasts (migration, proliferation, attachment, protein synthesis, etc.) toward changes in their environment. In addition to these cell–cell and cell–ma-

Table 12.1 Influence of Cytokines and Growth Factors on Matrix Protein Synthesis

Cytokine	Collagen synthesis	Collagenase synthesis	Fibronectin synthesis	Proteoglycan synthesis
TGF-ß	↑	±	↑	↑
PDGF	↑	(↑) ± (↓)	±	?
IFN-γ	↓	(↑)	↑	↑
IL-1	(↑) ±	↑	↑	↑
IL-6	↑	(↑)	↑	±
EGF	(↑) ±	↑	?	?
TNF-α	↓	↑	↓	↑

trix interactions, soluble mediators (cytokines and growth factors) play an outstanding role in the regulation of fibroblast metabolism.

The effect of a given cytokine on the metabolism and function of its target cells cannot be discussed on its own because there exists a network in space and in time of antagonistic and synergistic interactions of different mediators with each other. Moreover, interactions of mediators with macromolecules of the ECM must be taken into consideration.

The processes occurring during wound healing very clearly demonstrate how the timing of the effects of a certain cytokine (e.g., on gene expression) is responsible for the tuning the different phases of healing. A cytokine is capable of mediating both biosynthetic and biodegradative reactions. The effect of TNF-α on the metabolism of fibroblasts is a good example of this dual role. This cytokine stimulates the synthesis of proteoglycans and inhibits the formation of collagen and fibronectin. At the same time it stimulates a degradation of collagen by inducing collagenase. The selective induction of protease inhibitors (e.g.,

Table 12.2 Influence of Cytokines and Growth Factors on Proliferation and Chemotaxis of Fibroblasts

Cytokine	Proliferation	Chemotaxis
TGF-ß	↑	↑
PDGF	↑	↑
IFN-γ	↓	↓
IL-1	↑	↑
IL-6	↑	(↑)
EGF	↑	(↑) ±
TNF-α	↑ (↓)	±

TIMP) by cytokines is an other mechanism by which these mediators may exert their effects on the regulation of fibroblast metabolism.

Other cytokines, (e. g., IL-6 and IL-1), also show such pleiotropic effects, for they stimulate both matrix-forming and matrix-degradative processes. At first view, this is a contradiction in terms. However, these apparently inconsistent effects are due to the concentration-dependence (a cytokine may act at low concentrations as stimulator and at higher concentrations as inhibitors), the different timing of the effects, and synergistic or antagonistic interactions with other mediators. Therefore, a complex network of regulatory mechanisms and mutual interactions must be assumed to act in the connective tissue. A disturbance of this network due to a change in one component causes corresponding changes of all the other components and may result in either an insufficient response of fibroblasts (prolonged wound healing) or an overactivation leading to uncontrolled formation of ECM (e.g., fibrosis).

At present, our knowledge of autocrine regulatory mechănism is limited, although the first results demonstrate that disturbances of such control circuits may be important in some pathologic mechanisms. PDGF and IL-6 are produced by the fibroblast and their secretion is among others controlled by these cytokines themselves. Both mediators possess the potency to overstimulate the fibroblasts permanently.

Almost all available data on the regulation of fibroblast activity by cytokines and growth factor originate from in vitro experiments by studying the effects of a certain mediators alone or in combination with others on fibroblast in monolayer cultures. More recently, a number of such investigations was carried out with fibroblast cultures using a dermal equivalent such as a three-dimensional collagen lattice. These experiments demonstrated that the effects of cytokines and growth factors depend strongly on the condition of cell culture (medium, fetal calf serum, etc.), the cell density and the number of passages, the cell cycle, origin of the fibroblasts (tissue-specific effects and age of the donor), and the differentiation state of the fibroblast used (artificial selection of cell subpopulation with high proliferation rates).

Today, we are only at the beginning of elucidating the mechanisms by which cytokines and growth factors regulate the biological activity of fibroblasts and other cells. Further studies are necessary if we are to understand these physiological processes. The available techniques of molecular biology (transfection experiments, transgenic animals, etc.) raise the hope of a better understanding of the basic regulatory mechanisms in connective tissue formation and degradation as well as the identification of crucial steps that may be important in the development of connective tissue diseases.

REFERENCES

1. Rodland KD, Muldoon LL, Magun BE. Cellular mechanisms of TGF-beta action. J Invest Dermatol 1990; 94: 33S–40S.
2. Lyons RM, Moses HL. Transforming growth factors and the regulation of cell proliferation. Eur J Biochem 1990; 187: 467–73.
3. Antonelli OA, Saunders KB, Smith SR, D'Amore PA. An activated form of transforming growth factor beta is produced by cocultures of endothelial cells and pericytes. Proc Natl Acad Sci U S A 1989; 86: 4544–8.
4. Rossi P, Karsenty, G, Roberts AB, Roche NS, Sporn MB, de-Crombrugghe B. A nuclear factor 1 binding site mediates the transcriptional activation of a type I collagen promoter by transforming growth factor-beta. Cell 1988; 52: 405–14.
5. Overall CM, Wrana JL, Sodek J. Transforming growth factor-beta regulation of collagenase, 72 kDa-progelatinase, TIMP and PAI-1 expression in rat bone cell populations and human fibroblasts. Connect Tissue Res 1989; 20: 289–94.
6. Fukamizu H Grinnell F. Spatial organization of extracellular matrix and fibroblast activity: effects of serum, transforming growth factor beta, and fibronectin. Exp Cell Res 1990; 190: 276–82.
7. Kulozik M, Hogg A, Lankat-Buttgereit B, Krieg T. Co-localization of transforming growth factor beta 2 with alpha 1(I) procollagen mRNA in tissue sections of patients with systemic sclerosis. J Clin Invest 1990; 86: 917–22.
8. Kähäri VM, Chen YQ, Su MW. Tumor necrosis factor alpha and interferon-gamma suppress the activation of human type I collagen gene expression by transforming growth factor-beta 1. Evidence for two distinct mechanisms of inhibition at the transcriptional and posttranscriptional levels. J Clin Invest 1990; 86: 1489–91.
9. Coustry F, Gillery P, Maquart FX, Borel JP. Effect of transforming growth factor beta on fibroblasts in three-dimensional lattice cultures. FEBS Letts. 1990; 262: 339–41.
10. Heldin C-H, Claesson-Welsh L, Westermark B. Platelet-derived growth factor and its receptor. In: Sara VR, Hall K, Low H, eds. Growth factors: from genes to clinical applications. Raven Press, New York, 1990: 41–50.
11. Schlessinger J. Allosteric regulation of the epidermal growth factor receptor kinase. J Cell Biol 1986; 103: 2067–72.
12. Geppert TD, Lipsky PE. Dissection of the antigen presenting function of tissue cells induced to express HLA-DR by gamma interferon. J Rheumatol 1987; 14: 59–62.
13. Dustin ML, Rothlein R, Bhan AK, Dinarello CA, Springer T. Induction by IL 1 and interferon-gamma: tissue distribution, biochemistry, and function of a natural adherence molecule (ICAM-1). J Immunol 1986; 137: 245–54.
14. Czaja MJ, Weiner FR, Eghbali M, Giambrone M-A, Eghbali M, Zern MA. Differential effects of γ-interferon on collagen and fibronectin gene expression. J Biol Chem 1987; 262: 13348–51.
15. Rosenbloom J, Feldman G, Freundlich B, Jimenez SA. Transcriptional control of human diploid fibroblast collagen synthesis by gamma-interferon. Biochem Biophys Res Commun 1984; 123: 365–72.
16. Scharffetter K, Heckmann M, Hatamochi A, Mauch C, Stein B, Riethmüller G, Ziegler-Heitbrock H W, Krieg T. Synergistic effect of tumor necrosis factor-alpha

and interferon-gamma on collagen synthesis of human skin fibroblasts in vitro. Exp Cell Res 1989; 181: 409–19.
17. Duncan MR, Berman B. Differential regulation of glycosaminoglycan, fibronectin, and collagenase production in cultured human dermal fibroblasts by interferon-alpha, -beta, and -gamma. Arch Dermatol Res 1989; 281: 11–8.
18. Majewski S, Hunzelmann N, Schirren CG, Mauch C, Aumailley M, Krieg T. Increased adhesion of fibroblasts from patients with scleroderma to extracellular matrix components: in vitro modulation by IFN-gamma but not by TGF-beta. J Invest Dermatol 1992; 98: 86–91.
19. Giri SN, Hyde DM, Marafino BJ Jr. Ameliorating effect of murine interferon gamma on bleomycin-induced lung collagen fibrosis in mice. Biochem Med Metab Biol 1986; 36: 194–7.
20. Adelmann-Grill BC, Hein R, Wach F, Krieg T. Inhibition of fibroblast chemotaxis by recombinant human interferon gamma and interferon alpha. J Cell Physiol 1987; 130: 270–5.
21. Elias JA, Reynolds MM, Kotloff RM, Kern JA. Fibroblast interleukin 1 beta: synergistic stimulation by recombinant interleukin 1 and tumor necrosis factor and posttranscriptional regulation. Proc Natl Acad Sci. U S A 1989 86: 6171–5.
22. Varga J, Diaz-Perez A, Rosenbloom J, Jimenez SA. PGE2 causes a coordinate decrease in the steady state levels of fibronectin and types I and III procollagen mRNAs in normal human dermal fibroblasts. Biochem Biophys Res Commun 1987; 147: 1282–8.
23. Kähäri V-M, Heino J, Vuorio HJ. Interleukin-1 increases collagen production and mRNA levels in cultured skin fibroblasts. Biochim Biophys Acta 1987; 929: 142–7.
24. Postlethwaite AE, Raghow R, Stricklin GP, Poppleton H, Seyer JM, Kang AH. Modulation of fibroblast functions by interleukin 1: increased steady-state accumulation of type I procollagen messenger RNAs and stimulation of other functions but not chemotaxis by human recombinant interleukin 1 alpha and beta. J Cell Biol 1988; 106: 311–8.
25. Zhang YH, Lin JX, Yip YK, Vilcek, J. Enhancement of cAMP levels and of protein kinase activity by tumor necrosis factor and interleukin 1 in human fibroblasts: role in the induction of interleukin 6. Proc Natl Acad Sci U S A 1988; 85: 6802–5.
26. Dayer J-M, de Rochemonteix B, Burrus B, Demczuk S, Dinarello CA. Human recombinant interleukin 1 stimulates collagenase and prostaglandin E2 production by human synovial cells. J Clin Invest 1986; 77: 645–8.
27. Circolo A, Welgus HG, Pierce GF, Kramer J, Strunk RC. Differential regulation of the expression of proteinases/antiproteinases in fibroblasts. Effects of interleukin-1 and platelet-derived growth factor. J Biol Chem 1991; 266: 12283–8.
28. Taga T, Hibi M, Hirata Y, Yamasaki K, Yasukawa K, Matsuda T, Hirano T, Kishimoto T. Interleukin-6 triggers the association of its receptor with a possible signal transducer, gp130. Cell 1989; 58: 573–81.
29. Katz Y, Revel M, Strunk, RC. Interleukin 6 stimulates synthesis of complement proteins factor B and C3 in human skin fibroblasts. Eur J Immunol 1989; 19: 983–8.
30. Duncan MR, Berman B. Stimulation of collagen and glycosaminoglycan production in cultured human adult fibroblasts by recombinant interleukin 6. J Invest Dermatol 1991; 97: 686–92.

31. Kupper TS, Kronberger E, Bauer EA. Induction of collagenase gene expression in dermal fibroblasts by recombinant and purified fibroblast derived interleukin 6 (IL-6): a potential autocrine pathway for fibroblast collagenase production (abstr). Clin Res 1989; 37: 529A.
32. Lotz M, Guerne PA. Interleukin-6 induces the synthesis of tissue inhibitor of metalloproteinases-1/erythroid potentiating activity (TIMP-1/EPA). J Biol Chem 1991; 266: 2017–20.
33. Yarden Y, Ullrich A.Growth factor receptor tyrosine kinases. Ann Rev Biochem 1988; 57: 443–78.
34. Margolis B, Rhee SG, Felder S, Mervic M, Lyall R, Levitzki A, Ullrich A, Zilberstein A, Schlessinger J. EGF induces tyrosine phosphorylation of phospholipase C-II: a potential mechanism for EGF receptor signaling. Cell 1989; 57: 1101–7.
35. Huey J, Narayanan S, Jones K, Page RC. Effect of epidermal growth factor on the synthetic activity of human fibroblasts. Biochim Biophys Acta 1980; 623: 227–33.
36. Hiramatsu M, Kumegawa M, Hatakeyama Y, Yajima T, Minami N, Kodama H. Effect of epidermal growth factor on collagen synthesis in osteoblastic cells derived from newborn mouse calvaria. Endocrinology 1982; 111: 1810–6.
37. Buckley A, Davidson J, Kamerath CD, Wolt TB, Woodward SC. Sustained release of epidermal growth factor accelerates wound repair. Proc Natl Acad Sci U S A 1985; 82: 7340–4.
38. Laato M, Niinikoshi J, Lebel L, Gerdin B. Stimulation of wound healing by epidermal growth factor. A dose dependent effect. Ann Surg 1986; 203: 379–81.
39. Colige, A, Nusgens B, Lapiere CM. Effect of EGF on human skin fibroblasts is modulated by the extracellular matrix. Arch Dermatol Res 1988; 280: S42–6.
40. Hardouin S, Hossenlopp P, Segovia B, Seurin D, Portolan G, Lassarre S, Binoux M. Heterogeneity of insulin-like growth factor binding proteins and relationships between structure and affinity. 1. Circulating forms in man. Eur J Biochem 1987; 170: 121–3.
41. Hossenlopp P, Seurin D, Segovia-Quinson B, Binoux M. Identification of insulin-like growth factor binding protein in human cerebrospinal fluid with a selective affinity for IGF-II. FEBS Lett 1984; 208: 439–42.
42. Froesch ER, Schmid C, Schwader J, Zapf JA. Actions of insulin-like growth factors. Ann Rev Physiol 1985; 47: 443–67.
43. Old LJ. Tumor necrosis factor. In: Granger BB, ed. Tumor necrosis factor: structure, mechanism of action, role in disease and therapy. Karger, Basel, 1990: 1–30.
44. Duncan MR, Berman B. Differential regulation of glycosaminoglycan, fibronectin, and collagenase production in cultured human dermal fibroblasts by interferon-alpha, -beta, and -gamma. Arch Dermatol Res 1989; 281: 11–8.
45. Mauviel A, Heino J, Kähäri V-M, Hartmann D-J, Loyau G, Pujol J-P, Vuorio E. Comparative effects of interleukin-1 and tumor necrosis factor-alpha on collagen production and corresponding procollagen mRNA levels in human dermal fibroblasts. J Invest Dermatol 1991; 96: 243–9
46. Brouckaert PG, Libert C, Everaerdt B, Takahashi N, Fiers W.A role for interleukin 1 in the in vivo actions of tumor necrosis factor. Lymphokine Res 1989; 8: 269–74.
47. Delaporte E, Croute F, Vincent C, Fertin C, Bonnefoy J-Y, Gaucherand M, Nicolas

J-F. Keratinocyte–fibroblast interactions: effect of keratinocyte cytokines on fibroblast proliferation. Eur J Dermatol 1991; 1: 117–23.

48. Vilcek J, Palombella VJ, Henriksen-DeStefano D, Swenson C, Feinman R, Hirai M, Tsujimoto M. Fibroblast growth enhancing activity of tumor necrosis factor and its relationship to other polypeptide growth factors. J Exp Med 1986; 163: 632–43.
49. Gospodarowicz D, Ferrera N, Schweigerer L, Neufeld G. Structural characterization and biological functions of fibroblast growth factor. Endocrinol Rev 1987; 8: 95–114.
50. Dubertret L, Brunner-Ferber F, Misisti J, Thomas KA, Dubertret M-L. Activities of human acidic fibroblast growth factor in an in vitro dermal equivalent model. J Invest Dermatol 1991; 97: 793–8.
51. Engel J. EGF-like domains in extracellular matrix proteins: Localized signals for growth and differentiation? FEBS Lett 1989; 251: 1–7.
52. Burgess W-H, Maciag T. The heparin-binding (fibroblast) growth factor family of proteins. Ann Rev Biochem 1989; 58: 515–606.
53. Yayon A, Klagsbrun M, Esko JD, Leder P, Ornitz DM. Cell surface, heparin-like molecules are required for binding of basic fibroblast growth factor to its high affinity receptor. Cell 1991; 64: 841–8.
54. Roberts R, Gallagher J, Spooncer E, Allen TD, Bloomfield F, Dexter TM. Heparan sulphate bound growth factors: a mechanism for stromal cell mediated haemopoiesis. Nature 1988; 332: 376–8.
55. Perin J-P, Bonnet F, Maillet P, Jolles P. Characterization and N -terminal sequence of human platelet proteoglycan. Biochem J 1988; 255: 1007–13.
56. Yamaguchi Y, Mann DM, Ruoslahti E. Negative regulation of transforming growth factor-beta by the proteoglycan decorin. Nature 1990; 346: 281–4.

13

Aging and Premature Aging Syndromes

Charles M. Lapière
University of Liège, Sart Tilman, Belgium

Most connective tissues in humans are targets of the aging process leading to major pathologic conditions, such as osteoporosis and arteriosclerosis. The most striking clinical manifestations of aging of the skin also result from alterations in its connective tissue support. One can estimate the age of individuals at dawn or in counterlight not by the color of the skin or the texture of the epidermis but by the irregularity of the contour. The changes in the physical characteristic of the dermis provide the image reflected by the epidermal cover. Atrophy and wrinkling are the two main modifications affecting the dermis.

It is known that cells derived from the dermis age in vitro. The macromolecules forming the connective tissue are also modified as a function of time by external or internal factors, such as solar irradiation and metabolites. The aging of the dermis results from the combined action of these processes.

FIBROBLAST AGING IN VITRO AND IN VIVO

Two different approaches can be adopted for investigating the aging process in vitro. The first considers the phenotypic modifications of the skin-derived cells as a function of replication in vitro, (i.e., increasing population doubling). It is referred to as replicative senescence in vitro. The second approach, which is probably more relevant to the aging process in vivo, consist of evaluating the phenotype of skin-derived cells arising from individuals of varying age. It provides some indication about the state of the cells at the time of their collection from the tissue.

All normal cells age in vitro and display a finite proliferative capacity limited to around 50 population doublings at least for the skin-derived cells. The aging of the human skin fibroblasts in vitro proceeds by a mechanism of differentiation along a terminal cell lineage [1]. The cells isolated from the dermis are composed of a heterogeneous population of mitotic and postmitotic fibroblasts with distinct morphotypes in a proportion depending on the age of the donor. They will eventually differentiate along a seven-stage terminal cell lineage. This ends with the degenerating fibroblast with its characteristic flat aspect in vitro. This explains why the replicative lifespan of fibroblasts in vitro is inversely proportional to the age of the donor [2], although a large potential of replication remains even for the cells from the eldest individuals. However, the proportion of cells participating in mitosis decreases and the average cell cycle time increases in such conditions. These modifications are accompanied by a reduction in responsiveness to growth factors [3]. It is worth noting that newborn human fibroblasts age in vitro without ever acquiring the adult growth factor requirement. The information controlling cell multiplication seems to be contained in membrane proteins coded by mRNAs that are found in greater abundance in senescent human diploid fibroblasts [4]. Work is progressing to seek aging and longevity genes and the identification of sequences controling the life span of cells in vitro [5].

Several metabolic processes are modified in senescent fibroblasts in vitro. The synthesis of macromolecules is increased or altered, including that of collagen, proteoglycan, and fibronectin. Aged fibroblasts in culture produce a fibronectin that binds poorly to collagen type I, which perhaps explains the loss of organization of this glycoprotein at the surface of aged cultured fibroblasts. The most striking and perhaps significant modification is represented by an overexpression of collagenase activity and a loss of its regulation in the course of replicative senescence of human skin fibroblasts [6]. In addition, senescent human fibroblasts express relatively small amounts of collagenase inhibitor (TIMP), which is no longer inducible upon serum stimulation. Phenotypic modifications can likewise be related to the age of the donor. Elastin biosynthesis tested by measuring the steady-state level of its mRNA is reduced in fibroblasts collected from the skin of aged individuals [7], while collagen type III is known to be produced in larger proportion in fibroblasts of fetal skin than in cells collected from adult skin.

AGING OF MACROMOLECULES

Some macromolecules such as collagen and elastin that normally display a very low rate of turnover will accumulate in vivo alterations due to chemical modifications. Some of these depend on physiological maturation of the polymers. Others are nonenzymatic and known to depend upon various mechanisms [8].

Collagen is synthesized under the form of a precursor and is posttranslationally processed by several enzymes including lysyl-oxidase, giving rise to lysyl aldehydes that are responsible for the formation of covalent crosslinks. These crosslinks are first reducible before becoming spontaneously more stable. Their formation is accompanied by a progressive reduction in the extractibility of collagen monomers upon cooling in neutral salt solution. During aging of the polymers in vivo, other types of crosslinks also form. The accumulation of these intermolecular bonds induces a progressive insolubilization of the collagen polymers of the dermis [9]. Glycation of the collagen molecule also modifies its properties. This nonenzymatic addition of glucose increases with time and depends on the concentration of the sugar. It is increased in patients with diabetes. It is interesting to note that glycation of collagen disturbs its capacity to act as a substratum for cells [10]. Collagen and other stable macromolecules as elastin might also be the target of denaturing agents as, for example, ultra violet (UV) rays. The alterations induced by this radiation might be the cause of changes that occur more extensively in sun-exposed parts of the skin [11]

THE AGING DERMIS

Extrapolating the observations made in vitro on senescing cells to what occurs in the aging connective tissue in vivo is hazardous. There are indeed significant differences between the dermocyte, (the resident cell in the dermis) and the fibroblast (a cell derived from the dermis) that can be established in culture. Dermocytes barely divide in vivo while fibroblasts divide up to contact inhibition. The dermocyte is surrounded by a dense extracellular matrix and connected to a polymeric structure while the fibroblasts lie on a flat and inert surface and are immersed in a large amount of medium enriched with growth factors. Models of a reconstructed dermis can, however, provide some information. It is known that the responsiveness of fibroblasts in the dermal equivalent to growth factors differs from that of similar cells on plastic [12]. Collagen biosynthesis and production of collagenase are regulated in this system by contact of the cell with the support of fibrils and transfer of mechanical information. Tension stimulates the production of macromolecules and reduces the expression of collagenase, while relaxation has the reverse effect [13]. These mechanisms might be significant in the alterations observed during the aging process in humans.

Two types of aging will affect the skin. The first is chronologic, while the second is superimposed on the first in sun-exposed areas and is called photoaging. In the sun-protected dermis, the main morphologic alterations are a reduced density of the collagen fibrils in the bundles, an increased interfibrillar space, while cells display little rough endoplasmic reticulum and reduced contact with the bundles of polymers. Alterations in the network of elastic fibrils are characterized by a progressive reduction of the oxytalan fibers in the papillary dermis and degeneration of the elastic fibers of the reticular dermis [14]. In sun-exposed areas, alterations are similar but more pronounced and accompanied by a deposition of elastotic material mainly in the reticular dermis. Similar changes may be produced by chronic UV irradiation in the experimental animal [15].

Two main mechanisms, atrophy and changes in architectural organization, are involved in chronologic aging. They will affect with a different rate and extent the three parts of the dermis: the papillary and the reticular layer and the hypodermis. A genetic trait is probably responsible for the occurrence of atrophy at a different rate in specific individuals, as has already been demonstrated in some families for osteoporosis [16]. Environmental factors are superimposed on the evolution of this process in vivo. The susceptibility to sun exposure, toxic compounds such as industrial and cigarette smoke, the type of diet, and the production of free radicals as well as hormonal status will all contribute to modulating the changes occuring with time and regulated by the genome [17]. A most significant factor involved in the modifications of the architectural organization of the polymers is the mechanical forces. Modification of the papillary dermis is responsible for a change in the pattern of the primary lines of the skin [18]. Distention of the reticular dermis and the septa in the hypodermis causes larger folds. Gravity is responsible for the double chin, hanging cheeks, falling eyelids, and other changes. These alterations might occur through a remodeling of the connective tissue network progressively built under a larger frame due to the effect of the forces. Degeneration of the elastic fibers might also be involved. Distention of the septa in the hypodermis during a period of weight gain is also responsible for a similar process that results in contour deformation after weight loss. Mechanical forces are obviously also involved in the formation of facial frown lines. The mechanical stimulation of the connective tissue cells by the facial expression muscles induces the formation of thicker and shorter septa in the hypodermis, pulling on the reticular dermis and inducing the permanent depressions of the skin surface [19].

PROGERIA AND OTHER ACCELERATED AGING SYNDROMES IN HUMANS

Two genetic diseases in the human characterized by accelerated aging represent potential models for the investigation of aging in vivo and in vitro [20]. They are progeria of Hutchinson-Gilford and Werner's syndrome. There exist, however, differences that make these model diseases not the exact replication of the aging process at a faster than normal rate, even at the level of the clinical signs (Table 13.1).

Werner's syndrome is an autosomal recessive disease that is often diagnosed in early adult life and accompanied by death in the fifth decade mainly due to vascular disease. Besides a typical aspect of the face, cutaneous changes include

Table 13.1 Clinical Signs of Aging

	Physiological aging	Progeria Hutchinson-Gilford	Werner's syndrome
Skin atrophy	+ + +	+ −	+ −
Osteoporosis	+ + +	+ +	+ +
Arteriosclerosis	+ + +	+ + +	+ + +
Cataract	+ + +	−	+ + +
Brain	+ + +	−	−
Cancer	+ +	−	+ + +

a premature greying and loss of hair, chronic leg ulcers, poor wound healing, and an aged aspect of the skin, although the dermis is sclerotic as opposed to the classically observed laxity, atrophy, and wrinkling of the physiological aging process. Fibroblast-like cells isolated from the dermis of such patients display a short lifespan in vitro. They have a markedly reduced mitogenic response to Platelet-derived growth factor (PDGF) and fibroblast growth factor (FGF) and express a high constitutive level of collagenase, as do fibroblasts aged in vitro. They do not, however, increase collagenase activity upon stimulation by PDGF [21], indicating the existence of a disturbed intracellular control mechanism.

In patients with progeria of Hutchinson-Gilford, the diagnosis becomes evident during the second year of life by a striking retardation of growth. The face has also a typical aspect and the patient presents early alopecia, and a loss of soft tissue and skin changes characterized by either thinning and wrinkling or sclerosis. A mottled pigmentation is often present. These patients die prematurely during the second decade of life of vascular disease. Skin-derived cells also display signs of premature aging in vitro. They are difficult to propagate and grow poorly up to a maximum of 10-12 population doublings. Their mitogenic response to PDGF is compromised even though they respond normally to serum stimulation. The metabolic response to EGF is also much altered by a lack of collagenase-enhanced expression, while the reduction of collagen production by this growth factor is preserved. The phenotype of the cells is also disturbed since they display an increased production of elastin and collagen type IV (22).

Physiological aging of normal fibroblasts in culture and disturbed regulatory mechanisms affecting the cells of the premature aging syndromes point to an altered regulation of cellular oncogenes involved in the mitogenic response and in the control of the expression of collagenase.

PATHOMECHANISMS OF AGING AND THERAPY

The aging process, as well as the aging of the dermis, depend on complex mechanisms that involve a number of integrated parameters. The relationship between the aging cell in vitro and the age of the donor as well as the effect of the premature aging syndrome on the potential of cells to replicate in vitro support the concept of a genomic regulation of the process. Many other factors also influence the function of the aging genome in all types of cells. These include the production of free radicals under the influence of the diet and toxic compounds from the environment. Hormonal status is also specifically involved in the process. There seems to be a parallel between osteoporosis and skin atrophy. The beneficial effect of hormone replacement therapy on bone loss is also reflected in the skin. These environmental factors modulate the function of the aging genome characterized by defined inherited traits responsible for the heterogeneity of the aging signs observed in a population. Most of the therapeutic approach is preventive, such as protection from sun light, prevention of excessive weight variation, and the avoidance of toxic exposure. Topical therapy with retinoic acid has shown beneficial effects in aging human skin and in the experimental animal [15].

REFERENCES

1. Bayreuther K, Rodemann HP, Hommel R, Dittmann K, Albiez M, Francz PI. Human skin fibroblasts in vitro differentiate along a terminal cell lineage. Proc Natl Acad Sci 1988; 85: 5112–6.
2. Martin GM, Sprague CA, Epstein CJ. Replicative life-span of cultivated human cells: effects of donor's age, tissue and genotype. Lab Invest 1970; 23: 86–92.
3. Plisko A, Gilchrest BA. Growth factor responsiveness of cultured human fibroblasts declines with age. J Gerontol 1983; 38: 513–8.
4. Lumpkin CK, McClung JK, Pereira-Smith OM, Smith JR. Existence of high abundance antiproliferative mRNAs in senecent human diploid fibroblasts. Science 1986; 232: 393–5.
5. Vijg J, Papaconstantinou J. Aging and longevity genes: strategies for identifying DNA sequences controlling life span. J Gerontol 1990; 45: B179–82.
6. West MD, Pereira-Smith OM, Smith JR. Replicative senescence of human skin fibroblasts correlates with a loss of regulation and overexpression of collagenase activity. Exp Cell Res 1989; 184: 138–47.
7. Uitto J, Fazio MJ, Olsen DR. Molecular mechanisms of cutaneous aging—age-associated connective tissue alterations in the dermis. Jam Acad Dermatol 1989; 21: 614–22.
8. Harding JJ, Beswick HT, Ajiboye R, Huby R, Blakytny R, Rixon KC. Non-enzymic post-translational modification of proteins in aging. A review. Mech Ageing Dev 1989; 50: 7–16.
9. Legrand Y, Lapière CM, Pignaud G, Caen J. Microméthode d'extraction du collagène à partir de biopsie de peau humaine. Application à l'étude des maladies du saignement. *Pathol Biol* 1969; 17: 991–3.
10. Kawano E, Takahashi S, Sakano Y, Fujimoto D. Nonenzymatic glycation alters properties of collagen as a substratum for cells. Matrix 1990; 10: 300–5.

11. Yamauchi M, Prisayahn P, Haque Z, Woodley DT. Collagen cross-linking in sun-exposed and unexposed sites of aged human skin. J Invest Dermatol. 1991; 97: 938–41.
12. Colige A, Nusgens B, Lapière CM. The response to epidermal growth factor of skin fibroblasts from donors of varying age is modulated by the extracellular matrix. J Cell Physiol 1990; 145: 450–7.
13. Lambert CM, Soudant EP, Nusgens BV, Lapière CM. Pretranslational regulation of extracellular matrix macromolecules and collagenase expression in fibroblasts by mechanical forces. Lab Invest 1992; 66: 444–51.
14. Bouissou H, Pieraggi MT, Julian M, Savit T. The elastic tissue of the skin. A comparison of spontaneous and actinic (solar) aging. Int J Dermatol 1988; 27: 327–35.
15. Kligman LH, Duo CH, Kligman AM. Topical retinoic acid enhances the repair of ultraviolet damaged dermal connective tissue. Connect Tissue Res 1984; 12: 139–50.
16. Seeman E, Hopper JL, Bach LA, Cooper ME, Parkinson E, Mckay J, Jerums G. Reduced bone mass in daughters of women with osteoporosis. N Eng Med 1989; 320: 554–8.
17. Lapière CM. The ageing dermis: the main cause for the appearance of ''old'' skin. Br J Dermatol 1990; 122: (Suppl 35) 5–11.
18. Lavker RM, Kwong F, Kligman AM. Changes in skin surface patterns with age. J Gerontol 1980; 35: 348–54.
19. Pièrard GE, Lapière CM. The microanatomical basis of facial frown lines. Arch Dermatol 1989; 125: 1090–2.
20. Mills RG, Weiss AS. Does progeria provide the best model of accelerated ageing in humans. 1990; Gerontology 36:84–98.
21. Bauer EA, Silverman N, Busiek DF, Kronberger A, Deuel FT. Diminished response of Werner's syndrome fibroblasts to growth factors PDGF and FGF. Science 1986; 234: 1240–3.
22. Colige A, Roujeau JC, De la Rocque F, Nusgens B, Lapière CM. Abnormal gene expression in skin fibroblasts from a Hutchinson-Gilford patient. Lab Invest 1991; 64: 799–806.

14

Ehlers-Danlos Syndrome

Charles M. Lapière
University of Liège, Sart Tilman, Belgium

The Ehlers-Danlos syndrome is a family of related disorders characterized by abnormal rheologic properties, mainly elasticity and resistance of the soft connective tissues: skin, joints, fascia, blood vessels, hollow organs, ligaments, and tendons. It has to be differentiated from Marfan's syndrome in which the skin is grossly normal (except striae distensae); cutis laxa, characterized by laxity of the skin without hyperelasticity; and osteogenesis imperfecta in which the most striking alterations occur in bone.

Nine different subtypes of the Ehlers-Danlos syndrome have been reported that differ in terms of morbidity and mortality [1]. A correct diagnosis relies on genetic transmission and the nature of the clinical signs in terms of location and intensity, morphologic characterization of abnormal polymers in one form (type VII C), and biochemical markers in selected forms of the disease (IVA, B and C, VIA, VIIA, B, C, and X).

TYPES AND INHERITANCE

Nine different types of Ehlers-Danlos syndrome are accepted at the present time. They are numbered from I to X, the type IX being now classified as x-linked cutis laxa. Each of these nine types have received a clinical name (see Table 14.1). The inheritance is very important to consider. The most common types (I, II, and III), representing 90% of the syndrome, display an autosomal dominant

Table 14.1 Classification of Ehlers-Danlos Syndrome

Type	Clinical type	Inheritance
I	Gravis	A D
II	Mitis	A D
III	Hypermobile	A D
IV	Vascular	
	A: Acrogeric	A D
	B: Acrogeric	A R
	C: Ecchymotic	A D
	D: Other	A D
V	X-linked	X R
VI	Ocular scoliotic	
	A: Reduced hydroxylysine	A R
	B: Normal hydroxylysine	A R
VII	Arthrochalasis multiplex	
	A: Defect pro-alpha$_1$	A D
	B: Defect pro-alpha$_2$	A D
	C: Defective procollagen peptidase	A R
VIII	Periodontal	A D
X	Fibronectin abnormality	A R

A D, autosomal dominant; A R, autosomal recessive; X R, X-linked recessive.

inheritance. New mutation, (i.e., lack of familial history) is not unusual and reported to be higher than 50%. In type IV, the acrogeric type is either dominant or recessive. The ecchymotic type is dominant. Another form, less well characterized, also displays a dominant type of inheritance. The type V is the only form that is clearly x-linked. Only two families have been reported. Type VI with normal or reduced hydroxylysine is recessive. Type VII has been reported to be dominant when collagen genes are altered and recessive when procollagen peptidase activity is missing. Type VIII, which is very unusual, is dominant. Type X, only observed in two families, has been reported as recessive [2].

CLINICAL SIGNS

Skin

Alterations of the dermis exist in most types of the syndrome. With a little experience it is easy to recognize the characteristic feeling of a soft and velvety skin. Hyperelasticity but not laxity is also often recognized. The elastic skin can be pulled and recover its initial position rapidly as opposed to the lax skin that remains elongated when pulled away. Bruising is also a common characteristic related to the poor support of the blood vessels in the dermis. It is often located in front of the tibia. Abnormal scars are related to trauma, in which the extensibility of the skin induces larger than normal gaping wounds that will heal slowly to produce a thin scar resembling cigarette paper. Herniation of the adipose tissue also produces papules that are the so-called molluscoid scars. An additional sign is the thinness of the skin, mainly of the extremities and in front of the thorax. Its transparency allows one to view the underlying blood vessels. It is characteristic of the Ehlers-Danlos type IV. These skin signs occur with different intensities in various types of the syndrome (see Table 14.2).

Joints

Hypermobility of the joints depends on altered rheologic properties of the capsules, ligaments, and tendons. Its intensity varies in different types of the disease (Table 14.2). Major alterations occur in the Ehlers-Danlos type I, type III, and type VIIA and B. Scoliosis can be a significant problem in some of the types, while dislocation of the hips and knees is most common in type VIIA and B. Hypermobility has to be sought at the level of the knees, the elbows, and the shoulders. The small joints of the hands are also often affected. Combined with the softness and hyperelasticity of the skin, the hand of the patient with Ehlers-Danlos syndrome displays a rubbery texture when shaken. Rheologic signs are sometimes difficult to appreciate in young children and experience is needed to test them clinically.

Other Connective Tissues

The rheologic properties of one or several of other connective tissues can be defective in specific types of the syndrome (Table 2). Some of them are characteristic of a defined type. Ocular fragility and/or abnormal physical properties of the cornea occur in type VI. A special mention has to be given to the pinched face of the patient with Ehlers-Danlos type VI patient. Fragility of the blood vessels and spontaneous aneurysm or rupture testifies to the gravity of type IV. A very early, extensive, and progressive periodontitis accompanying other signs of the Ehlers-Danlos syndrome is the hallmark of type VIII. Many other defects have been reported, such as premature rupture of the fetal membranes in type I, varicose veins in type I and II. Hernia, striae distensae and petechiae, and short stature have been observed in some of the types. Abnormal cardiac valves are rarely found. This must be always investigated using noninvasive technologies.

MORPHOLOGIC, ULTRASTRUCTURAL, AND BIOCHEMICAL DEFECTS

Genes

Although the Ehlers-Danlos syndrome is one of the most frequent inherited disorders of the connective tissues, defective genes have only been found in a

Table 14.2 Clinical Signs of Ehlers-Danlos Syndrome

Type	Skin	Joint hypermobility	Other connective tissue
Most common types			
I	Soft, velvety	Large: + +	Premature rupture of fetal membranes
	Hyperextensible + + +	Small: + + +	Varicose veins
	Bruising + +		Hernia
	Abnormal scars	Scoliosis: +	Abnormal valves
II	Soft, velvety	Large: + +	Varicose veins
	Hyperextensible +	Small: + +	
	Bruising +	Scoliosis: + +	Abnormal valves
	Abnormal scars + +		
III	Soft	Large: + + +	
	Hyperextensible +	Small: + +	
		Dislocation: + +	
Types with high diversity			
IV A/B	Thin	Large: +	Pinched face
	Transparent	Small: +	Thin nose
			Prominent eyes
			Vascular rupture
			Gastrointestinal rupture (early)
			Thin extremities
			Short stature
C	Thin	Large: +	Same as above but milder
	Bruising + + +	Small: +	
	Abnormal scars + +		
D	Thin	Large: +	Normal face
		Small: +	No arterial problem
VI A	Soft, velvety	Large: + +	Ocular fragility
	Hyperextensible + +	Small: + +	Vascular fragility (late)
	Bruising +	Scoliosis: + + +	Myopia
	Abnormal scars + +	Dislocation: +	Hernia
B	Same as A, milder	Same as A, milder	Brittle cornea
			Blue sclerae
VII A/B	Soft, velvety	Large: + + +	Short stature
	Hyperextensible +	Small: + + +	
	Bruising +		
B		Dislocation: + + + (hips and knees)	
C	Soft, velvety		Hernia
	Bruising + +		Blue sclerae
	Fragility + + +		Vascular fragility
			Osteopenia

Table 14.2 Continued

Type	Skin	Joint hypermobility	Other connective tissue
Very rare types			
V	Soft, velvety Hyperextensible + + Bruising + Abnormal scars	Large: + Small: +	Intramuscular hemorrhage
VIII	Soft, velvety Hyperextensible + + Bruising + + Abnormal scars + +	Large: + Small: + +	Periodontitis juvenile
X	Hyperextensible + + Bruising + + Abnormal scars + +	Large: + Small: + +	Petechiae Striae distensae

+, Mild; + +, medium; + + +, severe.

few types of the disease. Mutation of the pro-alpha$_1$ III chain has been detected in type IV [3]. Splicing mutations causing exon skipping and deletions in the pro-alpha$_1$ or pro-alpha$_2$ chains of collagen type I have been shown to occur in type VII A and B, respectively [4]. These alterations suppress a sequence containing the site of cleavage of the amino propeptide extension and collagen is found in precursor form in the tissues.

Posttranslational Collagen Processing

The first biochemical markers of this syndrome have been found to be defective posttranslational enzyme processing as the lack of procollagen peptidase in dermatosparaxis [5] and in the form C of the Ehlers-Danlos type VII [6], and a defective hydroxylation of lysine by altered lysyl hydroxylase in type VI [7]. Another defect related to enzyme deficiency has been suspected in Ehlers-Danlos type V, the x-linked form of the disease. The suspected alteration of lysyl oxidase is no longer valid since the gene coding for this enzyme is located on chromosome 5 [8]. An altered biosynthesis of type III collagen is known to occur in Ehlers-Danlos type IV. The reduced proportion of collagen type III in the tissue is related either to an absence of synthesis or to intracellular storage by defective secretion [3]. A similar type of defective secretion has also been reported in one case of Ehlers-Danlos type II.

Abnormal Polymers

Most of the polymers of collagen in skin are made of large bundles of collagen type I associated with collagen type III and type V. Four types of alteration in

Table 14.3 Markers of Ehlers-Danlos Syndrome

Type	Gene	Processing	Abnormal fibrils	Occasional findings
I	?	?	Composite Large Unraveled	Disorganized collagen bundles Reduced type III Lack of expression of proα2 Increased hyaluronic acid Lack of decorin synthesis
II	?	?	Composite: large Granular Branched	Disorganized collagen bundles Lack of expression of proα2 Reduced secretion type III
III	?	?	Composite Large	
IV A	single base mutation Alpha$_1$ III	Absent or reduced secretion of type III	Small/large Branched	Thermal instability of type III
B	?	Same	Small/large Branched	
C	?	Same	Small/large Branched	
V	?	?	Composite	Abnormal relation of collagen–elastin
VI A		Defective lysyl hydroxylase	Composite	
B	?	?		‘‘holes’’ in collagen bundles
VII A	pro-alpha$_1$ (I)		Composite	
B	pro-alpha$_2$ (I)		Composite	
C		Defective procollagen peptidase	Hieroglyphic	
VIII	?		Composite Small/large	Disorganized collagen bundles
X	Fibronectin	?	Composite Large	Defective packing

the ultrastructure of the polymers have been recognized in the Ehlers-Danlos syndrome: composite fibers, large and/or small fibrils, granular branched or unwoven fibrils, and hieroglyphic fibrils [9]. These can be observed in skin of patients with different types of Ehlers-Danlos and do not represent a specific support for the diagnosis, since they are also found in other inherited diseases. The only exception is the observation of hieroglyphic fibrils resulting in the lack of activity of procollagen peptidase characteristic of Ehlers-Danlos type VII C in humans, or dermatosparaxis in animals [5,6].

Associated Biochemical Alterations

The primary defect of the most common types of Ehlers-Danlos patients (types I, II, and III) is not yet known and a variety of biochemical and morphologic alterations have been observed in selected patients (Table 14.3). An excessive synthesis of proteoglycans [10] and a deficient synthesis of the core proteins of dermatan sulfate [11] have been reported. Absent synthesis of collagen type III [12] also mentioned in the type II form [13] accompanied by a lack of synthesis of the alpha 2 chain were casual observations. Defective fibronectin is responsible for Elhers-Danlos type X [2]. Bundles of collagen fibrils interrupted by holes containing an amorphous material were recently reported in a patient presenting with clinical signs resembling EDS type VI but with a normal hydroxylysine level [14].

In Practice

Correct diagnosis of the Ehlers-Danlos syndrome to define the type of the disease relies on a good interpretation of the genetic transmission and of the clinical signs (Tables 1, 2). The diagnosis can be supported by morphologic and/or biochemical analysis of the tissues and enzyme in specific types (IV, VI, and VII) of the disease. A few isolated patients have been shown to display point mutations in the genes of procollagen type I [4]. The rheologic disorders observed in the Ehlers-Danlos syndrome are most probably related to abnormal structure and function of the collagen fibers. Polymer organization depends, however, on a variety of structural macromolecules including, besides the various forms of collagen, several glycoproteins and proteoglycans.

REFERENCES

1. Beighton P, de Paepe A, Danks D, Ginidori G, Gedde-Dahl T, Goodman R., Hall JG, Hollister DW, Horton W, McKusick VA, Opitz JM, Pope FM, Pyeritz RE, Rimoin DL, Sillence D, Spranger JW, Thompson E, Tsipouras P, Viljoen D, Winship I, Young I. International nosology of heritable disorders of connective tissue, Berlin, 1986. Am J Med Genet 1988; 29: 581–94.

2. Arneson MA, Hammerschmidt DE, Furcht LT, King RA. A new form of Ehlers-Danlos Syndrome: fibronectin corrects defective platelet function. JAMA 1980; 244: 144–7.
3. Pope FM, Nicholls AC, Narcisi P, Temple A, Chia Y, Fryer P, De Paepe A, De Groote WP, Mc Ewan JR, Compston DA, Oorthuys H, Davies J, Dinwoodie DL. Type III collagen mutations in Ehlers-Danlos syndrome type IV and other related disorders. Clin Exp Dermatol 1988; 13: 285–302.
4. Prockop DJ. Mutations that alter the primary structure of type-I collagen—the perils of a system for generating large structures by the principle of nucleated growth. J Biol Chem 1990; 265: 15349–52.
5. Lapière CM, Lenaers A. Kohn L. Procollagen peptidase: an enzyme excising the coordination peptides of procollagen. Proc Nat Acad Sci USA 1971; 68: 3054–8.
6. Nusgens B, Verellen C, Hermanns-Le T, De Paepe A, Nuytinck L, Piérard G, Lapière CM. Evidence for a relationship between Ehlers-Danlos type VII C in humans and bovine dermatosparaxis. Nature Genet 1992; 1: 214–7.
7. Wenstrup RJ, Murad S, Pinnell SR. Ehlers-Danlos syndrome type-VI—clinical manifestations of collagen lysyl hydroxylase deficiency. J Pediat 1989; 115: 405–9.
8. Hamalainen ER, Jones TA, Sheer D, Taskinen K, Pihlajaniemi T, Kivirikko KI. Molecular cloning of human lysyl oxidase and assignment of the gene to chromosome-5q23.3-31.2. 1991; Genomics 11:508–16.
9. Holbrook KA, Byers PH. Skin is a window on heritable disorders of connective tissue. Am J Med Genet 1989; 34: 105–21.
10. Shinkai H, Hirabayashi O, Tamaki A, Matsubayashi S, Sano, S. Connective tissue metabolism in culture fibroblasts of a patient with Ehlers-Danlos Syndrome type I. Arch Dermatol Res 1976; 257: 113–23.
11. Fushimi H, Kameyama M, Shinkai H. Deficiency of the core proteins of dermatan sulphate proteoglycans in a variant form of Ehlers-Danlos syndrome. J Intern Med 1989; 226:409–16.
12. De Paepe A, Nicholls A, Narcisi P, De Keyser F, Quatacker J, Van Staey M, Matton M, Pope FM. Ehlers-Danlos syndrome type I: a clinical and ultrastructural study of a family with reduced amounts of collagen type III. Br J Dermatol 1987; 117: 89–97.
13. Kojima T, Shinkai H, Fujita M, Morita E, Okamoto S. Case report and study of collagen metabolism in Ehlers-Danlos syndrome type II. J Dermatol 1988; 15: 155–60.
14. Royce PM, Steinmann B, Vogel A, Steinhorst U, Kohlschuetter A. Brittle cornea syndrome: an heritable connective tissue disorder distinct from Ehlers-Danlos syndrome type VI and fragilitas oculi, with spontaneous perforations of the eye, blue sclerae, red hair, and normal collagen lysyl hydroxylation. Eur J Pediat 1990; 149: 465–9.

15

Cutis Laxa

F. Michael Pope
M. R. C. Clinical Research Centre, Harrow, England

Cutis laxa, which is also called dermatomegaly, dermatochalasia, or chalasoderma, is a generalized abnormal looseness of skin that produces an appearance of premature aging. Such saggy skin is particularly noticeable over the neck, face, chin, earlobes, axillae, upper and lower arms, thighs, abdomen, and the dorsal of the hands. Sagging of the skin is a normal and natural result of the aging process. It is accelerated in certain abnormalities of connective tissue and there has been substantial semantic overlap between primary cutis laxa and the Ehlers-Danlos syndrome with cutis laxa. The best working classification includes primary inherited, secondary to diseases of connective tissue such as Ehlers-Danlos syndrome and pseudoxanthoma elasticum (PXE), and secondary to acquired diseases such as cutaneous amyloidosis, very severe sun-induced changes, and simple aging.

PRIMARY INHERITED CUTIS LAXA

McKusick [1] currently lists one autosomal dominant, four autosomal recessive, and one sex-linked recessive form of cutis laxa.

Autosomal Dominant Cutis Laxa

Although still confused with Ehlers-Danlos syndrome (EDS), the disease is excessively rare with less than 1% of the frequency of EDS, osteogenesis imperfecta, PXE, or Marfan's syndrome. Nevertheless the phenotype is a striking one and has been very clearly described in small families by Beighton (Fig. 15.1a–c). McKusick[1] records several dominant pedigrees (noting that male to male transmission is not strictly confirmed). The disease produces quite striking premature aging and skin laxity as shown in the mother and daughter illustrated by Beighton[2]: the daughter looks far older than her mother (and one might think the pictures had been mislabeled). Here the skin is inelastic and especially abnormal over the nasolabial folds and eyes, with a pointed chin, broadened nose, and long upper lip (Fig. 15.1a–c). The dominant disease is uncomplicated and does not usually produce either pulmonary emphysema or dilatation of the urinary tract, in contrast to several of the other varieties. The skin biopsy specimen shows normal elastic fibers on histologic examination.

Autosomal Recessive Cutis Laxa

Three forms occur under this heading: type I (219100), type II (219200), and a variant with corneal clouding and mental retardation (219180).

Type I Recessive Cutis Laxa

McKusick [1] reports the two brothers described by Goltz and also mentions other reported examples of either parental consanguinity or multiple affected siblings. In contrast to the autosomal dominant disease, the autosomal recessive form presents earlier skin signs and clearly is associated with a systemic connective tissue abnormality. Multiple diverticulae of the esophagus, duodenum, ileum, and bladder can occur and pulmonary emphysema and death from right heart failure are common (secondary to premature emphysema) (Fig. 15.2a–c). Deficiency of cutaneous elastic fibers has been described. This group could be genetically heterogeneous, since variations include a fatal infantile form with premature death from right heart failure (and severe emphysema), tortuous arteries, and arterial aneurysms with prenatal growth retardation, and congenital hip dislocation, dental caries, and a mild variable cutaneous form with lung, arterial, and renal tract abnormalities. The histologic differences between the autosomal dominant and recessive forms are subtle and depend upon the degree of elastic tissue change, which varies from slight prominence to complete deficiency. Cutis laxa with corneal clouding and mental retardation (De Barsey syndrome) was reported by McKusick (21915). De Barsey [3] described a 22-month-old girl with absent elaastin fibers and cutis laxa. She had cloudy corneas from a degenerated Bowman's membrane. Similar families have been described with other features such as athetosis, translucent skin, and dislocated thumbs, big toes, and hips. Collagen fibers were normal but elastic fibers were frayed and diminished in size and number in some of these patients.

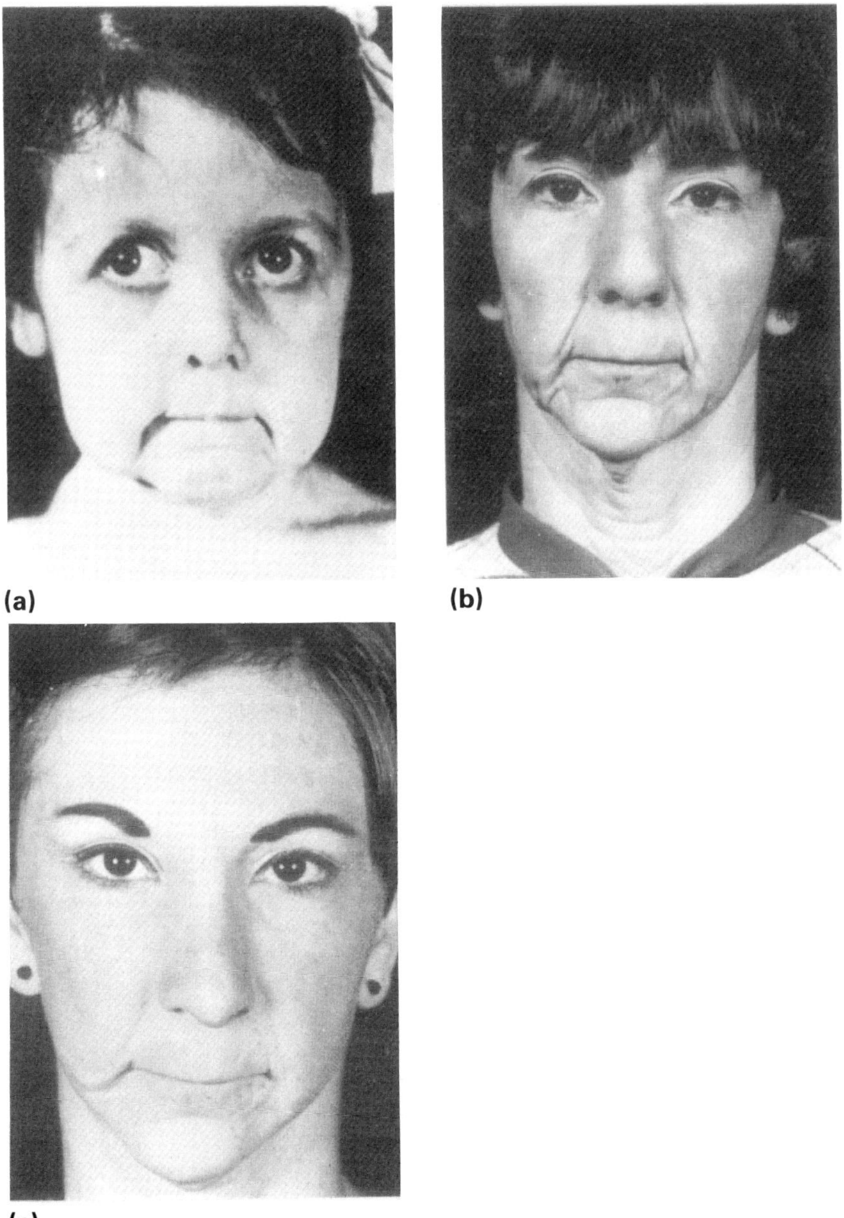

(a) (b) (c)

Figure 15.1 Original patients described by Beighton with autosomal dominant cutis laxa. (a) 9-year-old child. (b) 21-year-old woman. (c) Same woman after plastic correction of facial laxity.

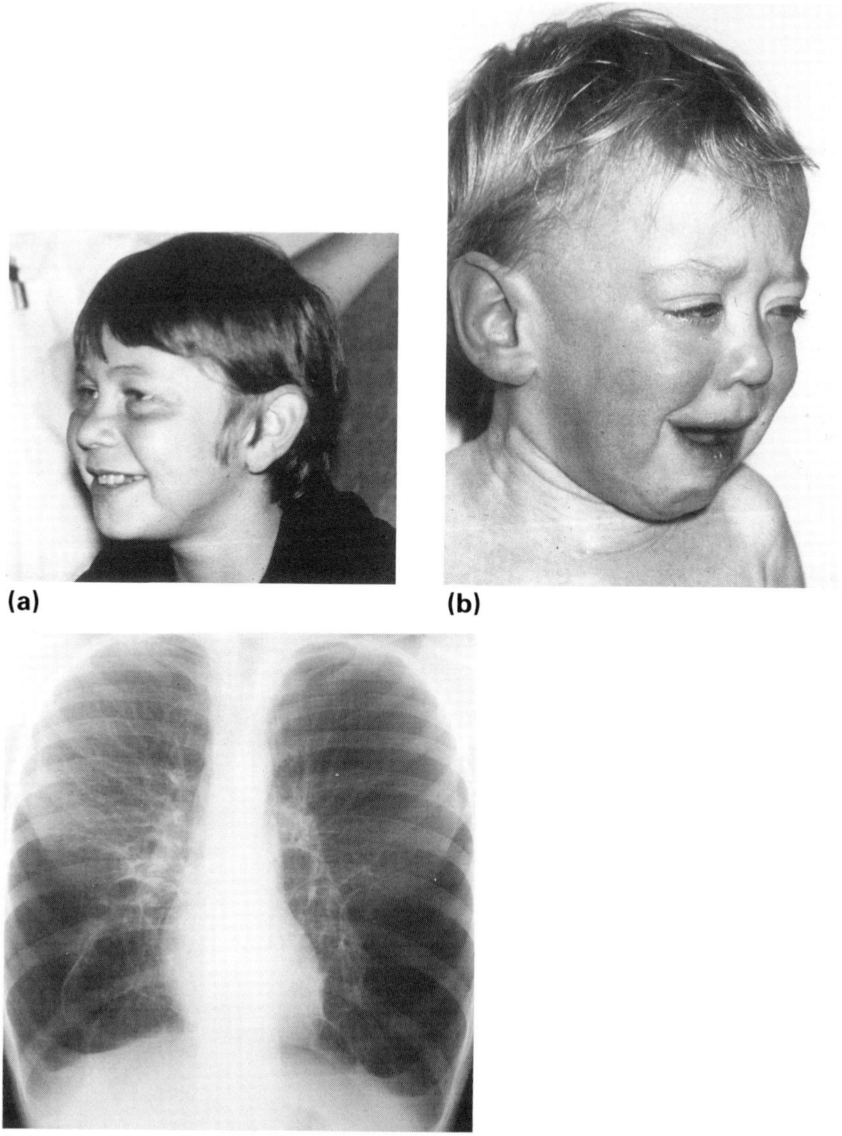

(a) (b)

(c)

Figure 15.2 Autosomal recessive cutix laxa. (a) 14-year-old boy with adolescent cutis laxa associated with pulmonary emphysema. (b) Face of 2-year-old boy with similar clinical phenotype. (c) Emphysematous bullae in chest x-ray of patient shown in (a).

Cutis Laxa with Bone Dystrophy and Joint Laxity: Recessive Type II Disease 21920

McKusick lists this variant in a 10-month-old girl with generalized congenital cutis laxa except in the face. Other associated features included persistent fontanelles, oxycephaly, and a dislocated hip. He also lists a form associated with severe intrauterine growth retardation that may possibly be x-linked dominant lethal in male babies and severely damaging in baby girls. Because of consanguinity in the Saudi Arabian population in which it mainly occurs, autosomal recessive inheritance is likely.

Sex-Linked Recessive Inheritance

Byers [4] in 1976 first described an x-linked form of cutis laxa with lysyloxidase deficiency. Five years later he described detailed changes in babies in whom electron microscopic examination showed large cutaneous collagen fibers [5]. In this form the skin is thin and lax (Fig. 15.3). This has been separately described as an x-linked disorder with occipital horns and cutis laxa, also known as EDS IX. It was removed from this category in the 1986 Berlin [6] classification and put instead into abnormalities of copper metabolism. Some families have a lifelong history of loose stools accompanied by urinary tract abnormalities such as bladder diverticula and bladder neck obstruction with hydronephrosis. Megaureters are common. Other associated clinical features include inguinal hernias and variable joint hypermobility and variable levels of ceruloplasmin and serum copper, implying a defect of copper metabolism. Copper concentrations can be elevated in cultured fibroblasts but decreased in serum and hair. McKusick considers it an allelic variant of Menke's syndrome. The latter does not produce cutis laxa, but is associated instead with growth retardation, peculiar steely hair, focal cerebral and cerebellar degeneration, and patchy stenosis and obliteration of peripheral arteries. Menke's syndrome and x-linked cutis laxa are therefore allelic copper metabolism abnormalities homologous to the lysyl-oxidase-deficient brindled mouse (Fig. 15.3b), which has a congenital propensity to ruptured aortic aneurysms. In humans the x-linked inheritance and lysyl oxidase deficiency together with abnormalities of copper metabolism produce a means of diagnosing affected males and carrier females by prenatal amniocentesis.

Cutis Laxa Secondary to Other Inherited Disorders

Ehlers-Danlos syndrome is a highly heterogeneous group of inherited disorders. Lax skin may be an early feature of types IV & VII EDS and it can and does occur later in surviving patients with Ehlers-Danlos types I, II, III, VII, normally as a late feature and then mainly affecting the face, forearms, dorsa of the hands, knees, and elbows (Fig. 15.4). Occasionally there is an association with extensive gastrointestinal diverticulae and families are encountered with recurrent and sometimes lethal peritonitis.

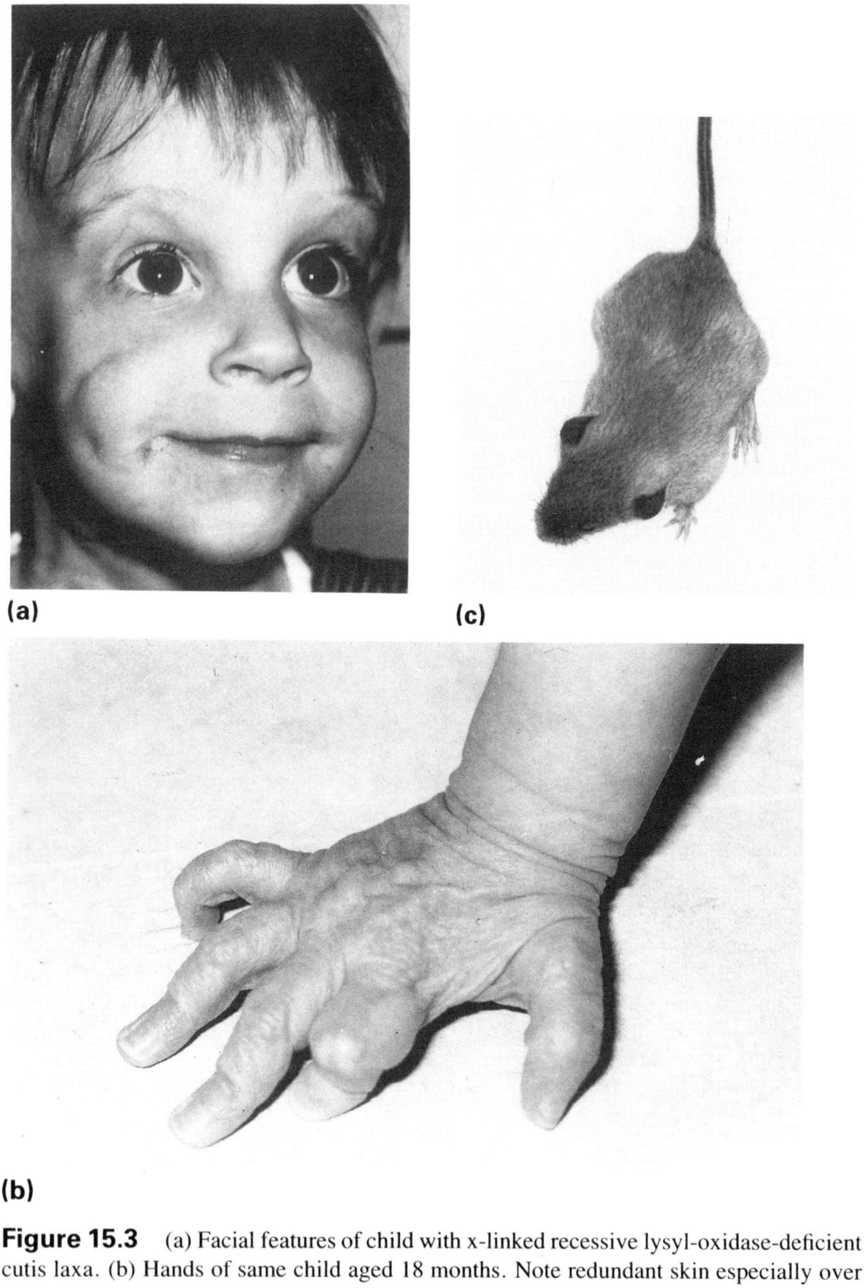

Figure 15.3 (a) Facial features of child with x-linked recessive lysyl-oxidase-deficient cutis laxa. (b) Hands of same child aged 18 months. Note redundant skin especially over wrists and dorsum of hands. (c) Brindled mouse with x-linked lysyl oxidase deficiency and homology to syndrome shown in (a) and (b).

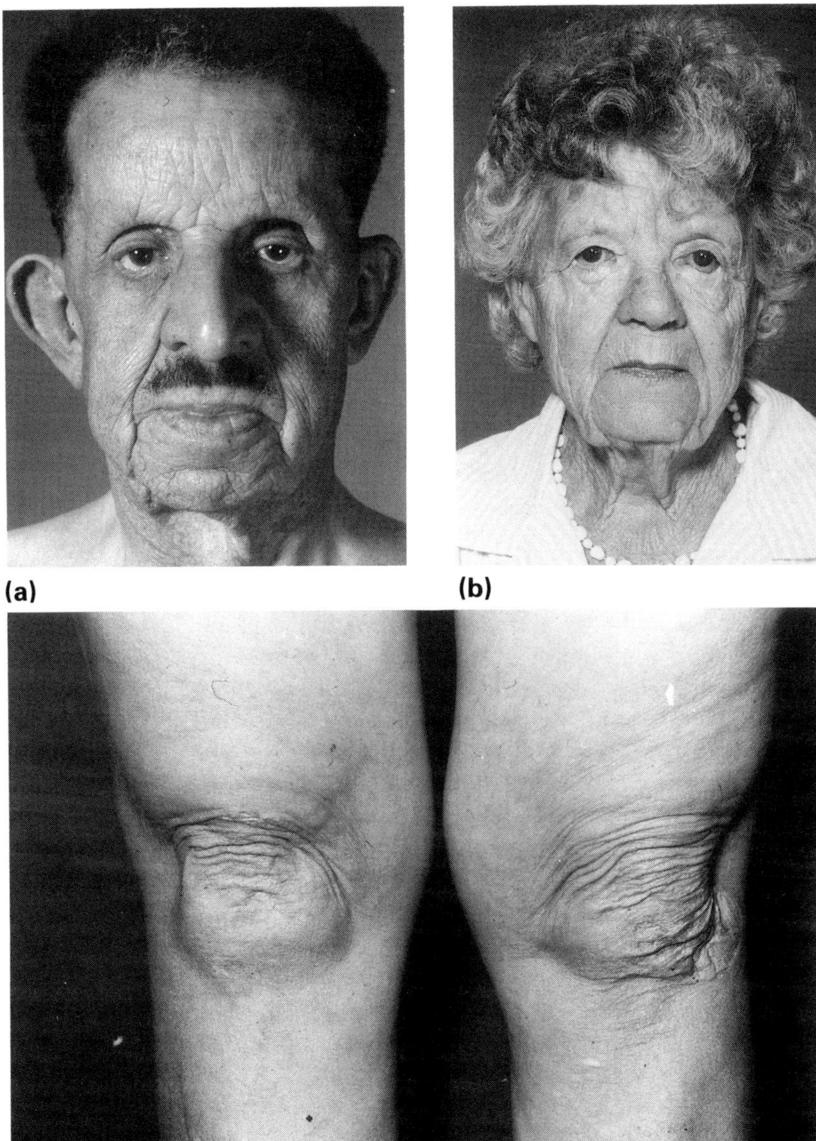

(a) (b) (c)

Figure 15.4 Cutis laxa in (a) 62-year-old man and (b) 63-year-old woman with Ehlers-Danlos syndrome. (c) Localized cutis laxa over the knees of patient with Ehlers-Danlos syndrome.

Other inherited diseases in which redundant skin occurs include neurofibromatosis, in which the skin is locally hypertrophic or nevoid but that has other important identifying features such as café-au-lait patches and pedunculated neurofibromas. Cutis verticis gyratum, although sometimes associated with joint laxity, presents with unmistakable infiltration of the forehead and scalp. Pachydermodactyly has infiltrative changes confined to the hands and feet and the wrinkly skin syndrome is largely limited to the dorsum and plantar/palmar aspects of the feet and hands, although thin skin with elastic fibril abnormalities has been described. The prune-belly syndrome can likewise be confused with x-linked cutis laxa but in the former there are no abdominal muscles. Both x-linked expression and autosomal recessive inheritance are possibilities. Posterior urethral valves, bilateral hydronephrosis, megaureter, and megalobladder without urethral stenosis are reported in patients with this syndrome. Leprechaunism is characterized clinically by severe intrauterine growth retardation, elfin face with protuberant ears and genital, hand, and foot enlargement with redundant and hypertrichotic skin without subcutaneous fat. It is associated with insulin receptor deficiency and hyperinsulinemia.

Acquired Cutis Laxa

This is a much less well defined group of disorders that, in contrast to the autosomal dominant, recessive, and sex-linked variants presenting in infancy or childhood, instead occur much later in life. Very probably there are both truly inherited varieties and those in which the mechanism is secondary to other pathologic processes and these in a sense fortuitous. In general, later-onset cutis laxa occurs under three circumstances: spontaneous or idiopathic, secondary to a persisting rash, and following generalized amyloidosis.

Idiopathic Cutis Laxa This is differentiated from the autosomal dominant and recessive types of cutis laxa only by its late onset. Generally once it begins progression is rapid and relentless, frequently ending with severe emphysema, right heart failure, and aortic dilatation. Spectacular examples were recorded separately by Reed[7] and by Bettman[8]. An excellent summary and review were produced by Tsuji and colleagues[9] who, in addition to their own patient, in whom the disorder had followed the nephrotic syndrome, reviewed 26 previously recorded examples.

Secondary to Persistent Cutaneous Rashes A second acquired group of variants follow various erythematous, eczematous, or vasculitic skin rashes that precede by variable periods the actual cutaneous degeneration. Fisher [10] and colleagues identify type I and type II variants of this sequence. Type I disease is identical to idiopathic generalized elastolysis (as described above) except for the preceding cutaneous changes. Type II disease is a more localized and discrete progress occurs without systemic complications but with patchy or extensive cutaneous changes. At one extreme the disorder resembles anetoderma being discrete and

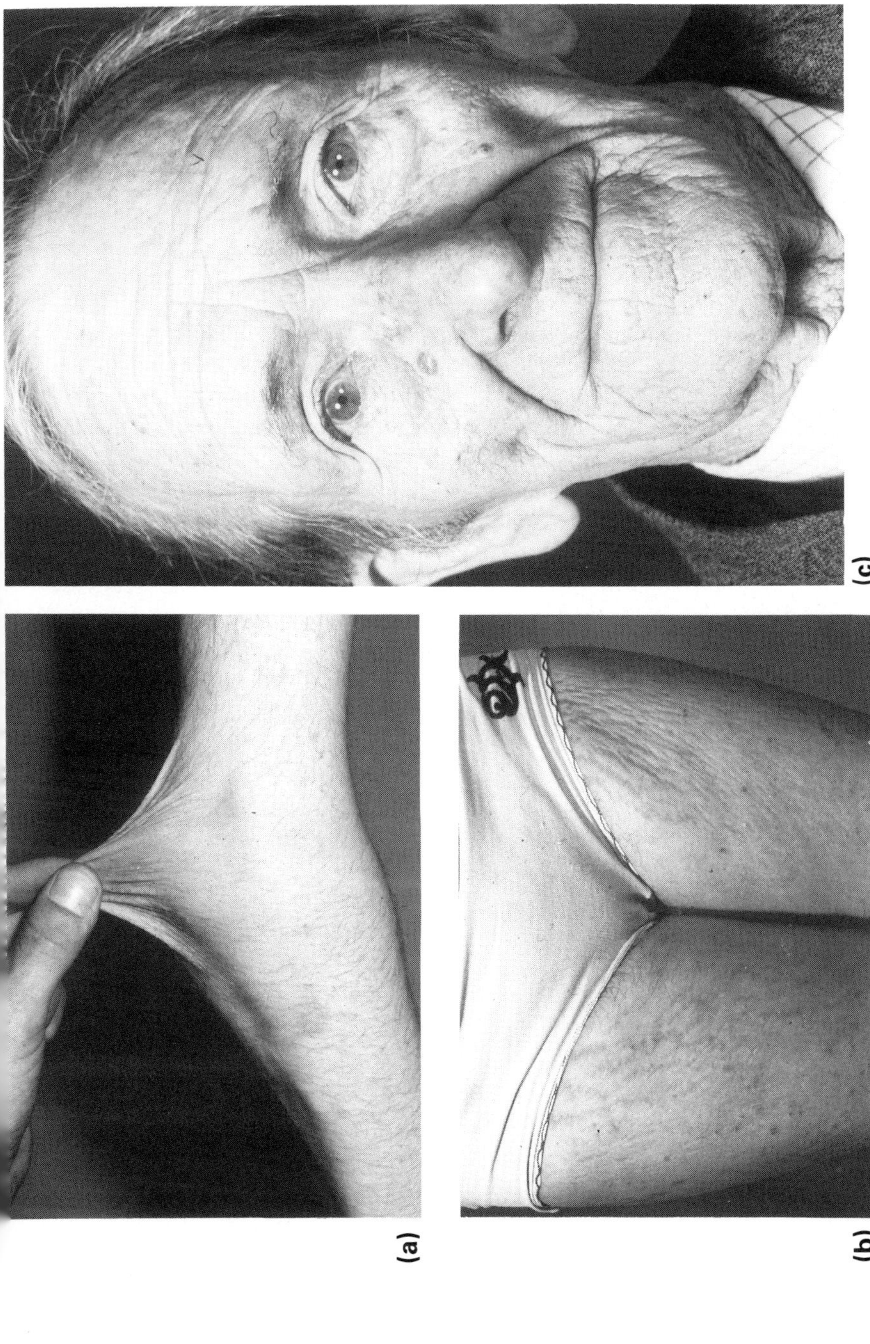

(a) (b) (c)

Figure 15.5 (a) Elbow from patient with benign hypermobile syndrome. (b) Upper thighs of patient after systemic steroids treatment. (c) Cutaneous atrophy and face of patient with cutis laxa and aging.

localized; at the other the spectrum of generalized cutaneous cutis laxa occurs. Verhagen and Woerderman [11] detailed the syndrome, which they also called inflammatory elastolysis, in Kenyan girls aged 5–11 years. Urticarial papules and plaques preceded the eventual atrophy. White patients have been occasionally described.

BIOCHEMICAL CHANGES

Even though connective tissue analysis and biochemical analysis are well advanced in diseases such as osteogenesis imperfect (OI), EDS, and Marfan's syndrome, the detection of mutations responsible for cutis laxa in its various forms is so far disappointingly rudimentary. Obvious candidates for change include collagen and various elastin components such as microfibrillar associated components such as collagen VI, lysyloxidase, fibrillin, fibronectin, and elastin.

Type VI collagen, for example, has three genetic components $\alpha1$, $\alpha2$, and $\alpha3$(VI) chains located on chromosomes 2 ($\alpha1$ and $\alpha2$[IV]) and 21 ($\alpha3$[VI]) collagen. We have observed consistently lower $\alpha1$ and $\alpha2$(VI) collagen chains in a family described by Fitzsimmons [12]. Crawford [13] and his colleagues have also suggested abnormalities of type VI collagen in autosomal recessive cutis laxa. Collagen $\alpha1$(I), $\alpha2$(I), and $\alpha1$(III) mutations have been associated with transient cutis laxa in EDS IV and VII, respectively, in which cases specific collagen fibril abnormalities also occur. A shortened $\alpha2$(I) collagen has been reported in an affected mother and daughter with cutis laxa and unspecified Ehlers-Danlos syndrome [14]. Lysyl-oxidase-deficient cutis laxa has been described in detail by Byers and colleagues [4,5] and although regarded as sex-linked recessive, may turn out to be autosomal recessive in view of the lysyl oxidase locus on chromosome 5 and not the X chromosome.

Defects of fibrillin staining have also been recorded in some patients with cutis laxa [15]. With the recent cloning, sequencing, chromosomal localization of fibrillin genes in chromosomes 5, 15, and 17 [16,17], and the detection of Marfan mutations in fibrillin 15 by SSCP [18], it will only be a matter of time before a systematic study of these components in the various forms of cutis laxa can be undertaken.

So far, despite the cloning and sequencing of the human tropoelastin [19] gene, no convincing abnormalities have been demonstrated in cutis laxa other than lowered mRNA levels [20].

Elastin-associated deposition of amyloid components occurs in acquired cutis laxa where amyloid P protein is deposited [21]. Other inherited abnormalities of amyloid deposition include Portuguese neuropathy (with defects of transthyretin or thyroxine-binding prealbumen). Furmar neuropathy (gelsolin) and Icelandic cerebral hemorrhage with cystatin C abnormalities, Alzheimer's β protein, and apolipoprotein AI substitutions have also been described [22]. There is therefore no shortage of candidate genes for study in the various inherited forms of cutis laxa.

STRUCTURAL ABNORMALITIES

The histopathologic examination of skin and internal organs such as lungs and arteries shows sparsity, fragmentation, and disruption of elastic fibers at the light level. Absence and fragmentation of elastic fibers in skin were first described by Variot and Cailliau [23] more than 30 years after Dubreuilh [24] first described cutis laxa. All forms of cutis laxa can show elastin fragmentation or depletion (including autosomal dominant) recessive and various late-onset forms. In other subsets of these groups elastic staining is normal. In amyloidosis amyloid P protein is associated with elastic fibers, while in PXE the elastic fibers are fragmented. Elastin fibers are normal in lysyl-oxidase-deficient cutis laxa. Fibrillin deficiency has also been detected in some patients with cutis laxa (category unspecified), although such changes are very typical of Marfan's syndrome [15].

Transmission electron microscopic examination shows a whole range of changes including microfibril proliferation, inmature elastic fibers with matrix deficiency, microfibril deficiency, and elastin amphorous accumulation [25]. Collagen fibril diameter enlargement has been well documented in lysyl-oxidase-deficient cutis laxa [5]. We have recently noted deficient microfibrillar and amorphous components in autosomal recessive cutis laxa and gross microfibrillar proliferation in late-onset blepharochalasis. Such a number of morphologic changes implies a range of biochemical abnormalities in connective tissue components that make up the various components of connective tissue matrix.

REFERENCES

1. McKusick VA. Mendelian inheritance in man. Catalogs of autosomal dominant, autosomal recessive and X-linked phenotype, 9th ed. Baltimore and London: Johns Hopkins University Press, Index number 12370, 21920, 219150, 219200, 304150, 1990.
2. Beighton PH. The dominant and recessive forms of cutis laxa. J Med Genet 1972; 9: 216–21.
3. De Barsy AM, Moens E, Dierckx L. Dwarfism, oligophrenia and degeneration of the elastic tissue in skin and cornea. A new syndrome? Helv Paediatr Acta 1968; 26: 397–402.
4. Byers PH, Narayanan AS, Bornstein P, Hall JG. An X-linked form of cutis laxa due to deficiency of lysyloxidase. Birth Defects 1976; 12(5): 293–8.
5. Byers PH, Siegel RC, Holbrook KA, Narayanan AS, Bornstein P, Hall JG. X-linked cutis laxa: defective collagen crosslink formation due to decreased lysyloxidase activity. N Engl J Med 1980; 303: 61–5.
6. Beighton P, De Paepe A, Danks D, Finidori G, Gedde-Dahl T, Goodman H, et al.

International nosology of heritable disorders of connective tissue, Berlin, 1986. Am J Med Genet 1988; 29: 581–94.

7. Reed WB, et al. Acquired cutis laxa: primary generalised elastolysis. Arch Dermatol 1971; 103: 661–9.
8. Bettman AG. Excessively relaxed skin and the pituitary gland. Plast Reconstr Surg 1955; 15: 489–501.
9. Tsuji T, et al. Acquired cutis laxa concomitant with the nephrotic syndrome. Arch Dermatol 1987; 123: 1211–6.
10. Fisher BK, et al. Acral localised localised acquired cutis laxa. J Am Acad Dermatol 1989; 21:33–40.
11. Verhagen AR, Woerdeman MJ. Post inflammatory elastolysis and cutis laxa. Br J Dermatol 1975; 92: 183–90.
12. Fitzsimmons JS, Fitzsimmons EM, Guibert PR, Zaldua V, Dodd KL. Variable clinical presentation of cutis laxa. Clin Genet 1985; 28: 284–95.
13. Crawford SW, et al. Characterisation of type VI collagen Mw 140,000 protein from cutis laxa fibroblasts in culture. Biochem J 1985; 227: 491–502.
14. Taieb A, et al. Collagen studies in congenital cutis laxa. Arch Dermatol Res 1987; 279–308.
15. Godfrey M, Manashe V, Weleber RG, et al. Cosegregation of elastin associated microfibrillar abnormalities with the Marfan phenotype in families. Am J Human Genet 1990; 46: 652–60.
16. Maslen CL, Cuson GM, Maddox BK, et al. Partial sequence of a candidate gene for the Marfan syndrome. Nature 1991; 352: 334–7.
17. Lee B, Godfrey M, Vitale E, et al. Linkage of Marfan syndrome and a phenotypically related disorder to two different fibrillin genes. Nature 1991; 352: 330–4.
18. Dietz HC, Cutting GR, Pyeritz RE, et al. Marfan syndrome caused by a recurrent *de novo* missense mutation in the fibrillin gene. Nature 1991; 352: 337–9.
19. Fazio MJ, Matter M-G, Passage E, et al. Human elastin gene: new evidence for localisation to the long arm of chromosome 7. Am J Human genet 1991; 48: 696–703.
20. Olsen DR, et al. Cutis laxa: reduced elastin gene expression in skin fibroblast cultures as determined by hybridisation with homologous cDNA and an exon 1 specific oligonucleotide. J Biol Chem 263, 6465–7.
21. Newton JA, et al. Cutis laxa associated with amyloidosis. Clin Exp Dermatol 1986; 11:87–91.
22. Zalin AM, Jones S, Fitch NJS, Ramsden DB. Familial nephropathic non-neuropathic amyloidosis: clinical features immunohistochemistry and chemistry. Q J Med NS 1991; 81: 945–56.
23. Variot, Cailliau. Peau ridée sénile chez une enfant de deux ans: agénésie des réseaux élastiques du derme. Arch Med Enfantes 1920; 106–11.
24. Dubreuilh W. Un cas de dermatolysis généralisé. Ann Dermatol Syphiligr 1887; 7(23): 529–31.
25. Pope FM. Cutis laxa. In: Beighton P, ed. McKusick's inherited disorders of connective tissue, 5th edition. In press.

16

Marfan's Syndrome

F. Michael Pope
M. R. C. Clinical Research Centre, Harrow, England

Unexpected aortic rupture from aneurysms of the ascending arch or descending aorta is a devastating complication of Marfan's syndrome. Abdominal aortic aneurysms can also occur but aneurysms elsewhere in the arterial tree are rare. The syndrome is otherwise characterized by tall stature, long thin extremities (especially the fingers and feet), skeletal abnormalities such as pectus deformities and kyphoscoliosis, lens dislocations from ruptured suspensory ligaments (Fig. 16. 1a-f), and rarer complications such as recurrent lung cysts (sometimes polycystic lung disease), pneumothoraces, various hernias, and cutaneous striae [1,2]. Other cardiac complications also occur, including mitral valve prolapse, aortic incompetence and stenosis, pulmonary stenosis, and coarctation of the aorta. Marfan [3] (Fig. 16.2a) first described a 5-year-old girl with slender extremities and kyphoscoliosis, and called her condition dolichostenomelia (thin long extremities) (Fig. 16.2b), but no other abnormalities were mentioned. Achard [4] in 1902 used the term *arachnodactyly* (spider fingers) (Fig. 16.2c) (see Fig. 4d, e). Mery and Babonneux [5] followed up Marfan's patient 6 years later and commented upon additional fibrous contractures of the fingers. By this time the x-ray changes in the fingers and lumbar spine had been recognized (Fig. 16.2e, f). Shortly afterwards Boerger [6] reported the association with dislocated lenses, but it was many years before the term Marfan's syndrome was used eponymously. Baer [7] and Etter and Glover [8] independently observed the cardiovascular complications particularly aortic dissection following aortic aneurysm formation.

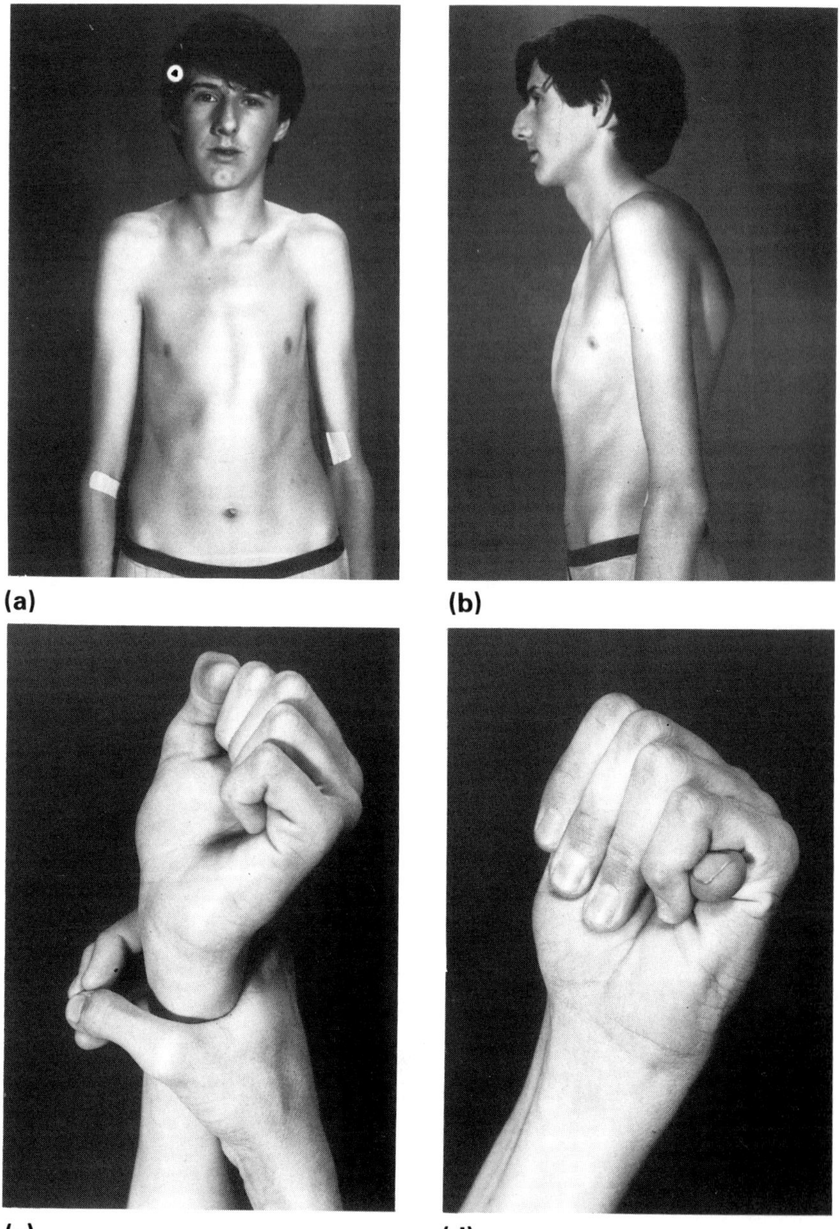

Figure 16.1 (a) Anterior and (b) lateral views of typical pectus carinatum, (c) wrist and (d) thumb signs typical of the long extremities, and (d) characteristic arachnodactyly of hands; (e) dislocated lens; and (f) high arched palate.

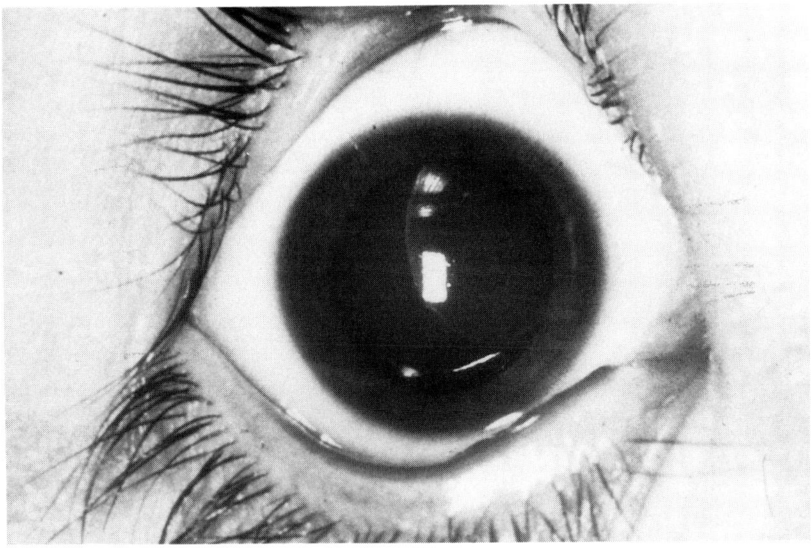

(e)

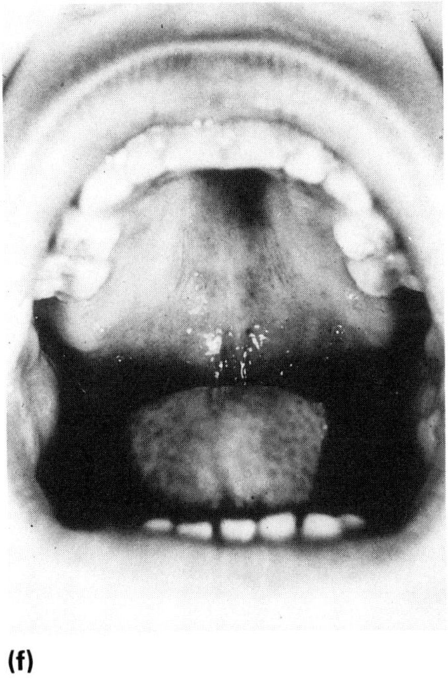

(f)

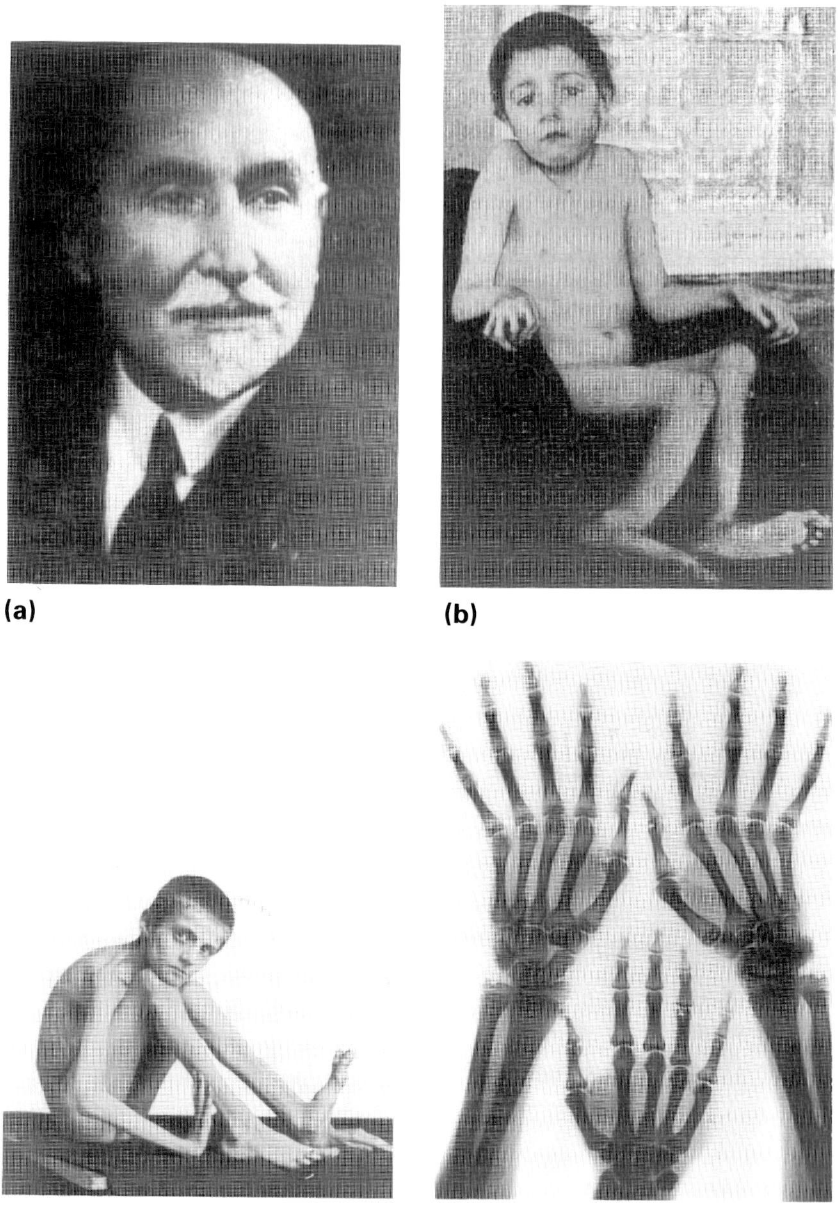

(a) (b) (c) (d)

Figure 16.2 (a) Marfan as illustrated by McKusick. (b) Marfan's original patient show long extremities, feet, and fingers. (c) Similar patient later described by Achard. (d) Roentgenogram of hands from patient with Marfan's syndrome compared with normal

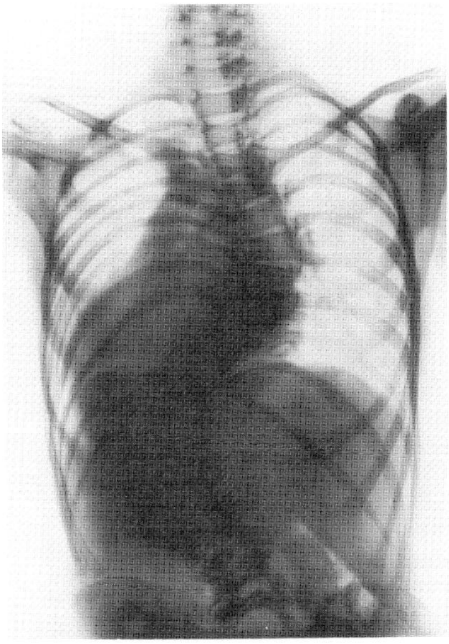

(e)

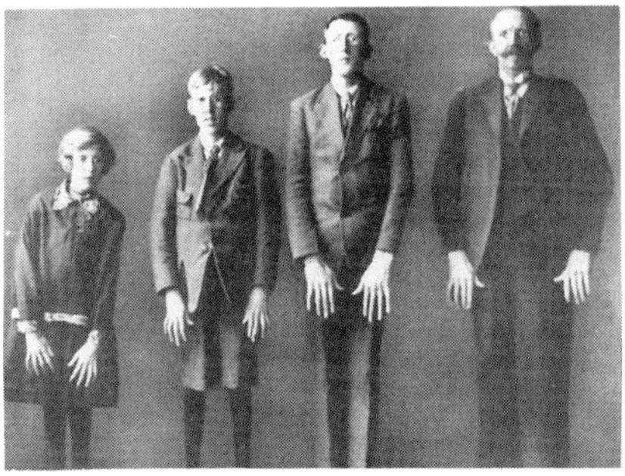

(f)

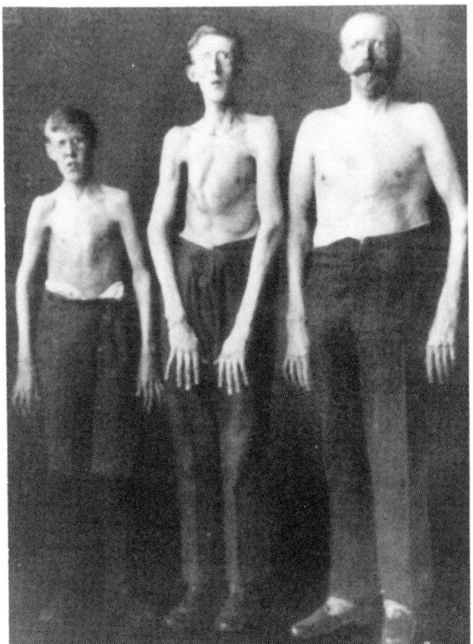

(g)

control. (e) Roentgenogram of kyphoscoliosis from same patient. (f, g) Original autosomal dominant family described by Weve shows father and three affected children with myopia, long extremities, and chest deformities.

Later other cardiac complications, such as mitral valve prolapse, aortic incompetence and stenosis, angina from a variety of causes, tricuspid regurgitation, pulmonary stenosis, and coarctation of the aorta became recognized complications. Then in 1931 Weve [9] clearly describe autosomal dominant inheritance of a syndrome with tall stature, myopia, long extremities, and pectus deformities in father, his two sons, and one daughter (Fig. 16.2g, h). He also attributed the disease to Marfan's syndrome for the first time and postulated a general mesenchymal abnormality.

From then on the essential elements and terminology of the disease were well defined and established but the cause remained mysterious. Any theory to explain it must account for the autosomal dominant inheritance and the curious combination of skeletal deformities (Fig. 16.3b), tall stature, aortic aneurysms with degenerated elastic tissue, fragile suspensory ligaments (Fig. 16.1e), loose-jointedness, and tendency to cutaneous striae (Fig. 16.3c). The combination clearly implies an abnormality of a structural connective tissue component.

GENETIC VARIABILITY

Genetic variability includes thin, heavy, and loose-jointed variants of families with ectopia lentis, aortic dilatation, and tall stature. McKusick [10] recognized skeletal, ocular, and cardiovascular elements of the disease, requiring at least two and preferably all three before diagnosis could be made (in the current absence of a measurable biochemical marker). He lists Marfan's syndrome as a single autosomal dominant disorder, and although he mentions an autosomal recessive form he considers this unlikely to exist. The marfanoid hypermobility syndrome is listed separately and includes tall stature, pectus excavatum, and joint hyperextensibility with excessively stretchy skin. Re-examination by McKusick of the original Walker patient 6 years later showed aortic incompetence but no ectopia lentis. Other similar clinical combinations occur and occasional examples of very tall Marfan's patients with a syndrome resembling Marfan's without ectopia lentis but with osteogenesis imperfecta or premature osteoporosis have been described. One of these patients had a transient defect of collagen $\alpha 2(I)$ production. We have observed a family with premature aortic dilatation and rupture, transverse cutaneous striae, joint hypermobility, pectus deformities, mitral valve prolapse, but without ectopia lentis who are variably type III collagen-deficient.

Contractural arachnodactyly, in addition to tall stature, flexion contractures of the fingers, kyphoscoliosis, and osteoporosis, is accompanied by crumpled ears without ocular and cardiovascular complications. Families have been described with both Marfan's syndrome and contractural arachnodactyly segregating in the same pedigree. We have also observed finger contractures in association with type III collagen-dependent Ehlers-Danlos syndrome type IV (Fig. 16.4e).

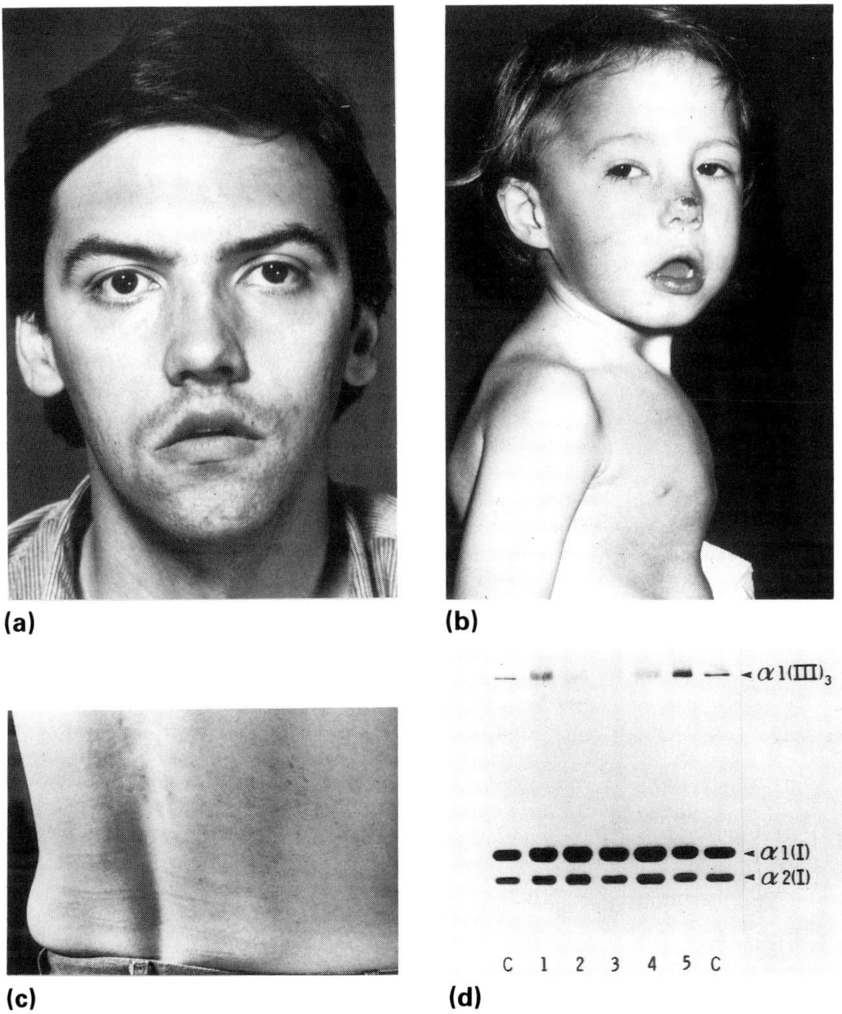

Figure 16.3 (a) Facial appearance of father and (b) pectus deformities of his affected son. (c) Transverse cutaneous striae of lower back. (d) Type III collagen profiles after pepsinization and without mercaptoethanol reduction show variable type III collagen bands.

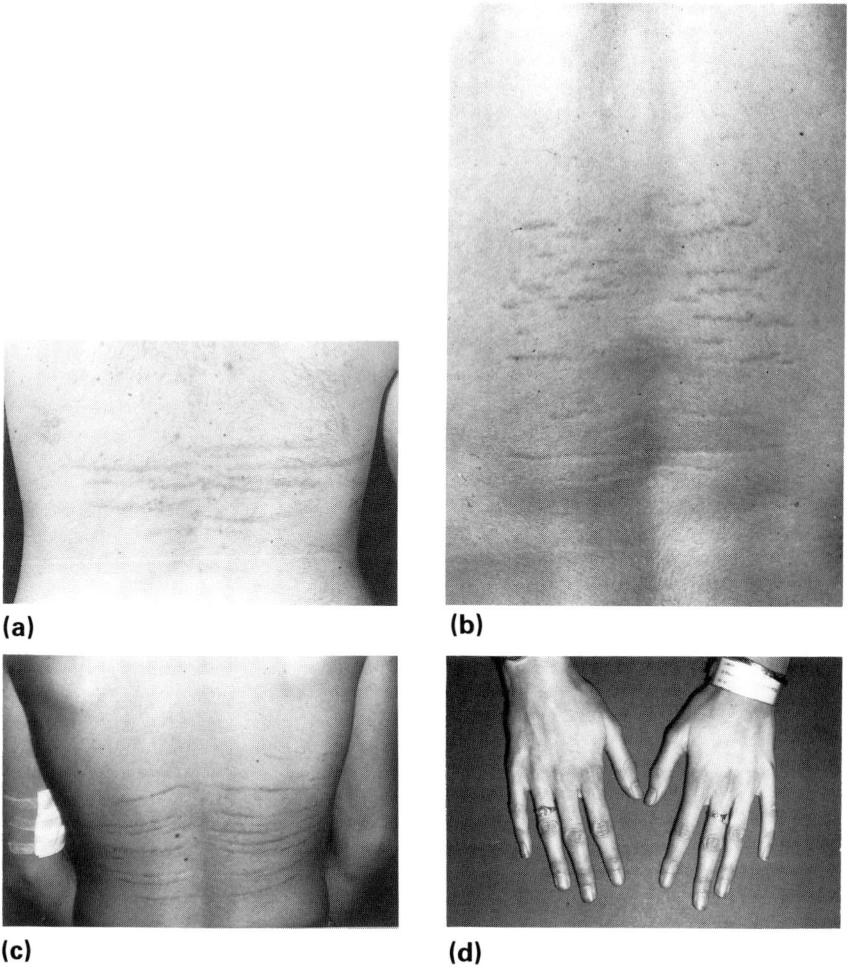

Figure 16.4 (a–c) Transverse cutaneous striae from three patients with typical Marfan's syndrome. (d, e) Arachnodactyly of hands and feet and (f) unusually contracted hands of patients with Marfan's syndrome.

DIFFERENTIAL DIAGNOSIS

The clinical phenotype of homozygous homocystinuria from cystathione synthetase deficiency produces a remarkably similar phenotype to Marfan's syndrome. Both disorders share tall stature, skeletal deformities, high arched palate, dental crowding, and ectopia lentis. Although the direction of lens dislocation is reported to differentiate between the two disorders (downward and outward in homocysti-

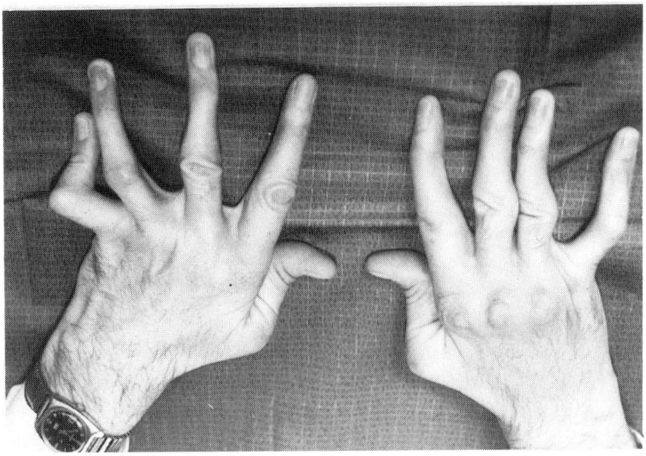

(e)

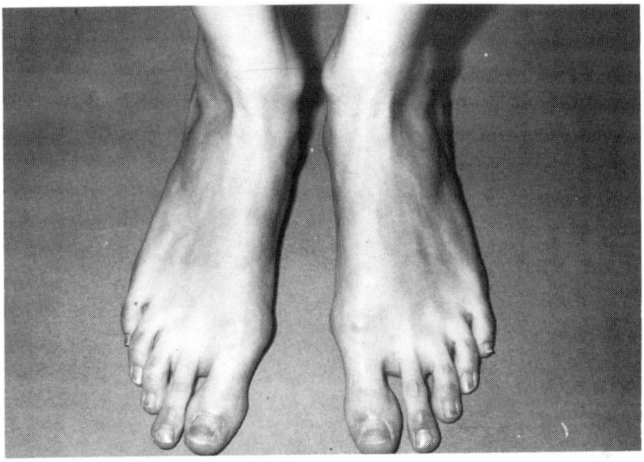

(f)

nuria, upward and inwards in Marfan's syndrome), this is unreliable. McKusick [1] comments that lens dislocation is universal (in patients over the age of 10 years) in homocystinuria and that two-thirds of such patients are mentally retarded. It can be excluded by measuring cystathione synthetase levels in skin fibroblasts. Patients heterozygotic for the condition develop homocystinemia after a methionine loading test. Other clinical possibilities in tall thin patients include a cutaneous neuronal thyroid carcinoma syndrome, nemaline myopathy, trisomy 8 syndrome, Klinefelter's syndrome, XYY syndrome, and familial idiopathic tall stature.

There is also substantial physical overlap with other inherited connective tissue disorders including acrogeric Ehlers-Danlos syndrome type IV with type III collagen abnormalities; some patients are tall, thin, loose-jointed, and have long, thin hands and feet. This disorder can also produce catastrophic aortic rupture and aneurysms elsewhere. Patients with lysyl hydroxylase deficiency (Ehlers-Danlos syndrome VI) can be tall, thin, loose-jointed, and develop ruptured aortic aneurysms as well as retinal detachments and global rupture of the eyes; some families with Ehlers-Danlos syndrome type III, benign hypermobile syndrome, are tall, loose-jointed, and have long thin hands and feet and heights in excess of their spans and may develop transverse cutaneous striae (Fig. 16.4a–c). As such they overlap with patients with marfanoid hypermobility syndrome. Ectopia lentis (Fig. 16.1e) occurs in Marfan's syndrome, homocystinuria, the Weil-Marchesani syndrome (which is easily separated by short stature and joint contractures), and as an idiopathic autosomal dominant characteristic with normal or short stature (occasional recessive forms have also been described). Persistent transverse cutaneous striae (Figs. 16.3c, 4a-c) are typical for Marfan's syndrome but can also occur in any other untreated defect of connective tissue with associated tall stature. Long hands and feet (Fig. 16.4d, f) can likewise also occur in patients with homocystinuria, Ehlers-Danlos syndromes III and IV, and tall stature.

PATHOLOGIC CHARACTERISTICS

Ruptured or dilated aortas from patients with Marfan's syndrome show an impressive consistent reduction in elastic fiber staining and its replacement by material with the staining properties of mucopolysaccharide. Alkali-resistant elastic proteins are depleted in such aortas although the primary mechanism is completely unclear. Dilatation at the aortic root is common and aortic dissection is a life-threatening complication (Fig. 16.5a, b). Mitral valves are often expanded but can show mucoid degeneration, while aortic valves are thinned and attenuated (producing mitral valve prolapse and incompetence and aortic incompetence) (Fig. 16.5c). Within arteries no consistent changes in collagen staining material are detected, despite the loss of elastic fibers (Fig. 16.5d), except for slightly increased collagen at the expense of smooth muscle and some degree of smooth muscle nuclear loss.

BIOCHEMICAL CHARACTERISTICS

Several different abnormalities of collagen, elastin, and proteoglycans have been identified in various (different) patients with Marfan's syndrome [2,10]. This

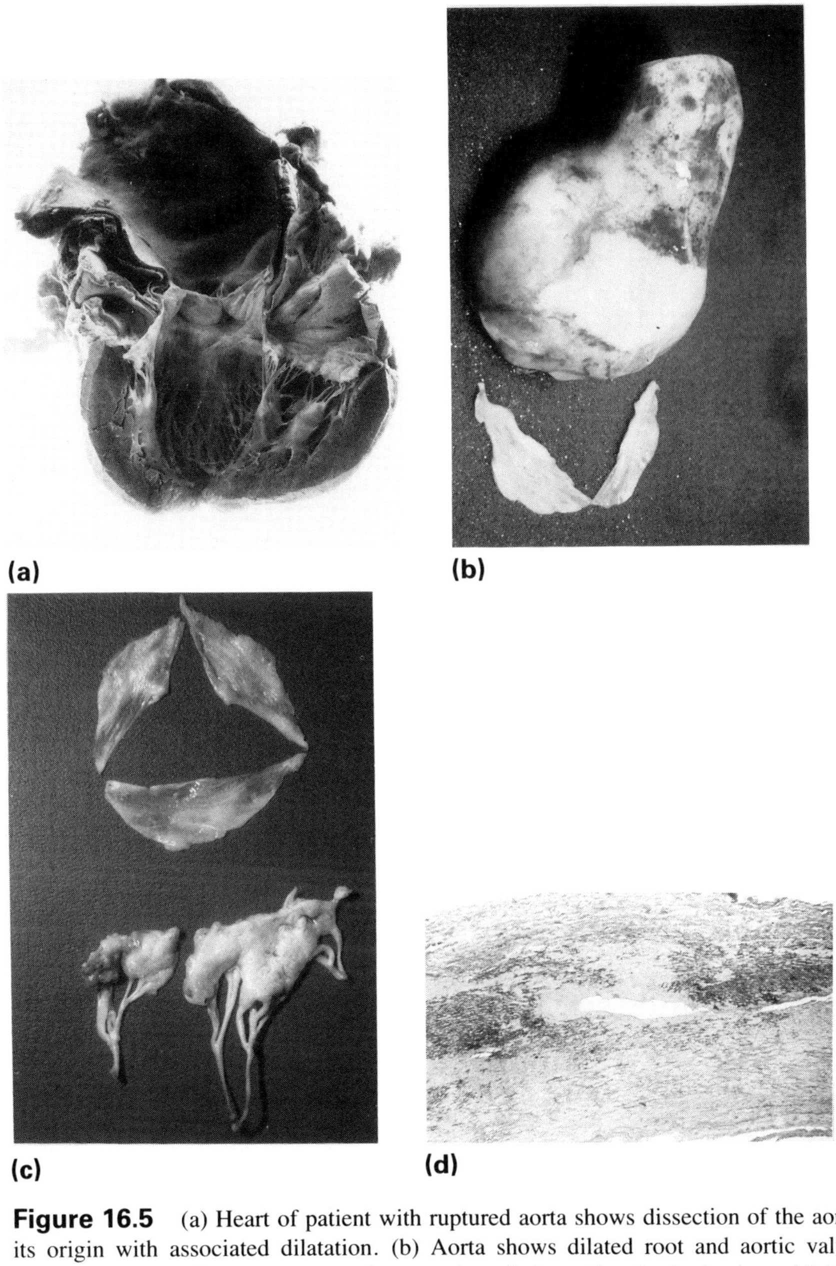

Figure 16.5 (a) Heart of patient with ruptured aorta shows dissection of the aorta at its origin with associated dilatation. (b) Aorta shows dilated root and aortic valvular incompetence. (c) Incompetence and attenuation of tricuspid and mitral valves. (d) Histologic appearance of expanded aorta shows elastic loss and medial degeneration.

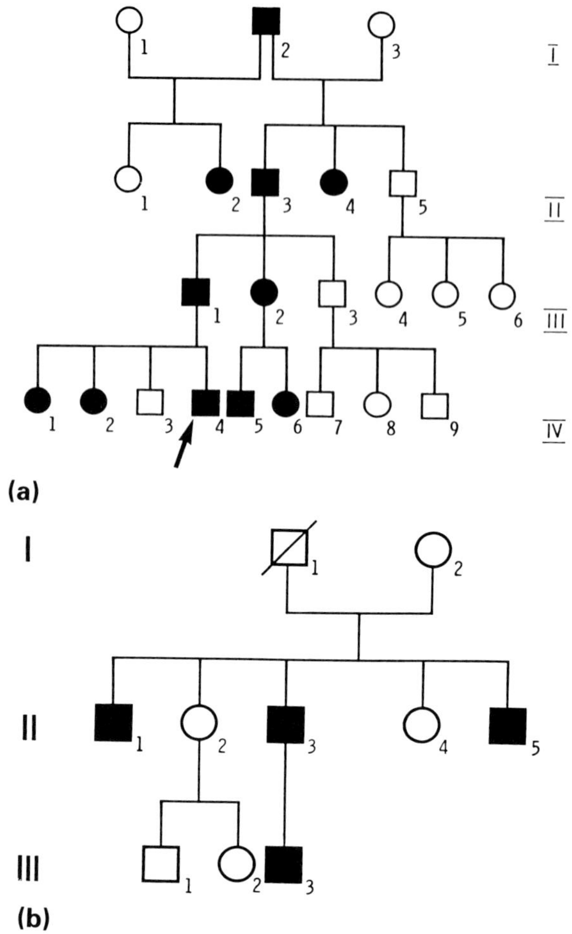

Figure 16.6 (a, b) Typical autosomal dominant pedigrees.

reflects the complexity of connective tissue components and interactions and the difficulty of excluding epiphenomena caused by other unidentified components. However, all the clinical and pathologic evidence strongly suggests that a defect of a structural protein or proteins causes this disease. For collagen alone there are 13 proteins coded by 20 or more genes and a host of posttranscriptional modifications involving 11 enzymes, 13 cofactors, and multistep changes. This takes no account of other components such as elastin (amorphous and microfibrillar components), proteoglycan, and other glycoproteins. Nevertheless the following changes have been noted by different authors at various times; a fivefold increase in hyaluronic acid synthesis, increased extractability of the collagen from skin and cultured fibroblasts of patients with Marfan's syndrome (implying unusual cross-linkage), decreased hydroxylysyl-derived cross-links in skin and aorta (with diminished hydroxylsinonorleucine in skin and 3-hydroxypyridinium in aorta). Specific collagen defects include alterations in type I/III collagen ratios and an insertion of 2–25 amino acids in the α2 chain of collagen I described by Byers [11]. McKusick thought this patient atypical since she had blue sclerae and no lens dislocations. Although the gene defect was thought to have been cloned (with a 38 base pair insertion), this later proved to be a normal collagen polymorphism.

Detailed re-examination mapped the original 20–25 aminoacid insertion to α2(I)CB3 or 5. PCR amplification of the appropriate gene fragment coding for this peptide shows the change of an arginine (GGC) to glutamine (GAC) at position 618 [12]. The proband's father also shares this mutation but it is still unclear whether he has Marfan's syndrome. In any case the effect of the amino acid change is uncertain but changes a basic amino acid to one without any charge.

This and the observation that clinical combinations closely resembling Marfan's syndrome can occur with type III collagen deficiency and EDS IV, and also with patients affected by lysylhydroxylase deficiency (with EDS VI), have strongly implied that molecular abnormalties of collagen might cause Marfan's syndrome and do cause Marfan-like disorders. Because of this possibility, all the relevant candidate collagen genes, including COL1A1, COL1A2, COL2A1, COL3A1, COL5A2, COL11A1, and collagen 11A2, which are distributed on chromosomes 2, 7, 10, 12, and 17, have been excluded by linkage analysis. Elastin has also been excluded. This strongly implied that for classic Marfan's syndrome some other connective tissue matrix protein is to blame.

IMPORTANT ADVANCES IN MOLECULAR ANALYSIS

Very impressive recent advances have occurred in the molecular analysis of Marfan's syndrome and are an object lesson in how modern recombinant DNA analysis provides real insight into the molecular diagnosis of various human diseases. It puts Marfan's syndrome efforts on a par with the very impressive analysis of diseases such as cystic fibrosis [13], Duchenne's muscular dystrophy [14], and neurofibromatosis [15]. Starting from a proven gene locus, the responsible genes have been located, sequenced, and used to provide real insight into protein structure and function.

Strategy

The successful combination of genetic linkage with a strong available candidate gene at that locus has obviated the need for the so-called reverse genetics approach used in Duchenne's muscular dystrophy and cystic fibrosis. In the latter, locating the mutant gene to a chromosomal region was followed by a highly labor-intensive and relatively difficult period of detailed gene mapping, followed by the convincing location of flanking gene markers and, finally, chromosome walking, hopping, and jumping until the mutant gene was finally recognized and characterized. In the case of Marfan's syndrome, two parallel and complementary approaches combined to a successful conclusion, including the accurate location of the mutant disease to chromosome 15 at DS15S45 [10,11].

In parallel to this work, a very strong candidate protein had been identified (fibrillin) [18] that was largely absent in skin biopsies or cultured fibroblasts from most biopsies from patients with Marfan's syndrome [19]. Very quickly following the confirmed location of the Marfan locus on chromosome 15 [16,20], fibrillin-specific protein sequence was used to detect a similar locus for one fibrillin gene [21], also at DS15S45. Other similar fibrillin genes were located on chromosomes 5 and 17 [22]. This was quickly followed by the clear demonstration of fibrillin point mutations and deletions in patients with classic Marfan's syndrome [23].

Linkage Studies

In 1989 an international consortium of interested researchers agreed to pool family data. Their combined evidence [20] strongly implicated chromosome 15 as the probable gene locus. Very quickly this was confirmed in several Finnish families [16]. When 17 families from 5 different American and Northern European groups were examined, there were no exceptions to this gene locus [17]. Using appropriate gene markers, the most likely gene locus was established at D15S45 [17].

Fibrillin Protein Data

In parallel to the gene linkage approach but preceding it by several years, convincing evidence emerged for an elastic-associated protein not previously described [18]. It was of much higher molecular weight than conventional connective tissue components such as collagen and elastin. Its tissue distribution in dermis, arterial wall, and suspensory ligament of the lens precisely matched the tissue changes of Marfan's syndrome, making it an extremely strong potential candidate for the faulty protein [18]. Furthermore, detailed preliminary studies of skin biopsies and cultured skin fibroblasts from patients with Marfan's syndrome showed a very close correlation between the absence of immunologic staining and the disease [19].

Combined Approach

In the summer of 1991, several very important pieces of evidence combined to clarify the precise molecular mechanism in certain patients with Marfan's syndrome and their families. First, two independant working groups identified the structure and sequence of the fibrillin gene and in one instance proved that three or more fibrillin genes at distinct gene loci existed [21,22]. Both research groups used portions of amino acid sequence obtained from purified fibrillin peptide fragments. The approaches by the two groups were slightly different.

The first group [21] screened a λgtll oligo dT-primed placental cDNA library using degenerate oligonucleotides (all possible combinations) for the 20 base pairs of a fibrillin peptide sequence. This yielded a large cDNA of 6.9 kb in 12 overlapping clones.

The second group [22] adopted a very similar strategy except that they used fibrillin peptide sequence for a subtraction cDNA approach from fibroblast and lymphocyte-derived cDNA. They detected a much smaller cDNA (1.6Kb) than the other group and also were able to isolate genomic clones that were more widely dispersed (on chromosomes 5, 15, and 17) than those of the first group, who isolated 15 specific sequences only. Both groups sequenced the cDNA and showed very similar physical properties including cysteine-rich sequences and EGF homology; the latter was possibly highly relevant to the unusually tall, thin Marfan phenotype. Furthermore, which was very important, the fibrillin 15 locus was exactly congruent with the Marfan's syndrome position at D15S45.

Study of Fibrillin Gene Markers

Two separate approaches were used. The first tested the segregation of PCR-amplifiable fibrillin sequence variations on appropriate families with Marfan's syndrome and other relevant and possibly related diseases such as annular aortic ectasia and congenital contractural arachnodactyly [22]. This proved several interesting facts. First reliable, easily amplifiable markers confirmed that fibrillin gene markers on chromosome 15 segregated with Marfan's syndrome. Second, none of the other disorders segregated in this way except that contractural congenital arachnodactyly (which has long been confused with Marfan's syndrome but is distinct from it) is not caused by a fibrillin abnormality but by the gene on chromosome 5. Furthermore, the other aortic fragility syndromes (annuloaortic ectasia, etc.) are not linked to this location.

The second approach by Maslen et al. [21] and their clinical collaborators Dietz et al. [23] directly examined fibrillin 15 mutations in Marfan's syndrome. Here the mutual strategy was to design primers to amplify the 6.9 kb mRNA in conveniently sized fragments and then to look for mutations (deletions or substitutions) using single-stranded conformational analysis with Marfan's syndrome sequences. Using this strategy, Dietz et al. detected mutations in those fragments amplifying amino acids 388–408 and 831–849. The protocol included mRNA extraction from cultured skin fibroblasts followed by single-stranded cDNA synthesis. A G–C transversion in nucleotide 716 of codon 239 substituted proline for arginine in two unrelated patients with sporadic Marfan's syndrome (with particularly severe joint laxity but otherwise typical features). No similar mutations in this region occurred in 19 patients with Marfan's syndrome or 24 single members of various families with Marfan's syndrome.

FUTURE ADVANCES

Even though much remains to be done once a full-length cDNA for fibrillin 15 is obtained, then all available patients with Marfan's syndrome abnormalities in the coding region will become detectable. Point mutations, deletions, splice junction defects, and regulatory mutations are all quite likely and prenatal diagnosis, prevention by chorionic sampling, and ovum and embryo selection are all within reach in the short-and medium-term future.

Detailed work remains to detect candidate diseases for the fibrillin genes on chromosome 17; contractural arachnodactyly has already been mapped to chromosome 15. Benign hypermobile syndrome, pseudoxanthoma elasticum, annular aortic ectasia, and certain forms of aortic aneurysm are all candidates for fibrillin-related mutations.

REFERENCES

1. McKusick VA. The Marfan syndrome, In: Heritable disorders of connective tissue, 4th ed, St. Louis: CV Mosby, 1972: 61–223.
2. Pope FM, Nicholls AC, Lewkonia RM, Halme T, Dorrance DE, Pomerance A. Clinical and genetic heterogeneity of the Marfan syndrome. Curr Probl Dermatol 1987; 17: 95–110.
3. Marfan AB. Un cas de déformation congénitale des quatre membres plus prononcée aux extrémités characterisée par l'allongement des os avec un certain degré d'amincissement. Bull Mem Soc Med Hop Paris 1896; 13: 220–1.
4. Achard C. Arachnodactylie. Bull Mem Soc Med Hop Paris 1902; 19: 834.
5. Mery H, Babonneix L. Un cas de déformation congénitale des quatre membres: hyperchondroplasie. Bull Mem Soc Med Hop Paris 1902; 19: 671.
6. Boerger F. Uber zwei Falle von Arachnodaktylie. Z Kinderheilkd 1914; 12: 161–84.
7. Baer RW, Taussig HB, Oppenheimer EH. Congenital aneurysmal dilatation of the aorta associated with arachnodactyly. Bull Hopkins Hosp 1943; 72: 309.
8. Etter LF, Glover LP. Arachnodactyly complicated by dislocated lenses and death from rupture of dissecting aneurysm of the aorta. JAMA 1943; 123: 88–91.

9. Weve A. Uber Arachnodaktylie (Dystrophia). Mesodermalis Typus Marfanus. Arch Augenheilkd 1931; 104: 1–46.
10. McKusick VA. Mendelian inheritance in man. Catalogs of autosomal dominant, autosomal recessive and x-linked phenotypes, 8th ed. Baltimore and London: Johns Hopkins University Press, 1989: 15470, 15475, 24875.
11. Byers PT, Siegel RC, Peterson KE, Rowe DW, Holbrook KA, Smith LT, Chang Y-H, Fu JCC. Marfan syndrome abnormal α2 chain in type I collagen. Proc Nat Acad Sci 1981; 781: 7745–9.
12. Phillips CL, Shrago AW, Pinnell SR, Wenstrup RJ. DNA sequence analysis of α2(I) collagen from an individual with the Marfan phenotype. Proc NY Acad Sci 1991;
13. Rommens JM, Iannuzzi MC, Kerem B, Drumm ML, Melmer G, Dean M, Rozmahel R, Cole JC, Kennedy D, Hidaka N, Zsiga M, Buchwald M, Riodan JR, Tsui L-C, Collins FS. Identification of the cystic fibrosis gene: chromosome walking and jumping. Science 1989; 245: 1059–65.
14. Monaco AP, Neve RL, Colletti-Feener C, et al. Isolation of candidate cDNAs for portions of the Duchenne muscular dystrophy gene. Nature 1986; 323: 646–50.
15. Fountain JW, Wallace MR, Bruce MA, Seizinger BR, Menon AG, Gusella JF, Michels VV, Schmidt MA, Dewald GW, Collins FS. Physical mapping of a translocation breakpoint in neurofibromatosis. Science 1989; 244, 1085–7.
16. Kainulainen K, Pulkkinen L., Savolainen A, Kailila I, Peltonen L. Location on chromosome 15 of the gene defect causing Marfan syndrome. N Engl J Med 1990; 323: 935–9.
17. Kainulainen K, Steinmann B, Collins F, Dietz C, Francomano CA, Child A, et al. Marfan syndrome: no evidence for heterogeneity in different populations, and more precise mapping of the gene. Am J Human Genet 1991; 49: 662–667.
18. Sakai LY, Keen DR, Engvall E. Fibrillin: a new 350Kd glycoprotein is a component of extracellular microfibrils. J Cell Biol 1986; 103: 2499–509.
19. Godfrey M, Menashe V, Weleber RG, Koler RD, Bigley RH, Lovrien E, Zonana J, Hollister DW. Cosegregation of elastin-associated microfibrillar abnormalities with the Marfan phenotype in families. Am J Human Genet 1990; 46: 652–60.
20. Blanton SH, Sarfarazi M, Eiberg H, de Groote J, Farndòn PA, Kilpatrick MW, Child AH, Pope FM, Peltonen L, Francomano CA, Boileau C, Keston M, Tsipouras P. An exclusive map of Marfan syndrome. J Med Genet 1990; 27: 73–77.
21. Maslen CL, Corson GM, Maddox BK, Glanville RW, Sakai LY. Partial sequence of a candidate gene for the Marfan syndrome.
22. Lee B, Godrey M, Vitale E, Hori H, Mattei M-G, Sarfarazi, et al. Linkage of Marfan syndrome and a phenotypically related disorder to two different fibrillin genes. Nature 1991; 352: 330–334.
23. Dietz HC, Cutting GR, Pyeritz RE, Marslen CE, Sakai LY, Corson GM, et al. Marfan syndrome caused by a recurrent *de novo* missense mutation in the fibrillin gene. Nature 1991; 352: 337–339.

17

Osteogenesis Imperfecta

F. Michael Pope
M. R. C. Clinical Research Centre, Harrow, England

In osteogenesis imperfecta (OI), skin is very much less affected than bone. The disease is considered here in detail since much of the basic protein chemistry and molecular biology have been worked out from the study of cultured skin fibroblasts. Almost all of the 80–90 known mutations prove to have defects of one of the two genes coding for type I collagen (COL1A1 and COL1A2). Even though the majority of them produce fragile osteoporotic bones, a minority spare the bones, producing instead easily torn hyperextensible skin, loose ligaments, and normal bones. These differences prove to be controlled by mutational position and type. The disease has a long history and has been clearly demonstrated in an Egyptian mummy of the 2nd century B.C. (Fig. 17. la, b), and also described in 9th century A.D. from Anglo-Saxon remains in Britain [1]. Decalcified bones are depleted in collagen-containing structures. These are distorted and badly organized with minor disturbance of the epiphyseal cartilage palisades (Fig. 17. 2a, b). Although the periosteum is normal, cortical bone is affected and perimedullary trabecular bone is almost completely absent in the more severe forms of the disease (Fig. 17. 2c-e). Sometimes membranous bones are very abnormal with accompanying skull deformities, wormian bones, abnormally persistent fontanelles, and facial dysmorphology. Anatomical changes range from minor bending and curvature of long bones to gross generalized disease in which no bone is normal. There is a clinical overlap with other connective tissue diseases such as Ehlers-Danlos syndrome, the benign hypermobile syndrome,

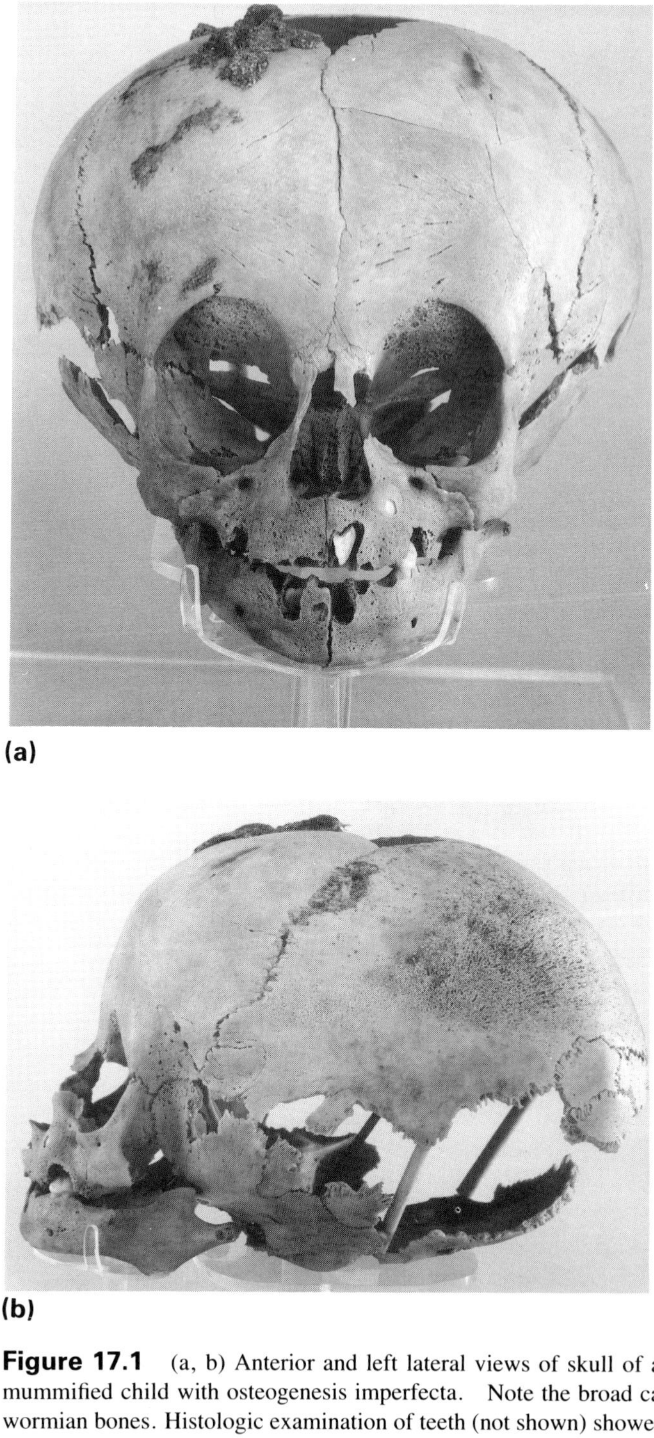

(a)

(b)

Figure 17.1 (a, b) Anterior and left lateral views of skull of a 4-year-old Egyptian mummified child with osteogenesis imperfecta. Note the broad calvarium and multiple wormian bones. Histologic examination of teeth (not shown) showed typical osteogenesis imperfecta.

and Marfan's syndrome, so that patients with brittle bones have features reminiscent of these other diseases. This essentially reflects some similarity in the underlying defect of the collagen molecule, and so will be discussed later. Since there are only a limited number of ways in which these changes can be expressed (with combinations of skin, ligamentous, and osseous changes in the case of type I defects), a clinical overlap and phenocopying are to be expected.

The spectrum of OI ranges from mild subclinical disease to lethal disease (Figs. 17. 3a; 4a, b; 5a–c). Between these extremes lie a variety of severely disabling and crippling phenotypes with both autosomal dominant and autosomal recessive inheritance [2–4] observed clinically and proved by genetic linkage to affect mainly collagen I $\alpha 1$ and $\alpha 2$ genes [5]. In general, diseases range from mild clearly autosomal dominant (Fig. 17. 3a–c), families with multiple affected generations [2] (with an excellent prognosis) to severely disabling lethal (Fig. 17. 4a, d–g) or crippling disorders (Fig. 17. 5a–c) that are frequently either autosomal recessive or lethal dominant diseases [3].

Apart from bones, abnormalities occur elsewhere including thin and stretchy skin, hyperextensible joints, blue sclerae, opalescent dentine and obliterated pulp cavities (Fig. 17. 3d, f, g), and dentinogenesis imperfecta. Inguinal, umbilical, and esophageal hernias can also occur. Calcified large peripheral arteries, dilated and stenotic aortic valves, and mitral valve abnormalities have been rarely observed. McKusick also records examples of combined aortic and mitral regurgitation [1] and an association with floppy mitral valve syndrome (mitral valve prolapse). All this suggests a generalized connective tissue defect.

HISTORY AND CLINICAL CLASSIFICATION

McKusick [1] lists the historical landmarks in the history of OI. It was first clearly described in 1790 by Ekman, who recorded it in a three-generation family. Vrolik in 1849 observed the first case in an infant, Spurway in 1896 recorded the blue sclerae, Looser in 1906 differentiated congenital and tarda forms of the disease, realizing that the infantile forms could progress to adult disease. Bell from the Galton laboratory in 1928 formally described autosomal dominant inheritance for the first time.

The best working classification is that devised by Sillence, who has clearly extended the genetic heterogeneity of the disease [2,3]. He proposed an initial classification into four genetic types, two of which are mild and autosomal dominant, the other two being much more severe and with autosomal dominant or recessive inheritance. In a later modification he expanded the classification of the lethal type II variants, which was itself later modified by Thompson [4]. Beighton [6], who has formalized the nosology of inherited defects of connective tissue has accepted the Sillence classification as a reasonable working framework for the disease [6].

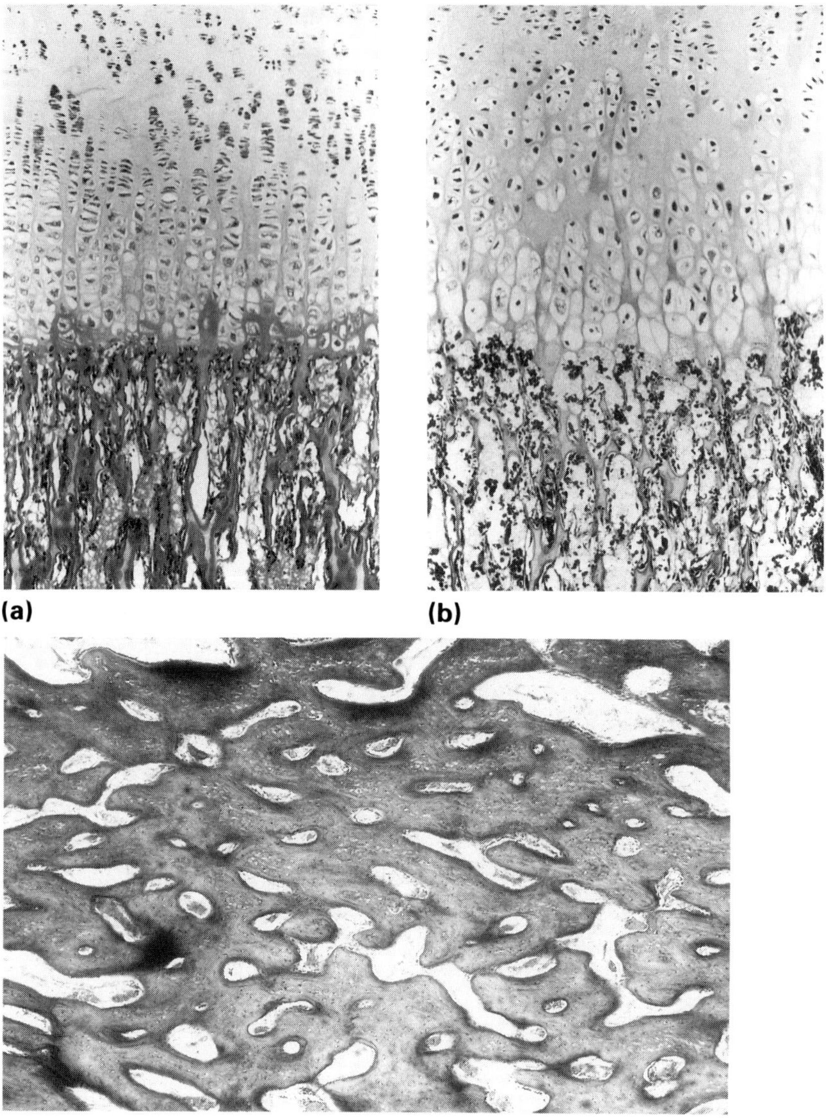

Figure 17.2 Cartilage–bone interface in (a) normal and (b) osteogenesis imperfecta. Note slight irregularities in cartilage columns of osteogenesis imperfecta bone compared with normal control. The trabecular bone is diminished in the OI sample compared with normal. (c) Midshaft cortical bone of normal control compared with (d) moderately severe OI patient and (e) lethal case.

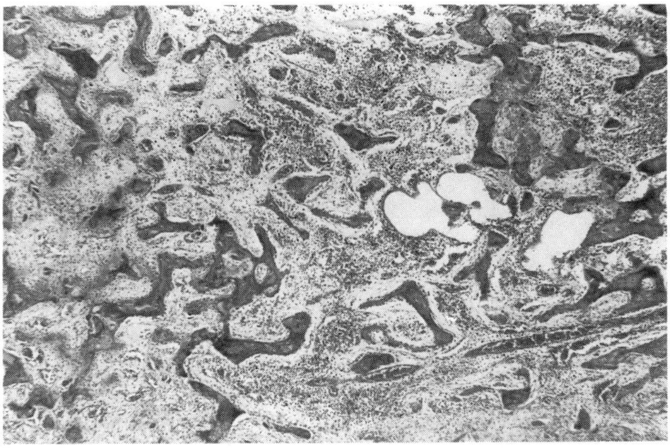

(d)

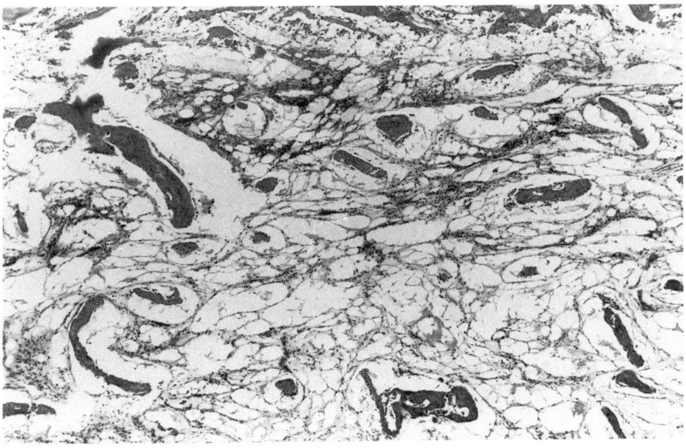

(e)

Sillence Type I OI

No problem exists with defining this form of the disease. In general, it is a mild condition except for occasional severely affected members in some pedigrees. Frequently, and not obvious until the child toddles, it is accompanied by other features including joint laxity, bright blue sclerae, deafness, and short stature. The x-ray changes are generally mild, showing wormian bones, osteoporosis, and sometimes dentinogenesis imperfecta (Fig. 17. 3a–f). Fractures can occur in infancy and recur throughout childhood until adolescence, when they often cease. Sometimes they recur in middle-aged menopausal women. The disease

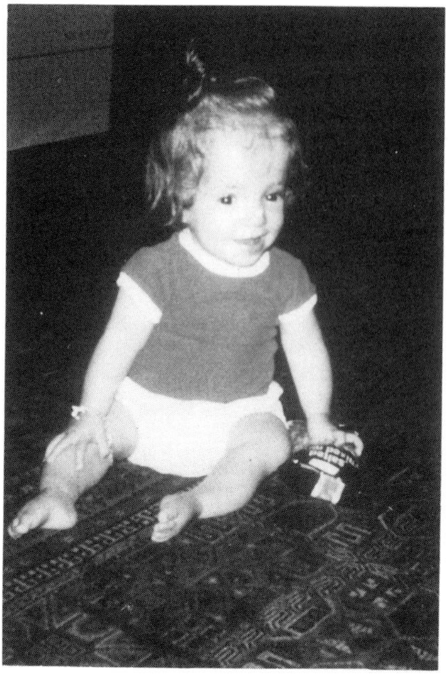

(a)

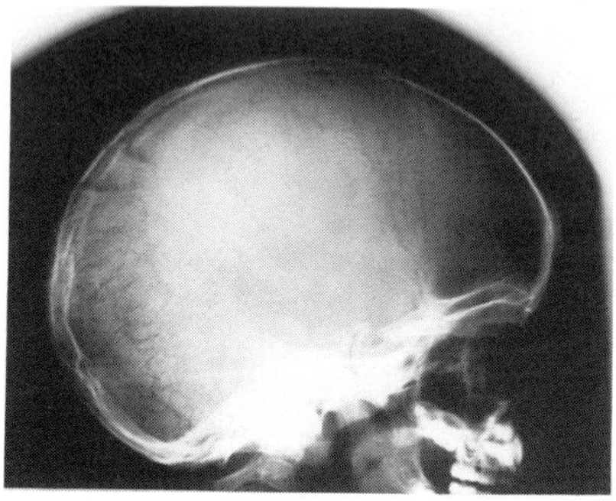

(b)

Figure 17.3 (a) Clinical appearance of child with mild Sillence type I OI. Notice the broad head and bowed tibiae. This particular clinical pattern carries an excellent prognosis. (b) Lateral view of skull shows typical wormian bones. (c) Lateral lumbar spine x-ray shows osteoporosis. (d) Typical dentinogenesis imperfecta of teeth that are irregularly opalescent. (e) Histologic section from normal tooth shows well-organized odontoblastic canals compared with (f) disorganized opalescent canals from patients with OI. (g) Pan-orthotomogram of OI teeth and (h) normal teeth: note difference between pulp cavities of (f) and (h).

can also be present perinatally or in infancy and merges imperceptibly in some families with more severe variations, especially Sillence type II OI. Dentinogenesis imperfecta usually breeds true in Sillence type I OI. Families with or without normal teeth can be identified (Fig. 17. 3d–f). Both genes ($\alpha 1[I]$ and $\alpha 2[I]$) of type I collagen have been unambiguously linked to Sillence type I OI [5].

Sillence Type II OI

Sillence in 1979 [2] defined the following features that comprised this group: a short-limbed dwarfism that is quickly fatal after birth or results in stillbirth (Fig. 17. 4a, d, e) with broadened continuously beaded ribs, marked tibial angulation,

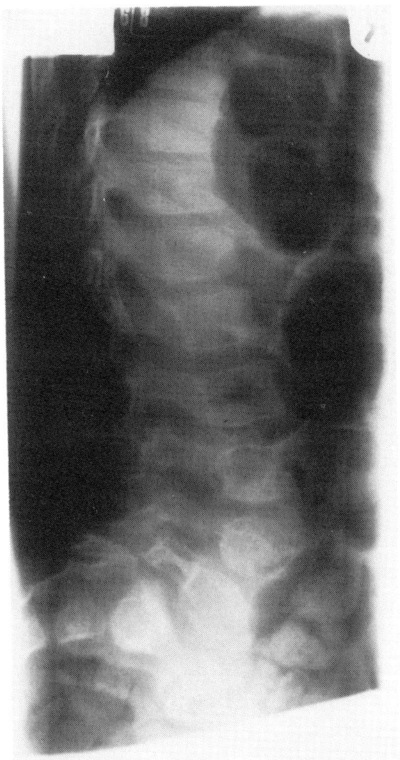

(c)

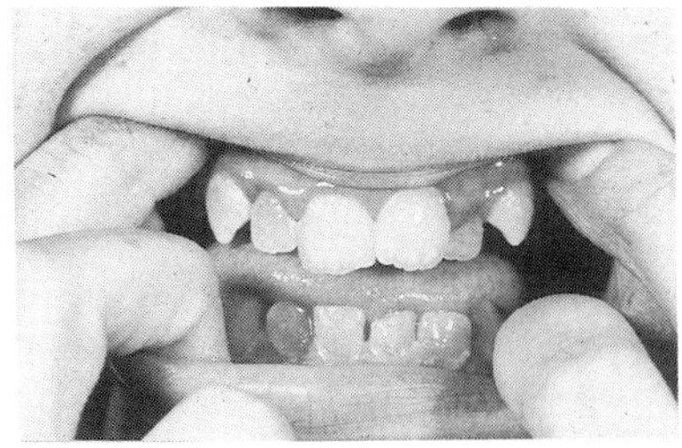

(d)

(e)

fractures of the shafts of upper limbs (Fig. 17. 6a), death usually occuring from asphyxia, chest infections, cerebral hemorrhage, or in rare cases, strangulated hernias. Five years later, Sillence [3] published a modification of this classification now describing IIa, IIb, and IIc phenotypes dependent upon x-ray findings.

Type IIa OI is characterized by broadened and shortened rectangular humeri and femora without modeling (Fig. 17. 4a, c, e). The ribs are also broadened due to multiple continuous fractures producing a finely striped appearance, the vertical axis of the ribs being wider than normal (Fig. 4e). Type IIb is similar to IIa except that the ribs show only occasional or sometimes no beading (Fig. 17.

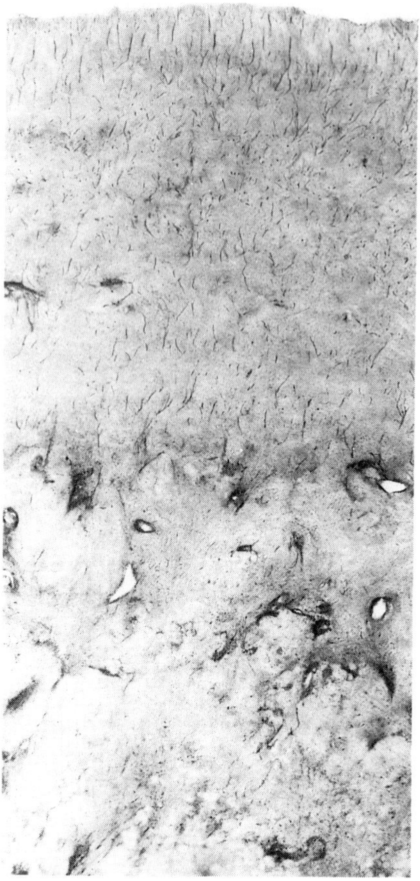

(f)

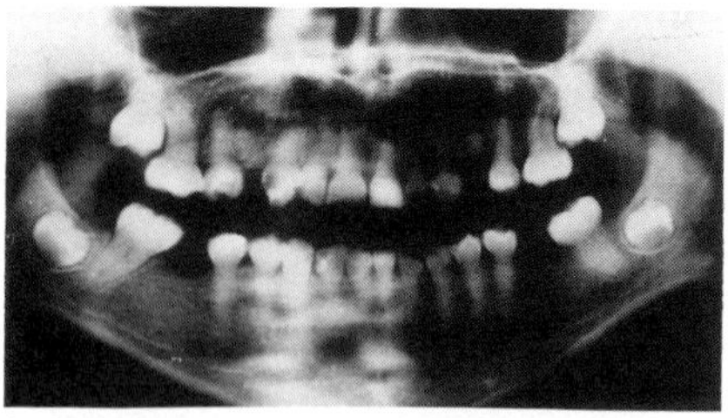

(g)

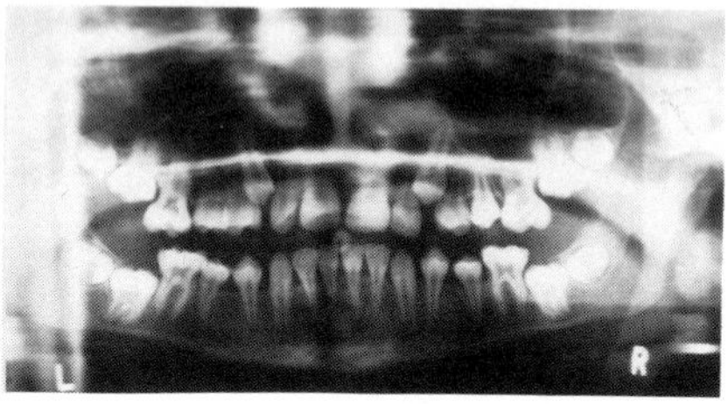

(h)

Figure 17.3 Continued

4b, d). The femora are unmodeled, as in type IIa. The type IIc phenotype shows slender long bones with inadequate modeling, although better than in IIa or IIb, and slender less uniformly beaded ribs than in IIb (Fig. 17. 4g). Sometimes there can be no beading of the ribs. He also described a type II OI in which the ribs can be fractured at birth in children who survive to adulthood. The classification is not completely comprehensive and does not fit all permutations of the physical signs. Thompson [4] has partially succeeded in resolving this situation. The classification should probably be extended to include several other phenotypes that can be accommodated in the present scheme. Radiologic pattern at birth is

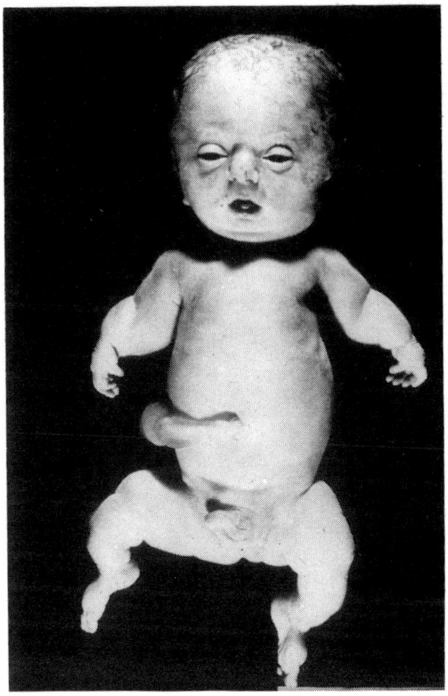

(a)

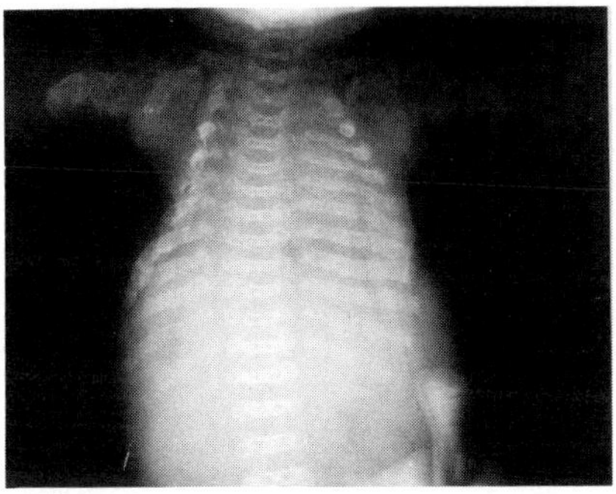

(b)

Figure 17.4 (a) Clinical appearance of child with Sillence type IIa OI. Notice distorted attenuated limbs and broad skull. (b) Chest x-ray from child with type IIa OI shows broadened, widened ribs with multiple fractures. (c) Nodular ribs from child with less severe type IIb OI. (d) Clinical appearance of child with type IIb OI. (e) Whole-body view of lethally affected fetus with Sillence OI type IIa. (f) Whole-body view of child described as type IIb by Sillence. (g) Whole-body view of fetus with OI type IIc.

an excellent indication of prognosis, genetics, and the likely type of mutation to be detected (see below).

Sillence Type III OI

Described by Sillence in 1979 [2] and associated with type IV OI by Thompson [4], the main features include fractures present at birth, grey, blue or white sclerae, with twisted long bones and progressive deformity (Fig. 17. 5a–f). Unlike Sillence type II OI, in which there is a very high frequency of prematurity, the majority of infants are born at full term. The radiologic changes at birth described by Sillence include multiple fractures of long bones and ribs. The femora can be shortened, broadened, or relatively normal and the ribs can be either normal or continuously beaded. Thompson's definition is much more precise but more limited than Sillence, and in the main describes a syndrome of

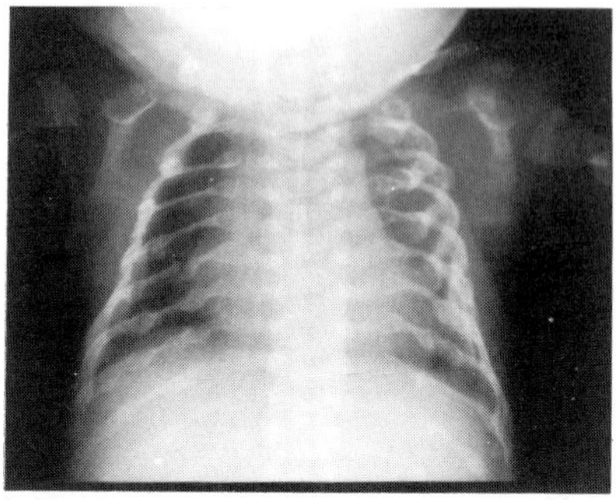

(c)

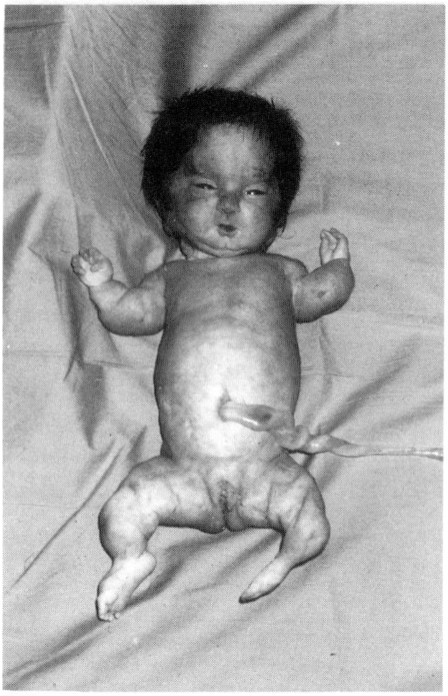

(d)

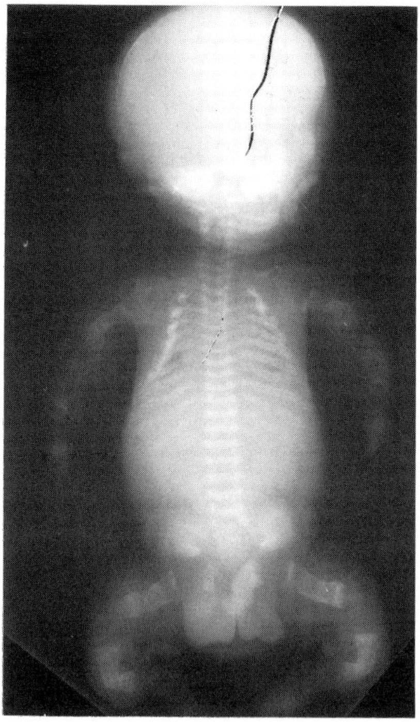

(e)

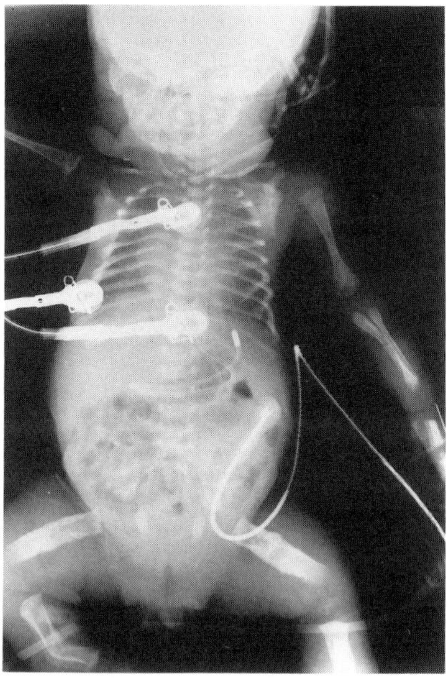

(f)

Figure 17.4 Continued

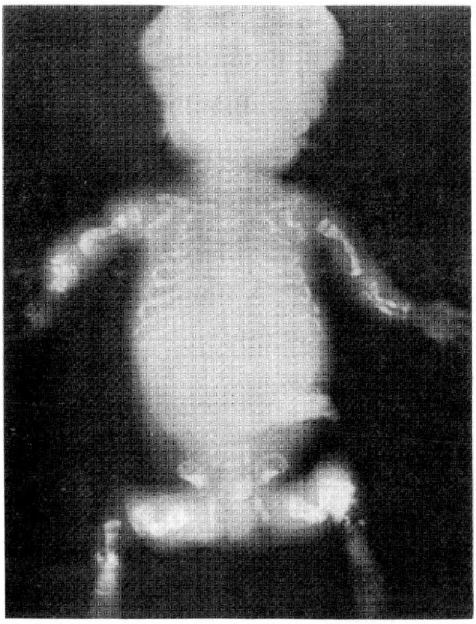

(g)

shortened femora with flared metaphyses and angulated diaphyses with mostly slender ribs (Fig. 17. 5d, f). Later the radiologic changes (Fig. 17. 5f) and popcorning of the lower ends of the femurs and upper ends of the tibiae are mainly characteristic. Sometimes clinically normal parents have premature osteoporosis (Fig. 17. 5e). Neither the Thompson or Sillence classification takes into account identical phenotypical changes (as described by both authors) but with blue sclerae. The most important feature of this subgroup is relentless progression and gross lower limb deformities that make walking impossible and limit the child's mobility to a wheelchair.

Sillence Type IV OI

Sillence's original description [2] was precise and well defined. This is an autosomal dominant multigenerational disease very like the type I phenotype (i.e., relatively mild), with the exception that the sclerae are white or grey rather than blue. Autosomal dominant inheritance is the rule and the prognosis is relatively good.

MOLECULAR PATHOLOGIC CHARACTERISTICS OF OSTEOGENESIS IMPERFECTA

Bones in patients with osteogenesis imperfecta are strikingly depleted in trabecular matrix, which in the most severe cases is almost absent (Fig. 17. 4a, b). The

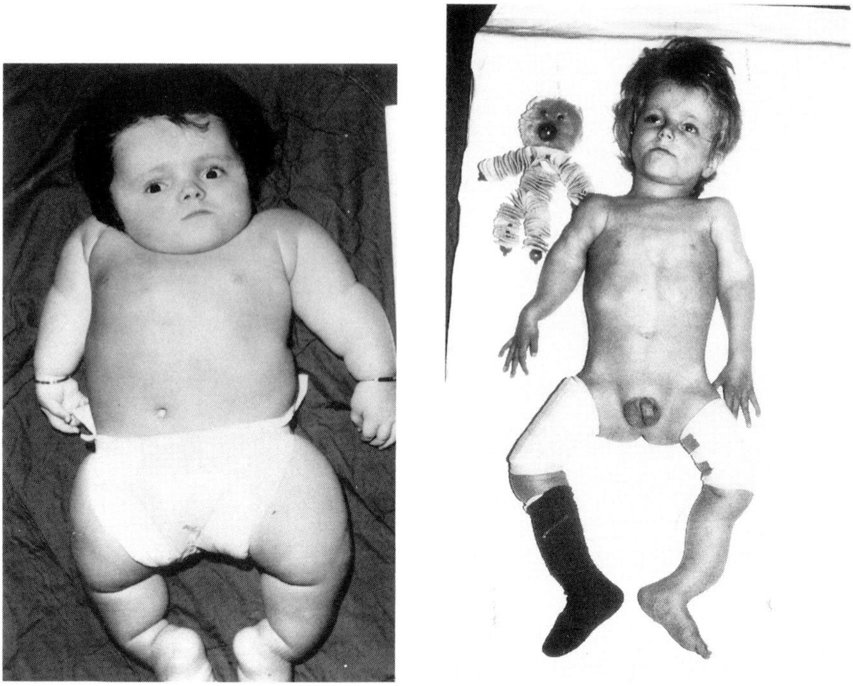

(a) (b)

Figure 17.5 (a–c) Typical clinical appearance of children with severe, progressively deforming Sillence type III OI. (d) Whole-body view of fetus with lethal Sillence type III OI. (e) Lateral lumbar spine of one heterozygous carrier parent of the fetus shown in (d). (f) Appearance of femora in surviving sibling of the lethally affected fetus in (d) as viewed at 12 months of age.

major protein of bone matrix is type I collagen with traces of collagen type III and V. Nearly all the molecular defects so far identified in OI affect one collagen gene (α1[I] or α2(I)], since Penttinen first described disturbed type I collagen synthesis in skin fibroblasts of lethal Sillence type IIa osteogenesis imperfecta. Many other abnormalities have been described, including various point mutations, small and large deletions, insertions, splice-junction and acceptor sites, substitutions, and regulatory mutations [6–10]. New dominant mutations and gonadal mosaicism have also been observed [11,12] and in some families there is preliminary evidence that genes other than α1(I) or α2(I) are to blame for the disease. Classic gene linkage studies in Sillence type I and type IV OI have confirmed the protein and gene data from individual cases and have basically shown type linkage to collagen α1(I) or α2(I) without exception [5].

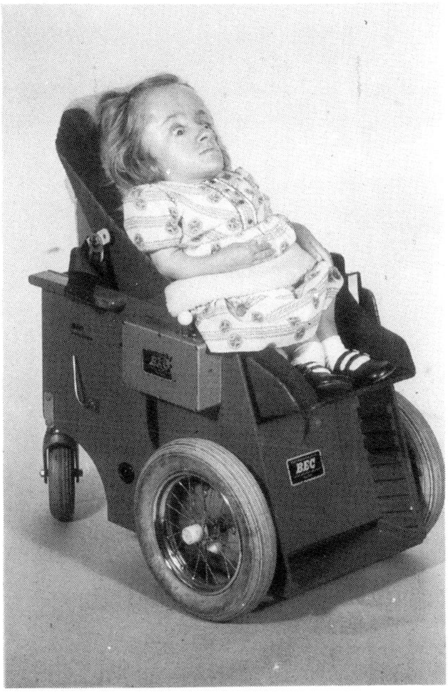

(c)

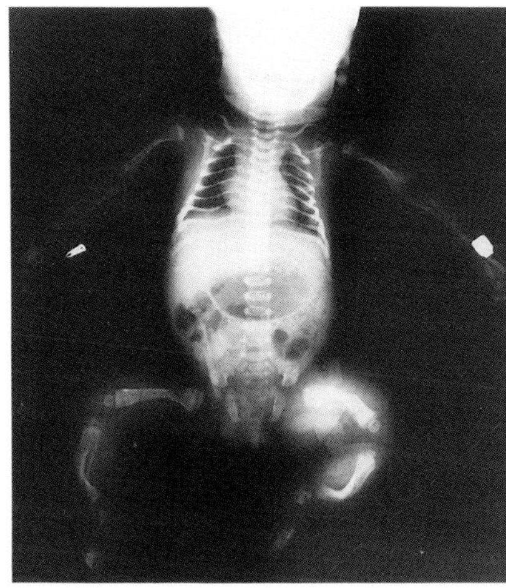

(d)

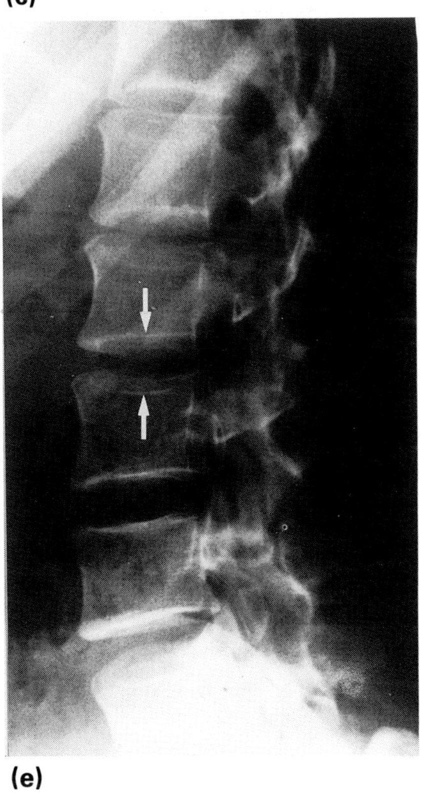

(e)

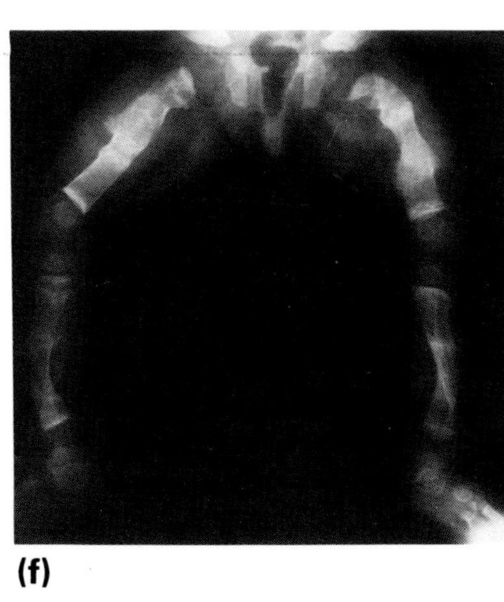

(f)

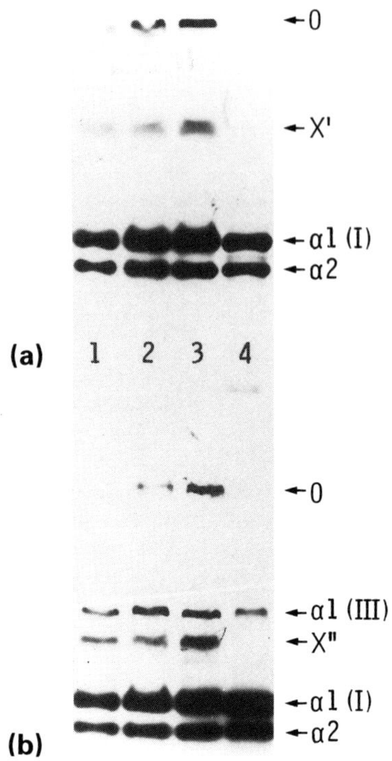

Figure 17.6 Five percent polyacrylamide gel electrophoresis of radiolabeled [^{3}H] collagen after pepsinization (a) unreduced and (b) reduced with mercaptoethanol. An unexpected disulfide linked dimer X^I is present and after reduction (X^{II}) runs below α1(III) and above α1(I). (c) Two-dimensional gel electrophoresis showing localization of the mutant cysteine to collagen peptide α1(I)CB6. (d) Normal melting profile of the mutant α1(I) dimer and normal α(I) and α2(I) chains from the radiolabeled collagens of this child. (e) Sequence of PCR amplified DNA covering the mutated region of α1(I)CB6 showing a glycine/cysteine mutation at position 1017. (f) Type I collagen profile of child with progressively deforming Sillence type III OI (shown in Fig. 5b) displaying electrophoretogram of radiolabeled collagens from upper control fibroblast line and lower patients' fibroblasts. (g) Sequence of amplified region of mutant α2(I) chain shows a four base pair deletion, reversing the whole sequence of the C terminus to an out-of-phase nonsense mutation.

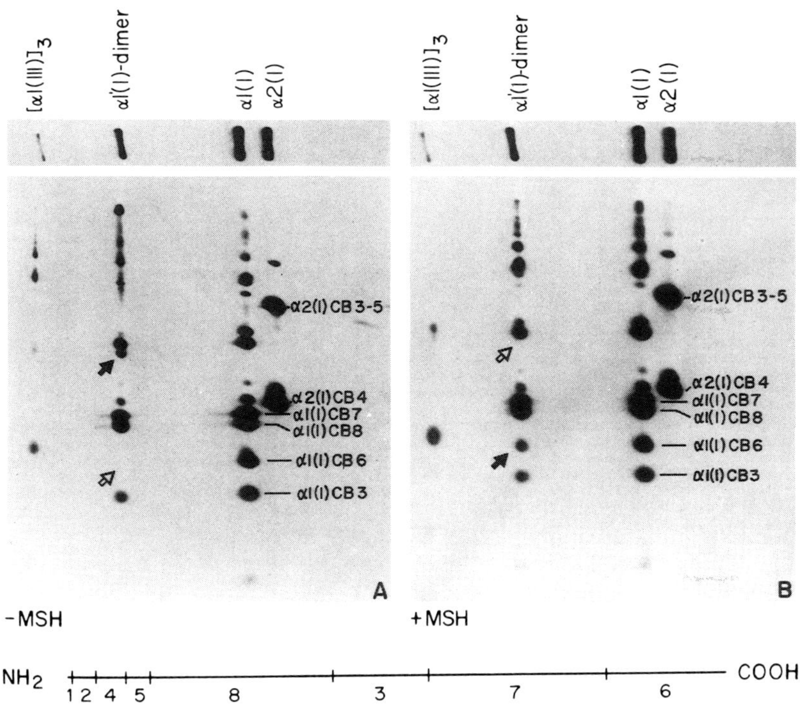
[α1(III)]3
α1'(I)-dimer
α1(I)
α2(I)
α2(I)CB3-5
α2(I)CB4
α1(I)CB7
α1(I)CB8
α1(I)CB6
α1(I)CB3
A
B
-MSH
+MSH
NH2
COOH
1 2 4 5
8
3
7
6

(c)

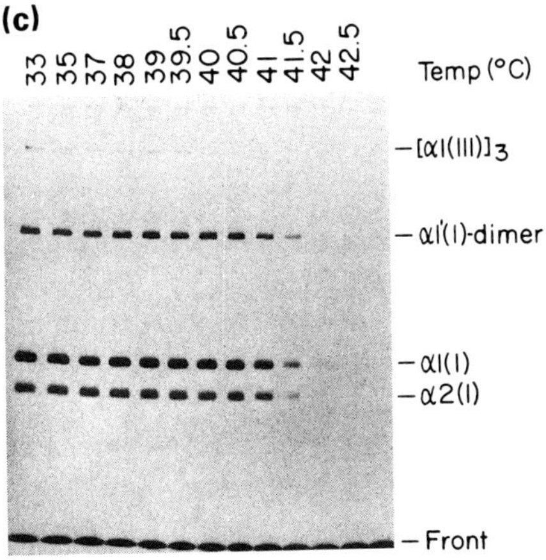
33 35 37 38 39 39.5 40 40.5 41 41.5 42 42.5
Temp (°C)
–[α1(III)]3
–α1'(I)-dimer
–α1(I)
–α2(I)
–Front

(d)

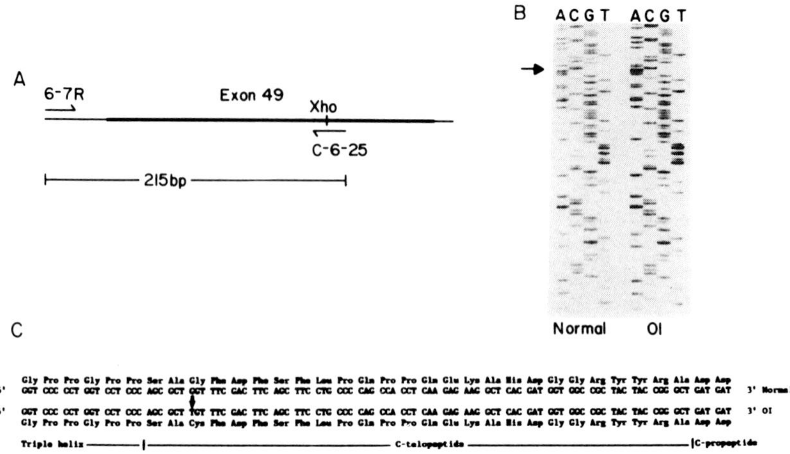

(e)

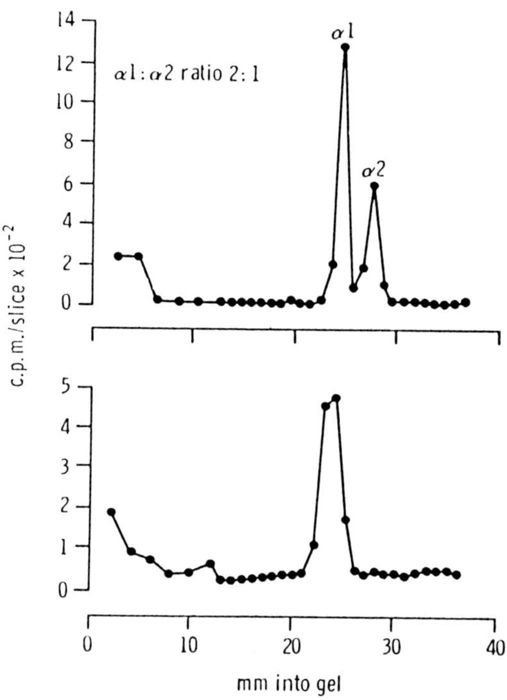

(f)

Figure 17.6 Continued

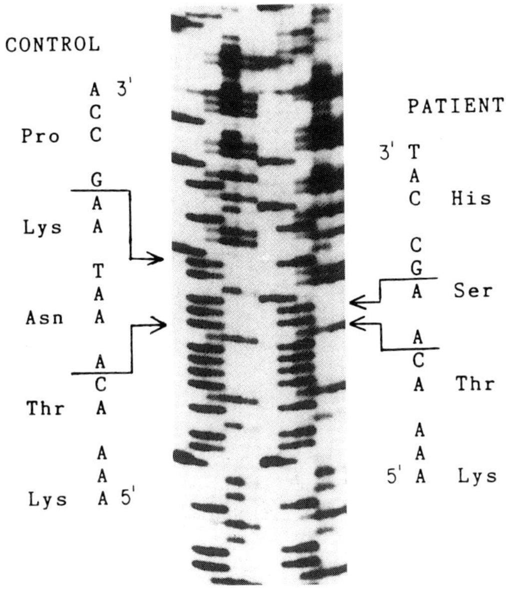

(g)

STRATEGY FOR MUTATION DETECTION IN OI

Skin fibroblasts, which are more convenient than osteoblasts can be used for the analysis of collagen mutations in OI. A 4 mm punch biopsy is used to establish primary fibroblast cultures which are conveniently stored in liquid nitrogen. With the use of $[^3H]$ or $[^{14}C]$proline, preferentially labeled procollagen can be examined by polyacrylamide gels using one-and two-dimensional electrophoresis for peptide mapping after treatment with cyanogen bromide (Fig. 17. a, b, c, e). In autosomal dominant mutations affecting helical winding, normal hydroxylation of lysyl and proline residues is exaggerated and overmodified from that point backwards to the N terminus (winding occurs from C–). Such changes are detectable as a diagonal retardation of the normally separated transverse peptide bands in two-dimensional preparations (smiling gels) [7]. The melting properties of collagen $\alpha 1$(I) or $\alpha 2$(I) chains are adversely affected by such mutations. This can be assessed by observing the susceptibility of separated $\alpha 1$(I) and $\alpha 2$(I) chains to trypsin over a range of temperatures near 37°C. The temperature at which the collagen helix is digested by trypsin indicates its conversion from a helical to a random coiled protein (Fig. 17. 6d). Accurate localization to a defined peptide (for which the published sequence is available on computerized data bases) allows the design of appropriate oligonucleotide gene sequences that flank the defect [11,13]. This can be followed by polymerase chain reaction (PCR) amplification of the mutant and wild-type gene fragments, which can either be cloned and sequenced or (Fig. 6e) sometimes sequenced directly, allowing the precise genetic defect to be defined. Prenatal diagnosis of that particular defect by chorionic villus biopsy is then possible either at the protein level by chorionic villus fibroblast culture and protein analysis or by RNA or DNA preparation and slot blot hybridization [11,12].

EXAMPLES OF MUTATION AFFECTING COLLAGEN TYPE I

Certain general rules emerge from the mapping of mutations by many different groups in the United States, Australia, Europe, and the United Kingdom [8–10]. Mutations within the C-terminal three-quarters of the molecule, including the C propeptide, are generally much more severe than those within the N terminal quarter of the molecule. Because of the specific biophysical effects of glycine occurring regularly at every third position of the collagen α helix $(glyxy)_{333}$, and the central positioning of glycines within the helix, their replacement by other larger amino acids (such as cysteine, alanine, arginine, valine, or serine) caused by a single base change, is severely disruptive.

Glycine mutations from residues 391 to 1003 are generally lethal while more N terminally placed cysteines, even when in the glycine position, produce rather mild disease. The cysteine mutation in the nonhelical globular C terminal portion of the molecule at position 1017 (Fig. 6a–e) produces remarkably mild OI (Fig. 6a–e). Yet only 28 aminoacids N terminal to this at position 998, the replacement of glycine by cysteine (within the helix) is lethal. Other similar mutations of glycine include arginine, alanine, serine, and asparagine. In brief, cysteine mutations have been recorded at positions 94, 175, 526, 691, 748, 904, 988, and 1017 ranging from mild at 94 and 1017 to severely crippling at 175 and 526 and lethal in all the rest. Similar considerations apply to a glycine to arginine mutations at positions 154, 391, 550, 667, 847, and 975. Fewer glycine to alanine (928) or serine (598, 637, 832, 964, and 1003) mutations have been detected; again the majority of them cause lethal Sillence type II OI. Other possible glycine mutations include tyrosine, valine, and stop codon changes and such alterations occur equally in $\alpha1(I)$, $\alpha2(I)$, or other collagens, producing various diseases [8]. A very useful and detailed clinicophysical mapping including all the recent point mutations and splice junction mutations has been published by Prockop and colleagues [9], and diagrammed by Byers [10]. Transgenic mice have now been created with glycine to cysteine or arginine substitutions at amino acid 859 of the mouse α1(I) protein [9] by using site-directed mutagenesis [14]. These animals have a stunted fetal phenotype very similar to osteogenesis imperfecta and represent good models for future studies in which other important collagen domains can be mutated. Obvious examples include 2nd position XY mutations, various cross-linking regions, and the N and C termini.

Deletions are relatively uncommon in OI, although a large 3-exon mutation of 84 aminoacids (600 base pairs [bp]) is omitted from the α1(I) triple helix of Pentinnen's original patient's cell line (ATC 1282). Other interesting mutations defined by Byers and his colleagues [10] include a 600 base pair insertion with a 3-exon duplication and a 7-exon 180 amino acid insertion in severe OI. A homozygous 4-bp deletion in the sequence of the collagen α2(I) and propeptide coding region produced a missense mutation in the remainder of this region and severely crippling Sillence type III OI in the affected proband [8] (Figs. 17. 5b, d; 6f, g). In general very similar changes to the α1(I) mutations can also occur in α2 chains.

Point mutations in splice donor or acceptor sites of intervening sequences cause missplicing of collagen exons that are frequently skipped. Thus collagen α1(I) or α2(I) chains produced in culture are usually short. One example is a deletion of exon 17 in father and son with OI. Fibroblast culture produced an abnormally short α1(I) chain [11]. An up-to-date splice junction map has been published by Byers [10]. Note that although exon 6 mutations invariably cause Ehlers-Danlos syndrome (EDS) VII without osteogenesis, splicing out of all exons from 8 to 47 cause variable severity of OI.

Very few mutations in the X or Y position of the collagen helix have so far been described and may be genetically neutral. Gonadal mosaicism is surprisingly common in recurrent lethal Sillence type II, IIb, IIc, and II/III OI and mixed gonadal/somatic mosaicism can produce great genetic variability between parent and child [11,12].

Several interesting clinical variations can result, including multiple recurrent lethally affected babies in whom the autosomal dominant pattern of the protein profiles suggests a low recurrence rate (two hits in a germ line mutation being very unlikely). In addition, mixed somatic and gonadal mosaicism is increasingly commonly detected especially using the new technique of DNA amplification by the polymerase chain reaction. Thus apparently mildly affected or normal-looking parents can produce lethally affected children. The latter have an easily mapped protein mutation that can then be cloned and sequenced at the gene level. Examination of DNA from various parental tissues such as fibroblasts, leukocytes, sperm or ovum samples, hair follicles, and others will show variable dosage of the mutant gene. Documented examples include a glycine to cysteine mutation at position 904 of collagen α1(I) chain with a mildly affected mother and lethally affected OI son, and a glycine to aspartic acid at position 988 of the collagen

$\alpha 1(I)$ chain in two infants with lethal perinatal OI whose clinically normal father showed varying gene dosage in fibroblasts, hair root bulbs, and lymphocytes [11].

Published gene linkage evidence shows that Sillence type I and IV OI are always caused by one or the other gene of collagen type I [i.e., $\alpha 1(I)$ or $\alpha 2(I)$] [5]. When individuals or small family groups are examined using specific protein alterations to map genetic defects, this also shows that OI is caused by either $\alpha 1(I)$ or $\alpha 2(I)$ changes. Sillence type IV is only associated with $\alpha 2(I)$ mutations while Sillence type I OI can be caused by $\alpha 1(I)$ or $\alpha 2(I)$ defects. So far no genetic compound of double $\alpha 1(I)/\alpha 2(I)$ mutations has been proved. Other evidence, however, suggests that genes other than type I may be involved in OI [15]. For example, we have recently studied severe autosomal recessive families with recurrent lethal OI occurring in consanguinous parents [15]. Although the protein data and peptide mapping clearly suggest a protein mutation localized to the region of $\alpha 1(I)$CB6 or $\alpha 2(I)$CB5 (at the extreme C terminal end of the protein and is followed by over hydroxylation of all subsequent N terminal peptides), the gene linkage data obtained by haplotyping the first-cousin parents show no shared $\alpha 1(I)$ or $\alpha 2(I)$ gene loci (RFLPs). Therefore, either a novel crossing-over or compound heterozygosity of the $\alpha 1(I)$ or $\alpha 2(I)$ genes has occurred or other genes are implicated in the pathogenesis of otherwise authentic osteogenesis imperfecta (with all the expected clinical, radiologic, and histologic features of this disease).

REFERENCES

1. McKusick VA. Osteogenesis imperfecta. In: Heritable disorders of connective tissue, 4th ed. St. Louis: CV Mosby, 1972: 390–454.
2. Sillence DO, Senn A, Danks DM. Genetic heterogeneity in osteogenesis imperfecta. J Med Genet 1979; 16: 101–16.
3. Sillence DO, Barlow KK, Garber AG, Hall JG, Rimoin DL. Osteogenesis imperfecta type II. Delineation of the phenotype with reference to genetic heterogeneity. Am J Hum Genet 1984; 17: 407–23.
4. Thompson EM, Young D, Hall CM, Pembrey ME. Recurrence risks and prognosis in severe sporadic osteogenesis imperfecta. J Med Genet 1987; 24: 390–405.
5. Sykes B, Ogilvie D, Wordsworth P, Wallis G, Mathew C, Beighton P, Nicholls A, Pope FM, et al. Consistent linkage of dominantly inherited osteogenesis imperfecta to the two collagen I loci:COL1A1 and COL1A2. Am J Hum Genet 1990; 46: 293–307.
6. Beighton P, De Paepe A, Danks D, et al. International nosology of heritable disorders of connective tissue (Berlin, 1986). Am J Med Genet 1988; 29: 581–94.
7. Bonadio JF, Byers PH. Subtle alterations in the chains of type I procollagen produce osteogenesis imperfecta type II. Nature 1985; 306: 363–6.

8. Pope FM, Daw SCM, Narcisi P, Richards AR, Nicholls AC. Prenatal diagnosis and prevention of inherited abnormalities of collagen. J Inherited Metab Dis 1985; 12 (Suppl.1): 135–173.
9. Kuivaniemi H, Tromp G, Prockop DJ. Mutations in collagen genes. Causes of rare and some common diseases. FASEB J 1991; 5: 2052–6.
10. Byers PH, Wallis GA, Willing MC. Osteogenesis imperfecta: translation of mutation to phenotype. J Med Genet 1991; 28:433–42.
11. Cohn DH, Starman BJ, Blumberg B, Byers PH. Germinal and somatic mosaicism for a mutation in a type I collagen gene (COL1A1) that produces lethal osteogenesis imperfecta. Am J Human Genet 1989; 45: 180–5. (abstr).
12. Constantinou CD, Pack M, Yang SB, Prockop DJ. Somatic cell mosaicism for a mutation in type I procollagen. The asymptomatic mother of a proband with lethal osteogenesis imperfecta is mosaic with a single base mutation that substitutes al (I) glycine 904. Am J Human Genet 1989; 45: 181. (abstr).
13. Cohn DH, Apone S, Eyre DR, Starman BJ, Andreassen P, Charbonneauh, Nicholls AC, Pope FM, Byers PH. Substitution of cysteine for glycine within the carboxyl terminal telopetide of the type I collagen produces mild osteogenesis imperfecta. J Biol Chem 1988; 263: 14605–7.
14. Stacey A, Bateman J, Choi T. Perinatal lethal osteogenesis imperfecta in transgenic mice bearing an engineered mutant proα1 (I) collagen gene. Nature 1986; 332: 131–6.
15. Nicholls AC, Daw SCM, Mitchell N, Levin LS, Green B, Mackenzie J, Evans DN, Chudleigh PA, Pope FM. Phenotypical features of an unique Irish family with severe autosomal recessive osteogenesis imperfecta. Clin Genet 1989; 35: 181–90.

18

Pseudoxanthoma Elasticum

F. Michael Pope

M. R. C. Clinical Research Centre, Harrow, England

Pseudoxanthoma elasticum (PXE) is an inherited disease of connective tissue characterized by elastic tissue deposition and degeneration in organs such as skin, arteries, buccal mucosa, the gastrointestinal tract, eyes, and lungs.[1]. The disease is generalized, commonly presenting with a variety of physical abnormalities mainly to dermatologists and ophthalmologists but sometimes to gastroenterologists, chest physicians, neurologists, surgeons, orthopedic surgeons, rheumatologists, pediatricians, general practitioners, and geneticists.

CLINICAL AND PATHOLOGIC SIGNS

The characteristic cutaneous lesion is widely distributed over the neck, axillae, groin, and flexures of the knees and elbows (Fig. 18.1). It is occasionally more widespread and generalized (Fig. 18.2a) but sometimes almost absent except for an occasional pinhead-sized papule or macule (Fig. 18.2b). Diagnostic changes are frequent over the buccal mucosa of the lower lip even when cutaneous changes are doubtful (Fig. 18.3a-c). The histologic changes in the yellow deposits are diagnostic with a wide band of fragmented calcified elastic fibers that stain specifically for elastin and calcium (Fig. 18.4c). Electron microscopic examination shows both normal and centrally calcified elastic fibers with occasional irregularities of collagen bundles forming rosettes (Fig. 4d, e). In apparently normal skin adjacent to typical elastin deposits there is only a slight overabun-

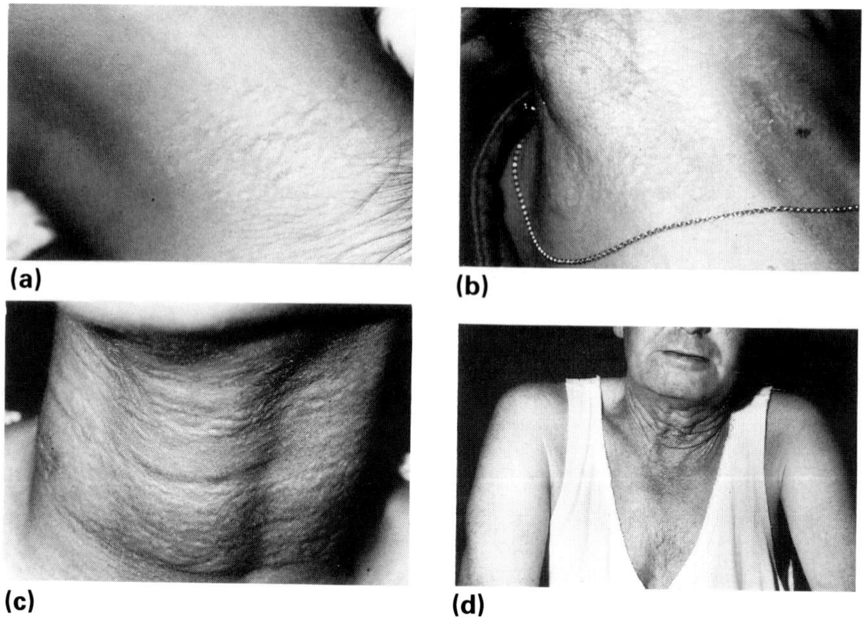

Figure 18.1 Typical cutaneous changes over the neck in various patients with PXE show (a) mainly localized papular rash, (b) more confluent changes over the posterior neck, (c) generalized peau d'orange infiltrates anteriorly, and (d) wrinkled redundant appearance over the anterior neck.

dance of elastin staining reminiscent of similar changes in acrogeric Ehlers Danlos syndrome type IV.

A distinctive elastic layer (Bruch's membrane) lies deeply to the retina and anterior to the choroid (Fig. 18.5a-e). Rents and irregularities of this membrane occur in areas of natural weakness such as around the optic nerve. This produces numerous radiating irregular cracks (angioid streaks) making the underlying choroid visible in contrast to the retina (Fig. 18.5a). Retinal blood vessels that lie anteriorly are more easily damaged with resulting microhemorrhages and scarring and visual impairment. When this coincides with the macula, central visual loss occurs; most typically in middle life and often after an identifiable injury (Fig. 18.5a–c). Pigmentation and proliferative scarring along the lines of the streaks are also common. Other typical ophthalmic changes include peau d'orange mottling of the posterior retinal poles, salmon spotting at which ill-defined but occasionally punched out discontinuities and pallor of the retina appear, thickening of the retinal basement membrane (drusen), which are common close to the optic disc. A snowstorm appearance with confluent salmon spotting and drusen (Doyne's choroiditis) (Fig. 18.5e) is a rare but spectacular complication (Fig. 18.4a–c). Visual acuity usually drops dramatically after the age of 40 years with a 30–40% frequency of acuities of 6/18 or below in a cross-sectional survey (unpublished data). Myopia, which has a 7–10% frequency in the British population was more than four times as common in the same series of patients with PXE.

Other complications of PXE include essential hypertension in some families and a low (10–15%) but dangerous frequency of gastrointestinal bleeding, which often recurs in pregnancy. No single cause of bleeding emerges and documented reasons include microaneurysms, aneurysms of medium-sized arteries, esophageal tears, arteriovenous malformations such as hematomas, and gastroduodenal ulcers. In rare cases no single source of bleeding is apparent and a generalized hemorrhagic catastrophy occurs that cannot be controlled by transfusions of fresh frozen plasma and more than 60 units of blood. Vigorous attempts should always be made to identify the source of bleeding including gastroscopy and high-resolution angiography despite which total gastrectomy is occasionally needed but is nevertheless life-saving. Bleeding from similar lesions lower down the gastrointestinal tract can also occur with a similar distribution of causes including bleeding from various diverticulae, angiomas, and microaneurysms. However, gastrointestinal bleeding affects only 10% of published cases and is probably substantially rarer in the general population of patients with PXE, many of whom go through a normal life undiagnosed and untroubled. On the other hand, obvious gastric irritants such as alcohol, aspirin or nonsteroid anti-inflammatory agents, and very hot spicy foods are best avoided.

VASCULAR DISEASE AND OTHER COMPLICATIONS

Since arterial media are so rich in elastin, especially in the larger vessels, and arterial calcification and intimal proliferation are relatively widespread in arteries of patients with PXE, strokes from cerebral thrombosis and peripheral arterial occlusion are only slightly more common than in the general population. Nevertheless, in cases, rare, spectacularly widespread coronary artery occlusion with angina and early myocardial infarction can occur in young adults. We have recently observed two women aged 22 and 32 years with severe occlusive disease. The former required triple bypass replacement and the latter has been successfully managed conservatively. In rare cases cerebrovascular complications including microaneurysms, aneurysms of the circle of Willis, and carotid aneurysms or transient ischemic attacks and occasional thrombosis have been documented. Yet the overwhelming impression gained in caring for several hundred patients with this disease is of a surprising lack of vascular thrombosis and occlusion despite the very widespread nature of elastic degeneration and arteriosclerosis in PXE arteries. Other minor complications include nose bleeds, bruising, and hematuria.

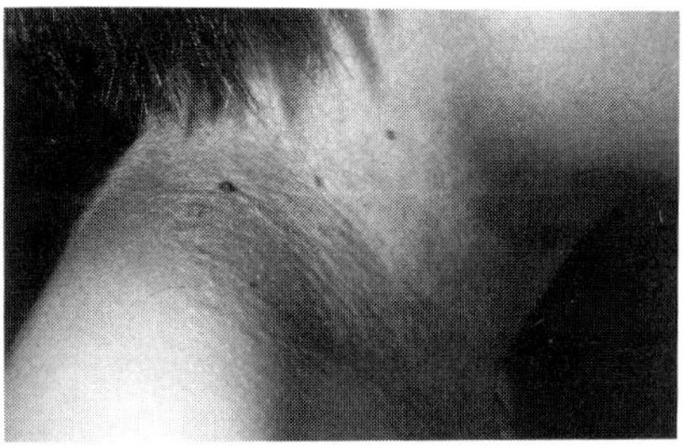

(a)

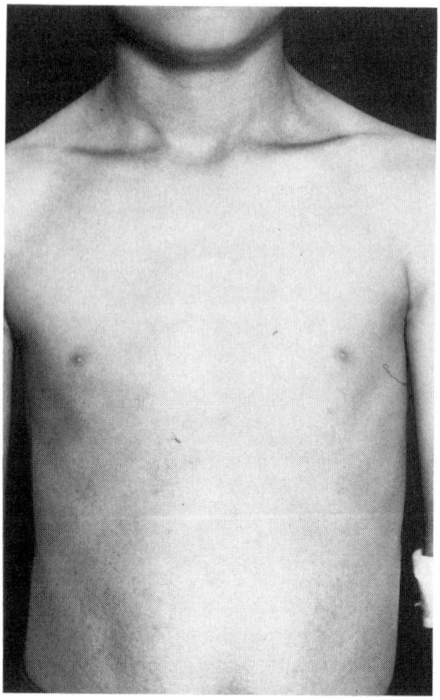

(b)

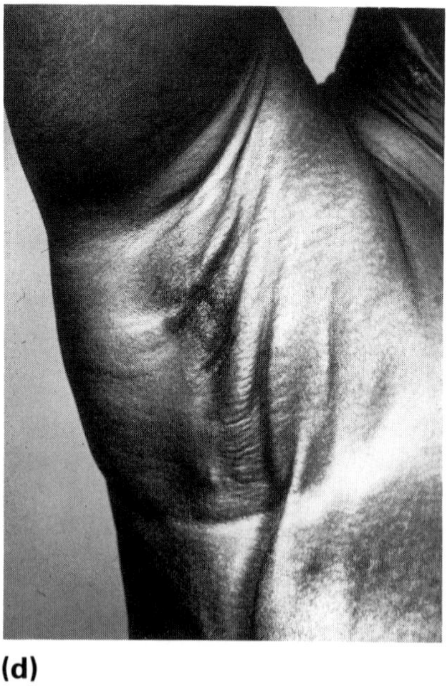

(d)

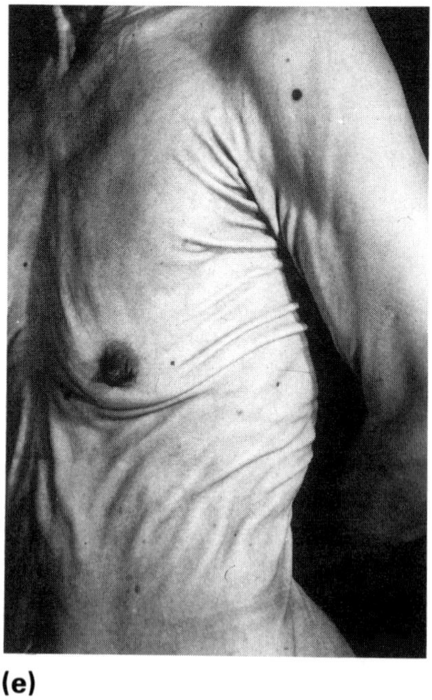

(e)

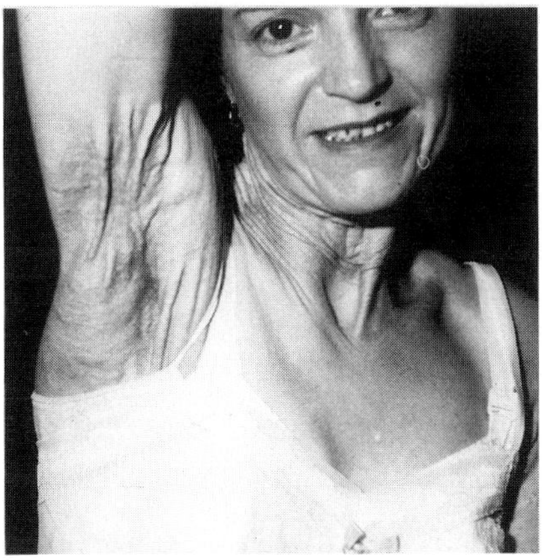

(c)

Figure 18.2 Range of clinical patterns varies from (a) few cutaneous papules, (b) generalized papular infiltrate, (c) widespread infiltration and cutis laxa of neck and axillae, to (d,e) complete cutaneous infiltration of entire skin.

Pregnancy, in the main, is safe except that difficulties with conception, recurrent prepartum hemorrhage, perineal tears necessitating mandatory episiotomy or low forceps delivery and postpartum hemorrhage are common. Also women with previous gastrointestinal bleeding frequently relapse during pregnancy, but such bleeding is rare for the first trimester. No problems occur with prematurity or postmaturity, 90% of patients with PXE having been born between the 39th and 41st week of pregnancy.

Other common associated features include hints of more generalized connective tissue features such as joint hyperextensibility (65%), increased cutaneous extensibility (86%), pectus excavatum (25%), high arched palate (52%), and long extremities (arachnodactyly; 17%).

EPIDEMIOLOGIC CHARACTERISTICS AND GENETICS

Population estimates of incidence vary from 1:70,000 to 1:1000,000 [1–3]. For example, Berlyne estimated a frequency of 1:160,000–1/1,000,000 in England and Wales, McKusick 1:60,000 in the United States and Altman and his colleagues 1:70,000 in Seattle. Neldner's estimate in Denver, Colorado, was 1:100,000. My own estimate in an attempted complete ascertainment in the United Kingdom was more than 1:200,000, although, depending upon the efficiency of ascertainment and the difficulty in diagnosis. It may have been as low

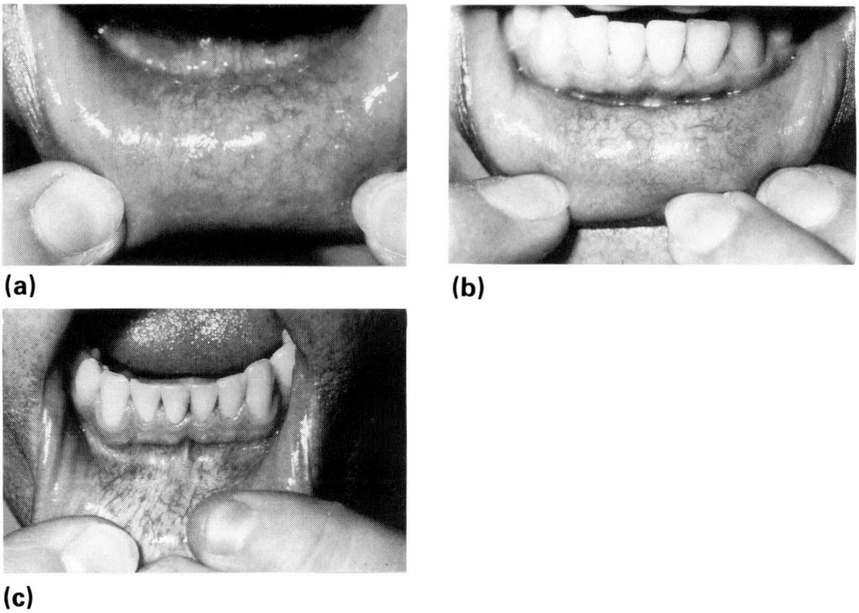

Figure 18.3 Typical submucosal infiltration of lower lip shows (a) barely detectable, (b) obvious, and (c) florid elastic infiltration.

as 1:40,000 (assuming one-fifth ascertainment). This compares closely with similar estimates for Marfan's syndrome, osteogenesis imperfecta, and Ehlers Danlos syndrome but is very much less common than the benign hypermobile syndrome, which is as frequent as 10% in the white population of the United Kingdom.

The genetics of PXE is controversial. Neldners position is that PXE is nearly always autosomal recessive [3] (over 90%) and that dominant disease is either nonexistent or extremely rare. My own view is that autosomal dominant disease occurs in a small but significant proportion of patients with PXE [4,6], but that recessive pedigrees are at least twice as common.[5] Sporadic cases in which the inheritance is unclear are the norm. Certainly there is good historical evidence for autosomal dominance (recent unpublished evidence), in which there were four convincing British pedigrees with three and possibly four-generation transmission of a typical PXE syndrome (and several smaller pedigrees with less impressive numbers). The autosomal dominant figures were swelled by another group of patients in whom PXE segregated in several generations with variable clinical features such as blue sclerae, pectus excavatum, joint and cutaneous

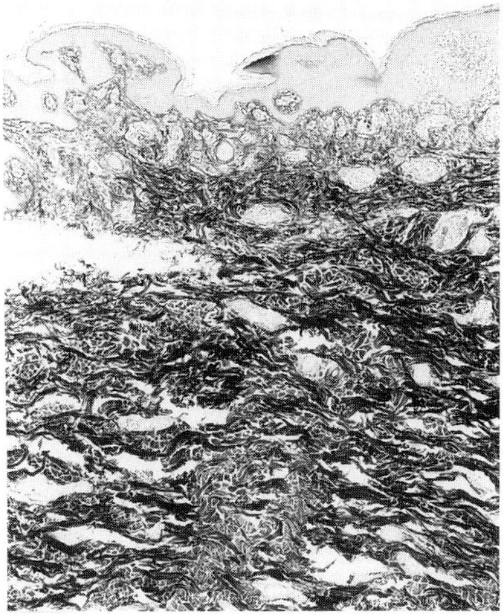

(a)

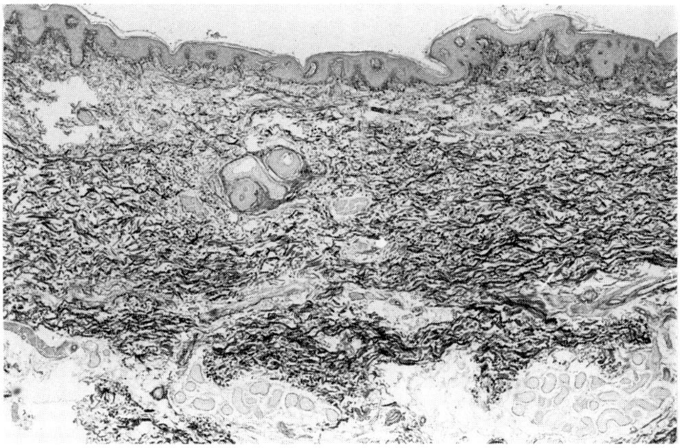

(b)

Figure 18.4 Typical histologic changes of orcein-stained skin sections (EVG × 65) for (a) normal control, (b) patient with typical EDS IV, (c) normal-looking skin from patient with PXE, and (d) typical biopsy specimen from elastic tissue infiltrate of PXE. Both EDS IV and normal-looking PXE skin display increased elastic staining but there is normal collagen staining in PXE compared with reduced quantities in EDS IV. An elastic papule from PXE skin shows typical clumping fragmentation of elastic fibers. (e) Electron microscopic examination of elastic fibers of PXE skin shows central calcium accumulation of otherwise normal-looking elastic fiber with normal, amorphous, and microfibrillar appearance. (f) Unusual rosette formation and variable collagen diameter are visible on skin from patient with PXE and joint hypermobility.

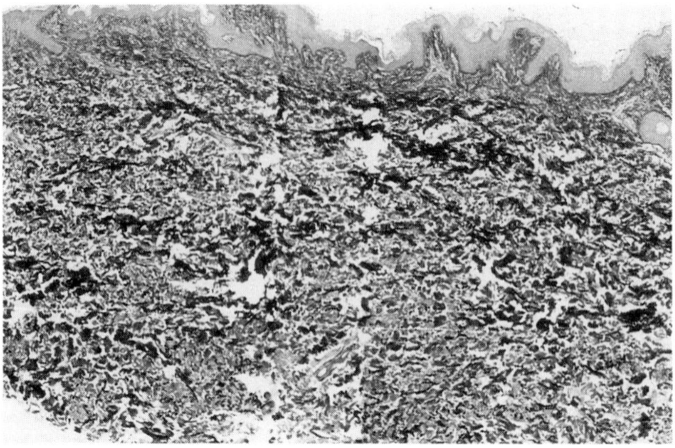

(c)

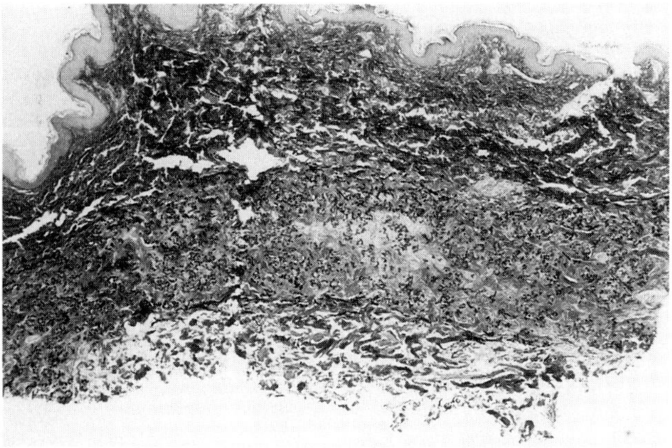

(d)

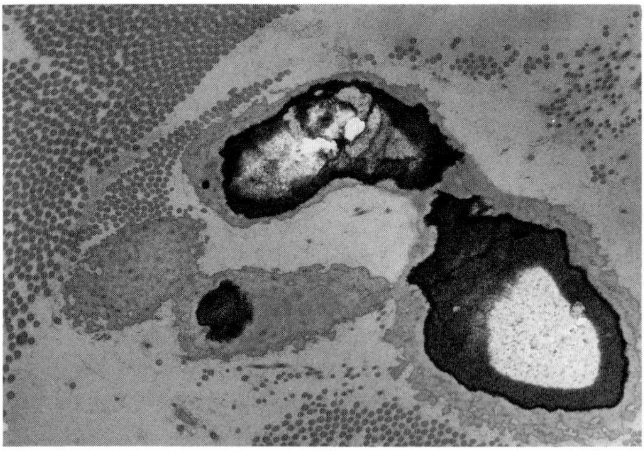

(e)

Figure 18.4 Continued

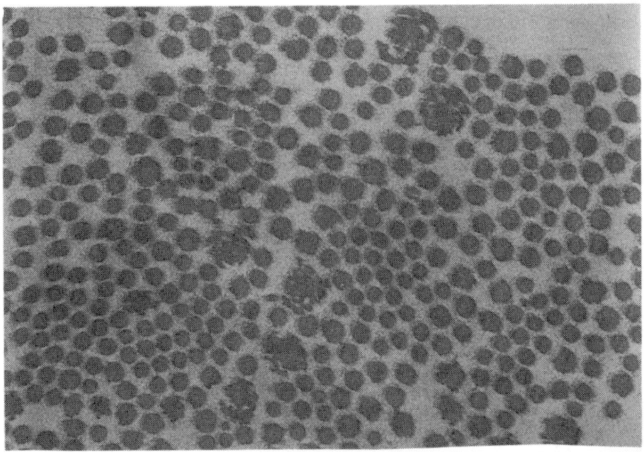

(f)

laxity, and rather variable elastic tissue changes including variable cutaneous pseudoxanthomas and angioid streaks. Possibly the compound interaction of two genes, one probably elastin and the other collagenous, may explain the high frequency of generalized joint laxity with elastin deposition in those single-generation PXE families with multiple affected siblings.

PREVIOUS EVIDENCE OF INHERITANCE

Very important families previously described in the literature and reviewed in previous publications include those described by Jones, and colleagues (two-generation families), Marchionini and Turgot (three affected children with unaffected mother), and the family of Cahill with five affected individuals in two generations. The families described by Collier (five affected children with an affected mother) and Goodman (three affected children with an affected father) are also impressive. Percival's family, in which PXE segregates with cutaneous elastosis in three generations, is also intriguing. There are also many published and convincing families in whom autosomal recessive inheritance is the most likely explanation. Included among them are those described by Batten (three of six affected siblings), Jones and colleagues, (four consecutively affected siblings), Goldblad (two of eight affected siblings in a first-cousin marriage), Lehrfield and Braun (three of nine affected siblings in one generation only). There are many other smaller affected families but Stegmaier's description of four affected siblings in one generation and an affected baby in the next generation from an affected/unaffected sibling mating is particularly interesting.

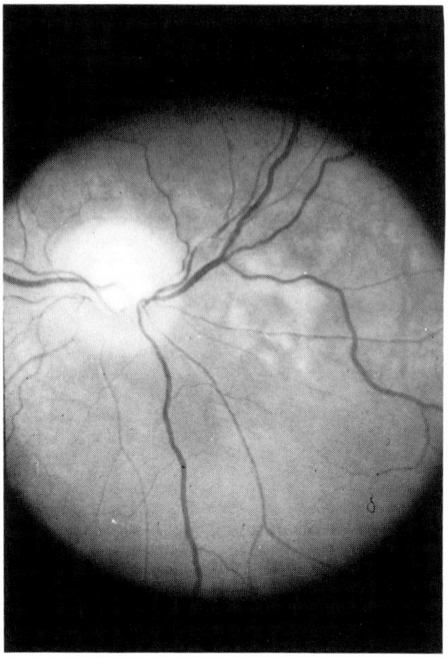

(a)

Figure 18.5 Typical ophthalmic changes include (a) infiltration close to macula, (b) wide angioid streaks radiating from optic disc, (c) thinner but more widespread angioid streaks, (d) macular scarring and degeneration, (e) peau d'orange infiltration of peripheral retina, and (f) generalized Doyne's choroiditis. Changes in (e) and (f) occurred in two Asian patients with florid generalized cutaneous infiltration.

MECHANISM

Any mechanism accounting for PXE has to explain all features of the disease, including several clinical forms and patterns of inheritance. It must also address the presence and absence of generalized connective tissue disorders such as joint laxity and blue sclerae and the various microscopical changes such as increased calcified and degenerated elastin, collagen depletion and elastin proliferation (in normal areas), and subtle changes in normal elastin components (at the electron microscopic level) despite overcalcification with irregularities of collagen fiber shape and form (twisting and rosette formation). The similarity of some changes to those of acrogeric Ehlers-Danlos syndrome (EDS) IV suggest a possible link with type III collagen mutations. The evidence here is contradictory and scanty. For example, gene linkage in one good autosomal dominant family excluded the type III gene as candidate, yet collagen and procollagen profiles can show apparent lowering of type III levels in some families but not in others. That PXE is a

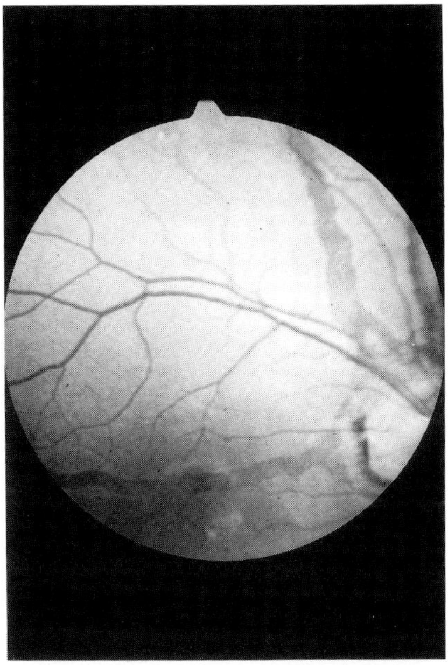

(b)

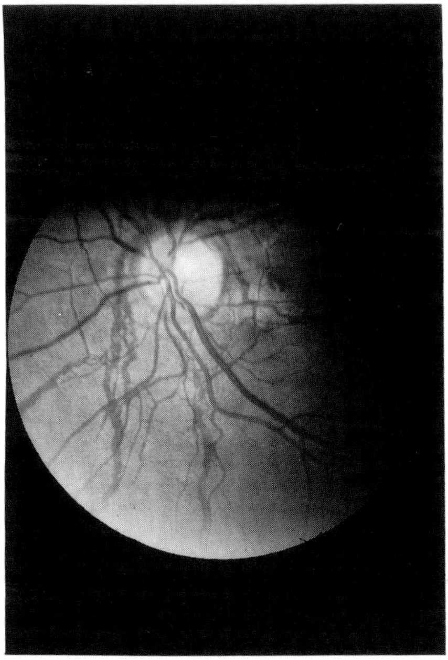

(c)

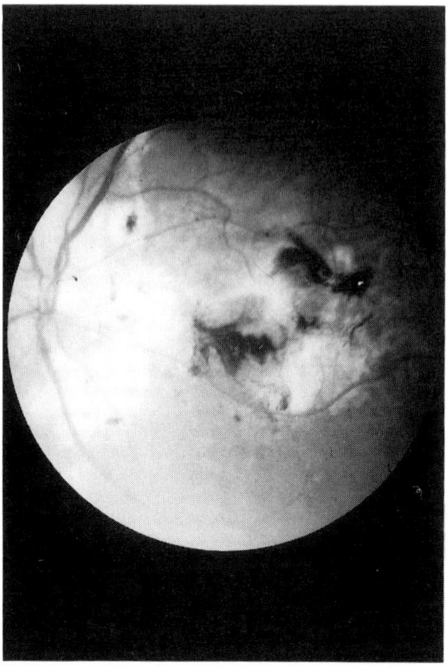

(d)

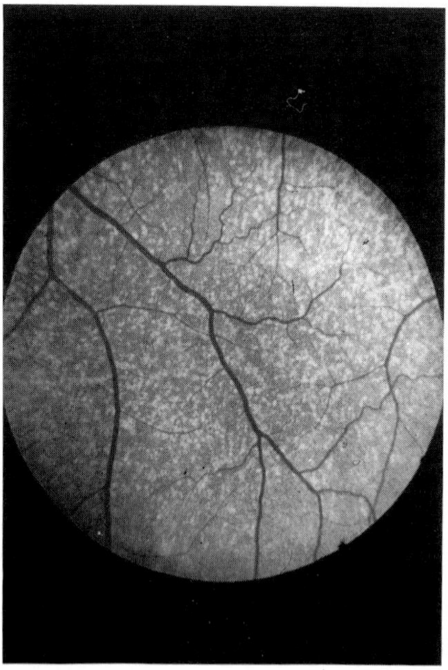

(e)

Figure 18.5 Continued

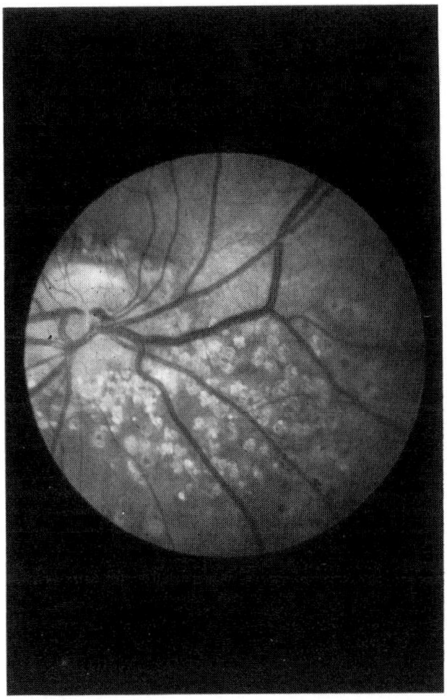

(f)

primary elastic fiber disease is by no means certain. It probably is genetically heterogeneous, with different mechanism for each chemogenetic subgroup and substantial variability within each subgroup.

Candidate genes worth excluding include collagens III and VI, elastin (microfibrillar and amorphous components), fibrillin, chondroitin sulfate, and hyaluronic acid. The best approach is a combined one of testing protein profiles in cultured fibroblasts in the various families and genetic subtypes. Then in a suitable pedigree and three-generation families, exclude linkage to the most likely candidate genes before using the candidate gene linkage approach to localize the mutant gene. These demanding studies of well-documented large families bear always the danger of missing the candidate gene by failing to recognize the possibility of genetic heterogeneity and causes.

From our own recent experience we can conclude the following:

1. Autosomal dominant PXE is an entity. Families with and without severe eye disease have been observed.
2. Autosomal recessive PXE also occurs with a phenotype indistinguishable from the autosomal dominant type.

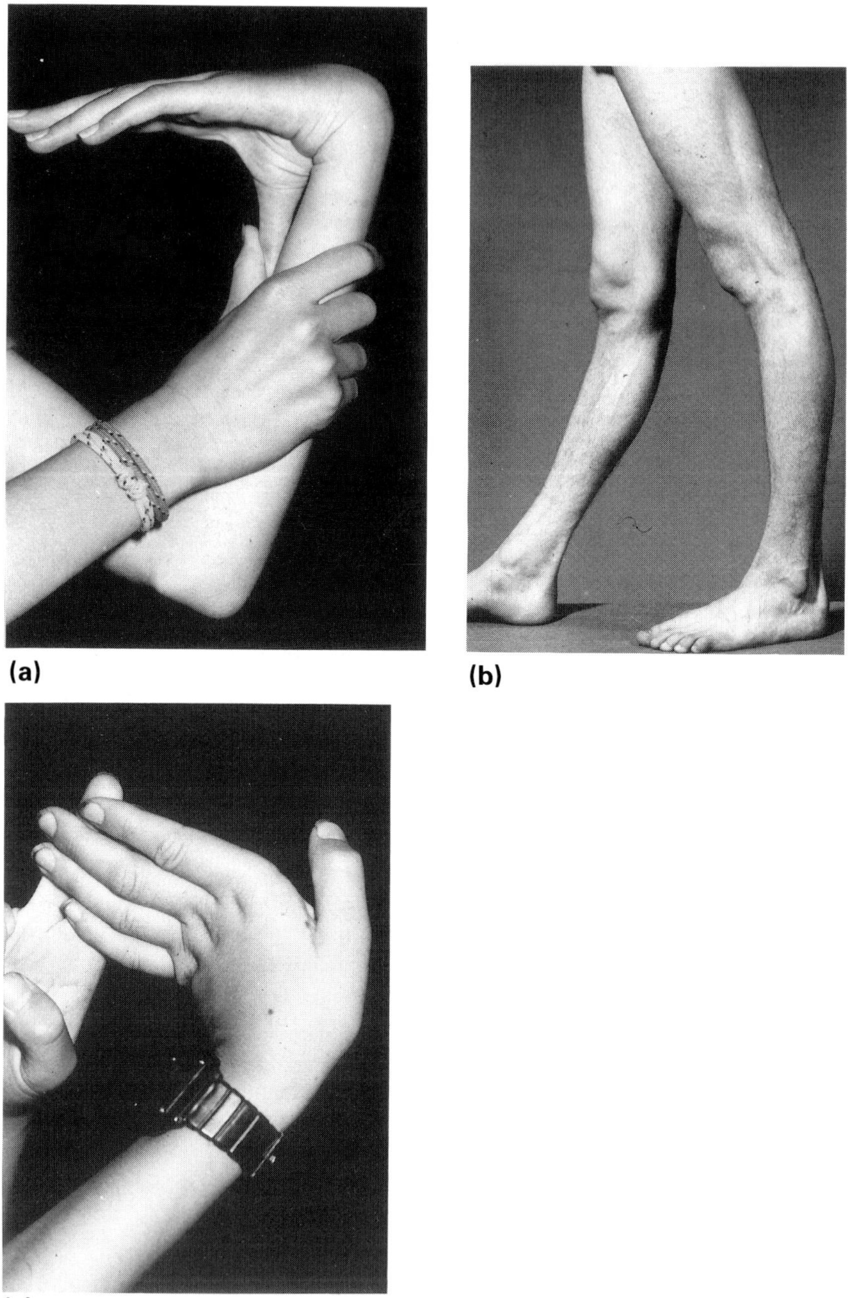

(a) (b) (c)

Figure 18.6 Generalized joint laxity of (a) thumb, (b) knees, and (c) metacarpophalangeal joints from patient with PXE and generalized connective tissue features.

3. In some families with many affected siblings and unaffected parents, gonadal mosaicism is a possibility.
4. A syndrome with combined benign hypermobile syndrome and PXE occurs and it is unclear whether this is a variable dominant, codominant, or chance association.
5. There are resemblances and possible overlap of PXE with type III collagen defects such as Ehlers Danlos syndrome type IV.
6. The majority of patients with PXE have sporadic disease and cannot confidently be designated as having autosomal dominant or recessive inheritance on clinical grounds. A priori recessive inheritance is at least twice as common as dominant inheritance, but the very careful examination of children and siblings by skilled ophthalmologists and dermatologists is desirable.
7. No good genetic markers for PXE presently exist, but elastin, collagen, and fibrillin are all good candidate genes, the importance of which can now be systematically tested.
8. Although gastrointestinal bleeding is relatively rare, when it does occur, it can be persistent (up to 50 pints blood transfused) and recurrent (especially in pregnant women with prepregnancy bleeding). Gastroscopy, angiography, measurement of plasma concentrates, partial and complete gastrectomy are all options to be considered and microaneurysms, angiomas, ulcers and hemorrhagic gastritis are the usual causes. Aspirin, alcohol, and gastric irritants should be avoided routinely.
9. Visual problems are rare in patients under the age of 40 years but regular follow-up by an interested ophthalmologist is desirable and mandatory if there is any sudden change in visual acuity.
10. Thrombotic occlusions of arteries are rare but smoking should be discouraged.
11. Hypertension and hypercholesterolemia should be vigorously controlled and treated when present.

CASE REPORTS

Case 1

A 33-year-old previously healthy woman with symptomless angioid streaks was referred by her optician to an ophthalmologist. Two years later she developed central chest pain radiating down the left arm on exertion and an exercise electrocardiogram and thallium 201 scan confirmed significant coronary artery disease. One year earlier endometriosis had been diagnosed on laparoscopy for evaluation of dysmenorrhea. Since then she has remained well and her condition is controlled with occasional sublingual administration of GTN. Clinical examination showed no visible cutaneous PXE, minor angioid streaks, and generalized joint laxity. Her pedigree was remarkable as she is 1 of 11 children. Of these only her younger sister was available for examination: she too was loose-jointed and had angioid streaks. She had scanty papular changes of PXE over the nape of the neck (Fig. 18.2b) and both sisters showed typical yellow infiltrates of the mucosal surface of the lower lips (Fig. 18.3a, b). Of her 9 other siblings the eldest had died of severe gastrointestinal bleeding, another brother had suffered severe vision loss at the age of 52 years, the third brother is developing visual impairment. Both parents were reputedly unaffected, the father is still alive aged 82 years; the mother died of a hypertensive stroke aged 79 years. Most of the third generation live in the Caribbean and are unavailable for examination, but two of them have the typical rash of the disease.

This is a family with multiple affected siblings in one and possibly two generations who have variable cutaneous changes ranging from typical to absent. In these circumstances lower lip infiltration was a helpful aid to diagnosis. Unfortunately the third generation lives abroad and was unavailable for examination. Nevertheless the disease apparently segregates as an autosomal dominant trait. Gastrointestinal bleeding and angina are irregular complications in this family, the former affecting only the eldest affected male and the latter the proposita.

Case 2

A 39-year-old man was referred from his general practitioner with a 3 year history of recurrent unexplained gastrointestinal bleeding. This had occurred in two phases: first in childhood between the ages of 6 and 11 years when he had bled and received transfusions on four separate occasions. Each time no obvious cause was found. After a trouble-free period of 19 years he again has had several episodes of gastrointestinal bleeding, sometimes associated with hematemesis and on other occasions with melena. On one of these latter occasions the cutaneous changes of PXE were noted for the first time. He had not been aware of them himself and considered all his relatives to be normal. Clinical examination showed the classic peau d'orange PXE of the neck, axillae, and flexures, a diastolic blood pressure of 100–111mm Hg, and minimal angioid streaking without macular changes. So far we have been unable to examine his family.

Case 3

A 53-year-old man presented to an opthalmologist after a routine eye test had shown angioid steaks and maculopathy. Clinical examination showed classic cutaneous PXE of the neck and flexures with buccal involvement. In addition he had blue sclerae and marked joint hypermobility. He knew that two of his three children, his brother, and his grandchildren were already affected since he had observed the typical cutaneous features. He considered his eldest child to be normal, but his elder son was particularly interesting since he had affected children from both his marriages. The younger son showed classic PXE of the neck and axillary fold, while the patient's mother was unaffected and his father dead.

This is a clear example of autosomal dominant transmission of typical PXE through three generations. Its origins in this family are obscure. In the absence of consanguinity and in view of its subsequent pattern, gonadal mosaicism is a possibility.

Case 5

A 9-year-old expatriate Vietnamese child was referred by his local dermatologist because of a widespread abdominal rash. Otherwise he was completely healthy and asymptomatic. Clinical examination showed unusually confluent PXE of the whole skin, which was especially obvious over the neck, flexures, abdomen, and groin (Figure. 18.1d). Routine histologic examination confirmed typical deposits of PXE. He had no other generalized connective tissue features. His fundi showed generalized peau d'orange mottling but no angioid streaks or maculopathy (Fig. 5d). His two siblings and parents were normal.

This is an example of an unusually severe widespread form of cutaneous PXE in the absence of connective tissue features such as joint laxity occurring in an unusually young patient. The fundal changes were similarly widespread and unusual without producing visual impairment. The features were similar to those families previously separated into a distinct autosomal recessive subgroup.

Case 6

A 24-year-old white man and his 27-year-old brother were diagnosed as having an unusual skin rash in early childhood. The older brother was otherwise asymptomatic until the age of 25 years, when a massive hematemesis was uncontrolled after 50 pints of blood and necessitated a complete gastrectomy. He successfully recovered but developed a troublesome dumping syndrome. Both he and his brother showed extensive cutaneous PXE of the neck, axillary, and flexures accompanied by capillary telangiectasia of the anterior chest. In addition both brothers had blue sclerae, loose-jointedness (Fig. 18.6), and cutaneous extensibility with transverse sacral striae. One of their siblings and both parents were similarly hyperextensible, with other features including blue sclerae, extensible skin, and flattened plantar arches. Electron microscopic examination showed rosette collagen fibers in one of the two brothers. Although unrelated, their parents' ancestors originated from the same small local rural community.

This family illustrates several important features of PXE: the difficulty of predicting the recurrence of gastrointestinal bleeding from other physical signs, the potentially catastrophic nature of this complication in some families, and the rarer occurrence in affected males. It is a good example of possible autosomal inheritance in a small (inbred) community. The cosegregation of a generalized connective tissue syndrome suggests various possibilities such as the coinheritance of two separate disorders of connective tissue, two separate but codominant disorders, or compound heterozygosity of two similar mutations. Resolution of these possibilities awaits the availability of appropriate polymorphic candidate gene probes for more detailed study.

REFERENCES

1. McKusick VA. Heritable disorders of connective tissue 4th ed. St Louis: CV Mosby 1972:475–520.
2. Pope FM. Pseudoxanthoma elasticum: an historical survey. Trans St. Johns Hosp Dermatol Soc 1972; 58:235–50.
3. Neldner KH. Pseudoxanthoma elasticum. In: Parish LC, ed. Clinics in dermatology, vol. 6. Philadelphia: JB Lippincott, 1988.
4. Pope FM. Autosomal dominant pseudoxanthoma elasticum. Med. Genet 1974; 11:152–7.
5. Pope FM. Two types of autosomal recessive pseudoxanthoma elasticum. Arch Dermatol, 1974; 110: 209–12.
6. Pope FM. Historical evidence of the genetic heterogeneity of pseudoxanthoma elasticum. Br J Dermatol 1975; 92: 493–509.
7. Doyne RW. Choroidal retinal changes: the result of blows on the eyes. Trans. Ophthalmol UK 1889, 9:128–9.
8. Darier J. Pseudoxanthoma elastique. Trans Third Int Congr Dermatol London.

19

Epidermolysis Bullosa

Leena Bruckner-Tuderman
University Hospital Zürich, Zürich, Switzerland

Epidermolysis bullosa (EB) describes a large group of genetic blistering disorders affecting most visibly the skin, but also other organs with stratified epithelia. All of these are characterized by epithelial–mesenchymal splitting and blister formation after minor trauma. The different clinical subsets of the disease are associated with a (presumably large) variety of molecular defects, of which only few have been characterized at the molecular level.

For a review of the structure of the dermoepidermal junction affected in EB, the reader is referred to Chapter 4.

CLASSIFICATION AND CLINICAL FEATURES

More than 20 different clinical and genetic subsets of EB have been described (for review, see [1–3]). These forms can be placed into three main categories: EB simplex (EBS), EB junctionalis (EBJ), and EB dystrophica (EBD), a division based on the level of blistering. EB simplex subtypes are characterized by blister formation inside the epidermis (i.e., true epidermolysis). Junctional EB results from separation of the epithelium between the lamina densa of the basement membrane and the basal keratinocytes (i.e., through the lamina lucida). Dystrophic EB demonstrates blisters that heal with atrophic scarring as a result of blister formation below the lamina densa. A more exact molecular characterization of the EB subtypes will show whether all of them represent independent genetic

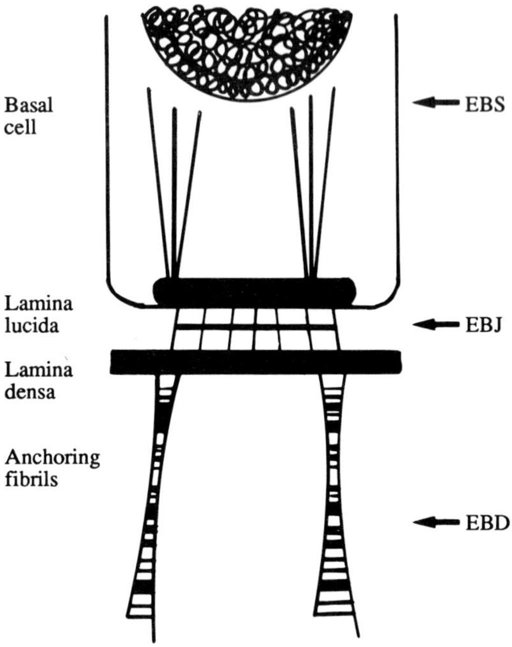

1 D-EBS generalisata
2 D-EBS localisata
3 R-EBS localisata
4 D-EBS Ogna
5 D-EBS with mottled pigmentation
6 D-EBS herpetiformis
7 D-EBS herpetiformis with mottled pigmentation
8 R-EBS with muscular dystrophy
9 R-EBS letalis
10 R-EBS Kallin
11 X-EBS Mendes da Costa

1 R-EBJ gravis
2 R-EBJ generalisata
3 R-EBJ localisata
4 R-EBJ inversa
5 R-EBJ progressiva
6 R-EBJ cicatricans

1 D-EBD generalisata
2 D-EBD localisata
3 R-EBD localisata
4 R-EBD inversa
5 R-EBD generalisata
6 R-EBD generalisata mutilans

Figure 19.1 Classification of epidermolysis bullosa according to the level of blistering. On the left, a schematic representation of the structural components of the dermo-epidermal junction zone. The arrows symbolize the splitting levels in the three major EB categories. On the right, the individual subsets of each major category are listed. D: dominant ; R: recessive; X: x-linked.

defects or whether they are differently expressed forms of the same disorder. In Fig. 1 the three main categories of hereditary EB and their subgroups are schematically represented along the level of blistering. The clinical features of the individual disorders will be reviewed in the following and examples are shown in Figures 19.2-4.

EB Simplex

All 11 subtypes show intraepidermal blisters and healing of the primary lesions without scars. However, after secondary traumatization or infection, scarring may occur. Blisters can be induced by heat and friction. The course of the disease is usually mild: blisters are present at birth or develop in early infancy but there

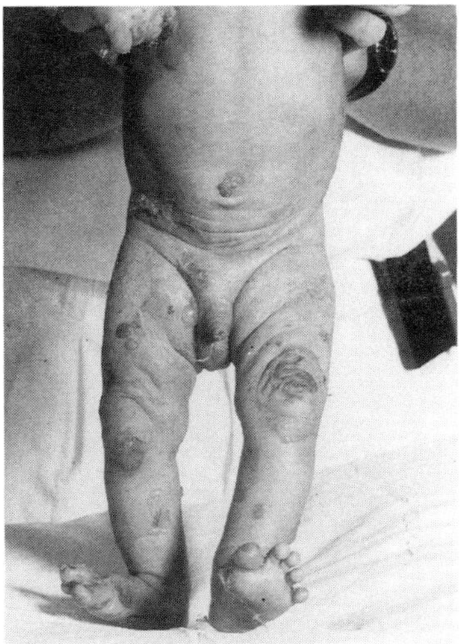

(a)

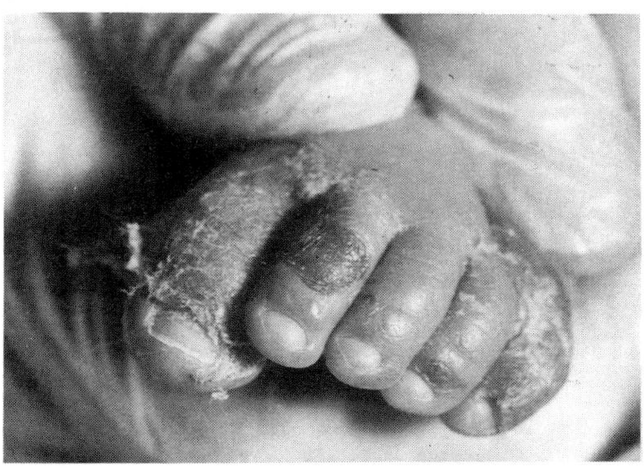

(b)

Figure 19.2 Epidermolysis bullosa simplex. (a) An infant with generalized blistering and healing without scars. (b) Detail shows the trauma-prone left foot with blisters, erosions, and crusts. The nails are normal.

is remarkable improvement after puberty. The phenotypic characteristics of each subtype are listed below.

EBS Generalisata (Koebner's disease)

Blisters occur on the whole integument but preferentially involve the skin of hands and feet, especially palms and soles. Diffuse palmar-plantar hyperkeratosis may be present. Nails and teeth are normal and oral mucous membranes are rarely involved. Inheritance is autosomal dominant.

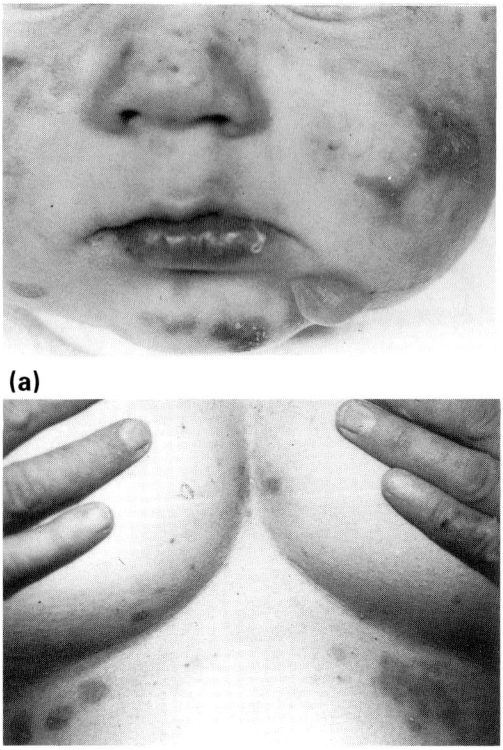

(a)

(b)

Figure 19.3 Epidermolysis bullosa junctionalis. (a) A child with generalized EBJ presents with numerous blisters on the face and head. (b) In a patient with the inversa subtype, blisters are localized in the submammary folds and on the fingers. Healing occurs without scars, but with slight skin atrophy and hyperpigmentation.

EBS Localisata (Weber-Cockayne Disease)

This is the most common variant of EBS. The recurrent, often painful, blisters are limited primarily to palms and soles. Onset is usually by toddler age, but can be as late as the twenties. Oral blisters are rare. Hyperhidrosis may be an accompanying symptom. Inheritance in most cases is autosomal dominant; one family has been documented with autosomal recessive inheritance.

EBS Ogna

In addition to seasonal acral blistering, patients exhibit tendency for skin bruising and often onychogryphotic nail changes. Thus far only Norwegian cases have been reported. A genetic linkage to glutamic–pyruvic transferase (GPT) polymorphism was demonstrated. Inheritance is autosomal dominant.

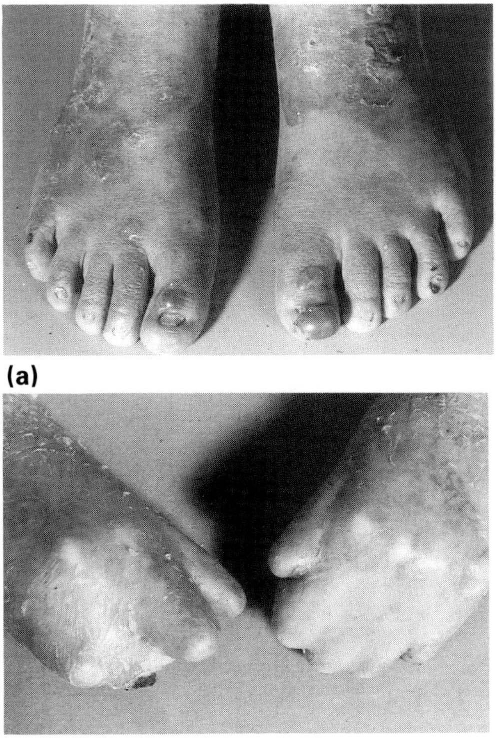

(a)

(b)

Figure 19.4 Epidermolysis bullosa dystrophica. (a) Typical blistering, nail dystrophy, and scarring of the feet in localized dystrophic EB. (b) Extensive mutilation of both hands as a result of repeated blistering and scarring in recessive generalized mutilating subtype.

EBS with Mottled Pigmentation

An asymptomatic, striking irregular mottled hyper-and hypopigmentation of the proximal extremities and the trunk accompanies blistering of trauma-exposed sites. Slight skin atrophy, palmar–plantar hyperkeratosis, onychodystrophy, mucosal blistering, and cariotic teeth can be part of this disease. Inheritance is autosomal dominant.

EBS Herpetiformis (Dowling-Meara Disease)

The outstanding clinical feature is the herpetiform distribution of the blisters on the whole integument. The blisters may spread in a centrifugal manner and heal rapidly leaving no scars but postlesional hyperpigmentation. Large blisters on palms and soles, oral blisters, palmar–plantar hyperkeratoses and repeated loss of nails are typical. No seasonal aggravation is found. The skin clears during high fever and rapidly improves around school age. Eye and tooth involvement may occur. Inheritance is autosomal dominant.

EBS Herpetiformis with Mottled Pigmentation

Herpetiform blistering is present at birth and is accompanied by postbullous hyperpigmentation as well as by a mottled, bizarre pigmentation of the neck and trunk from the age of 2–3 years. Plaquelike and punctate palmar–plantar hyperkeratoses are characteristic. Lost nails usually regenerate normally but sometimes become dystrophic. Inheritance is autosomal dominant.

EBS Associated with Muscular Dystrophy

Generalized blistering from birth is associated with progressive muscle dystrophy. Limited atrophic scarring, loss or dystrophy of nails, and loss of teeth are characteristic of the disease. Inheritance is autosomal recessive.

EBS Letalis

A large Sudanese family presented with generalized trauma-induced blistering with predilection for distal extremities, oral blisters, and erosions and postlesional dyspigmentation, but no involvement of nails, teeth, or hair. A considerable mortality rate within the first 2 years of life was associated with this disease. Inheritance is autosomal recessive.

EBS Associated with Anodontia, Hair, and Nail Disorders (Kallin syndrome)

Localized acral blistering of the palms and soles accompanied by anodontia, brittle hair, nonscarring alopecia, and onychogryphosis or curving nails was described in a Swedish family. Inheritance is autosomal recessive.

EBS Mendes da Costa

Trauma-induced blistering with predilection for the extremities during the first years of life is part of a complex syndrome including alopecia, dyspigmentation, and microcephaly. Inheritance is X-linked.

Extracutaneous involvement is not very common in EBS. However, blistering in the oropharynx and esophagus has been reported [4].

Junctional EB

The six subsets of junctional EB (EBJ) present with splitting through the lamina lucida and healing without scars and milia. The severity and course of the symptoms vary greatly: the most dramatic disease leads to death within the first year of life, but in the mild progressive subset the symptoms do not appear until the teens and show a very benign course. In the milder variants, gradually appearing atrophy of skin is typical, and nail deformities, hoarseness, and dysphagia may accompany the skin symptoms. Usually the blistering worsens in summer.

EBJ Gravis (Herlitz disease)

This is the most severe subtype of the whole EB family, also called EB letalis. Characteristics are extensive, progressive skin and mucosal blistering followed by erosions and infections. The prognosis is poor: most patients do not reach the age of 12 months, even though older survivors have been described. There are no definitive phenotypic characteristics to differentiate this from the more benign types in an early postnatal phase. Inheritance is autosomal-recessive.

EBJ Generalisata

This form is also called atrophicans generalisata mitis, referring to the mild course of generalized blistering from birth, which heals with mild skin atrophy. Nail dystrophy, hyperkeratoses, and hair loss are usual features. Inheritance is autosomal recessive.

EBJ Localisata

Blistering is limited to hands and feet with some involvement of proximal extremities. Nail loss, mucosal involvement, and enamel hypoplasia may occur. Usually the disease exhibits a mild course without systemic affection. Inheritance is autosomal-recessive.

EBJ Inversa

Generalized blistering at birth disappears after some months and recurs. After the teens, the blistering concentrates on the inversa areas: axillary and inguinogenital bends, neck, lower back, and buttocks. Sometimes oral blistering and dysphagia are found. Female sex hormones exhibit a positive effect: improvement of the symptoms during pregnancy and worsening after menopause are seen. Inheritance is autosomal-recessive.

EBJ Progressiva

Dystrophy and loss of nails are usually the first symptoms which appear late, between the ages of 5 and 15. Acral blistering, which can involve also palms and soles, follows often after years. Healing leads to gradual mild atrophy with loss of fingerprints. Oral blisters occur. Hypoacusia may accompany. Inheritance is autosomal-recessive.

EBJ Cicatricans

In this subset there is a discrepancy between the clinical appearance and the ultrastructural findings: despite junctional splitting with rudimentary hemidesmosomes, on electron microscopic (EM) examination, the blisters with acral predilection heal with scarring and syndactyly may occur. Oral blistering, tooth dysplasia, loss of nails, and stenoses of anterior nares are accompanying features. Inheritance is autosomal-recessive. Involvement of the digestive, pulmonary, and genitourinary systems and the eye has been documented [4].

EB Dystrophica

All six diseases of this subset present with dermal blistering below the basement membrane and subsequent scarring and milia formation. A great deal of clinical heterogeneity is observed. Two of the subtypes are inherited in an autosomal-dominant and four in an autosomal-recessive manner.

Dominant Traits

EBD Generalisata (Pasini disease)

This form is also called albulopapuloidea because of the whitish papules of the back that often accompany the disease. However, whitish papular lesions are found in patients with other subtypes of EB as well, and to date the albulopapuloid sign is no longer considered pathognomonic for EBD generalisata. Blistering appears in the first week of life and becomes generalized with involvement of the head and trunk. Healing occurs with larger areas of atrophic scarring. Oral blisters and nail dystrophy are observed.

EBD Localisata (Cockayne-Touraine disease)

Strictly acral blistering occurs from birth or from early childhood. Nail dystrophy is common but oral blisters or tooth abnormalities are rare.

Recessive Traits

In the past this group of syndromes has been considered to be one disease, often called recessive dystrophic EB of Hallopeau-Siemens. However, by now, after better pathophysiological, immunochemical and ultrastructural analysis, it has become obvious that several subtypes can be identified. Probably all of them represent distinct genetic disorders.

EBD Localisata

Acral blistering appears from birth. Atrophic scars resembling cigarette paper develop distally from the elbows and the knees. Nail and tooth dystrophy is common. It may be impossible to differentiate this type clinically from dominant EBD localisata. Inheritance is autosomal-recessive.

EBD Inversa

The neonatal generalized blistering and scarring concentrate on the trunk in childhood and in school aged children on the inversa regions: axillary, inguino-genital and submammary folds, lower back, neck, as well as hands and feet.

Esophageal involvement is often extensive, and as a typical sign the lingual frenulum is shortened as a result of early oral blistering and scarring. Teeth are normal.

EBD Generalisata, Non-mutilating

Generalized blistering is present at birth. Acral predilection is obvious; however, the patients have generalized traumatic blisters on the trunk as well. Mucosal blistering, dystrophy of teeth, and loss of nails almost always occur. Esophageal involvement may occur. Notably, there is no mutilation or syndactylies.

EBD Generalisata, Mutilating

This form belongs to the most severe subsets of the EB family. Generalized blistering is present at birth, extends progressively, and leads to remarkable scarring. Already in childhood syndactylies of hands and feet develop leading to the characteristic mitten-like hands and feet. Scarring causes joint contractures. Mucosal blistering is severe and esophageal strictures common. Teeth are severely affected and dental treatment may be difficult because of the mucosal involvement. Probably because of limited nutritional intake due to eating difficulties, the growth is retarded and anemia develops early. Eye involvement may be present.

Involvement of the respiratory, digestive, and genitourinary system has been described. The symptoms are found more often in the recessive than the dominant types [4].

The Bart syndrome, which is also known as congenital localized absence of skin, was believed to be a distinct entity of EB. To date this condition has been observed as an early symptom of several EB subtypes and should no longer be described as a separate disorder [2]. Epidermolysis bullosa acquisita is an acquired chronic bullous autoimmune disorder with EBD-like symptoms and autoantibodies against type VII collagen in the anchoring fibrils. It does not belong to the group of hereditary EB, despite its misleading name.

ULTRASTRUCTURAL ABNORMALITIES

Electron microscopic investigations of EB skin have been invaluable in determining the level of blistering and in classification of the disorders [5,6]. However, compared to the multitude of phenotypic expression of the subsets the ultrastructural analysis has yielded relatively little information about mechanisms leading to the dermoepidermal disintegration.

EB Simplex

In all EBS the blistering occurs as a result of cytolysis of the basal keratinocytes. The splitting takes place in the subnuclear space just above the hemidesmosomes.

In two subtypes, an additional structural abnormality can be observed: EBS herpetiformis shows a characteristic clumping of tonofilaments in the basal cells [5] and EBS with mottled pigmentation presents with focally interrupted and discontinous basement membrane [7].

EB Junctionalis

There is separation through the lamina lucida in all subtypes. A hemidesmosome hypoplasia, reduction in number of hemidesmosomes, and rudimentary attachment plaques and subbasal plates is seen in many but not all patients. No ultrastructural characteristics to differentiate between the individual disorders of the EBJ group have been found [6]. An exceptional form is EBJ progressiva, in which deposits of electron-dense material in lamina lucida were observed in some patients who had normal hemidesmosomes [5].

EB Dystrophica

This group has been the object of intensive ultrastructural study, and some confusion. There are still differences of opinion as to the extent of involvement of anchoring fibrils. Most studies point out that anchoring fibrils are absent in the recessive EBD generalisata, mutilating, despite the fact that some patients exhibited reduced numbers of normal anchoring fibrils [5, 6]. Immuno-electron-microscopic studies with antibodies to collagen VII, the main structural protein of anchoring fibrils, demonstrated an absence of staining in this subtype [8]. We recently examined two patients with EBD inversa and found no intact anchoring fibrils (Fig. 19.5) whereas other investigators recorded some poorly structured fibrils. Localized forms of EBD, both dominant and recessive, present with a variably decreased number of normal anchoring fibrils. In the generalized dominant EBD the anchoring fibrils may be qualitatively abnormal and reduced in number [5, 6]. The interpretation of the ultrastructural findings is complicated by the normal variation of density of anchoring fibrils in different locations.

Little functional information can be gained from morphologic analysis alone. A combined approach using immuno-electron-microscopy with specific antibodies and biochemical characterization of the involved structures of the dermoepidermal junction zone will yield relevant new structural information in the next few years.

IMMUNOCHEMICAL ABNORMALITIES

Several monoclonal or polyclonal antibodies against antigens of the dermoepidermal junction demonstrate selective abnormal staining patterns in EB skin [6, 9]. The localization of the antigens was determined by immunofluorescence and

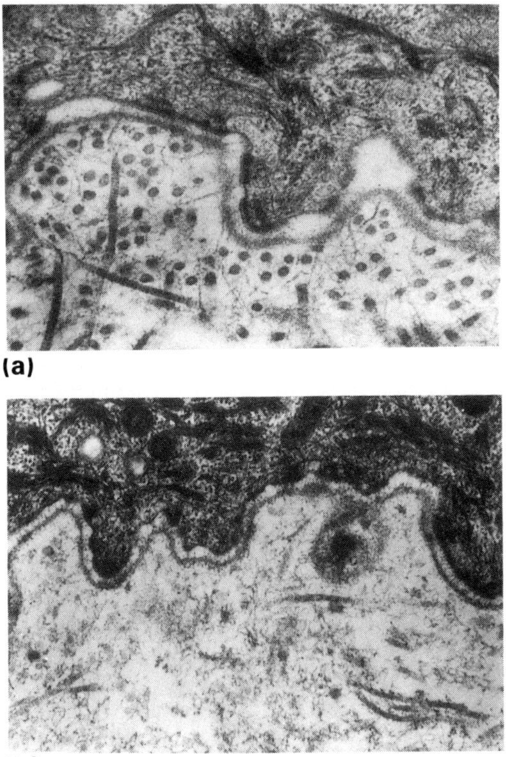

Figure 19.5 Ultrastructure of the dermoepidermal junction zone in (a) normal skin and (b) recessive EBD inversa. Note the absence of intact anchoring fibrils in (b).

immuno-electron-microscopy on salt-split skin, but the biochemical characteristics of most of these proteins are not known. The only exceptions are collagen VII, the major structural protein of anchoring fibrils, and the GB3 protein [10], which may be associated with hemidesmosomes. Both of these have been extensively characterized. Collagen VII is absent from skin in most patients with generalized mutilating dystrophic EB [8] and reduced in some patients with recessive localized dystrophic EB [6]. GB3 is absent from all patients with EBJ gravis. Figure 19.6 summarizes the localization of the antibodies and the EB subsets with abnormal staining patterns. Based on these data alone, it is unfortunately not possible to hypothesize about the molecular mechanisms leading to the abnormalities. For further progress to occur, it is of pivotal importance that the molecular characteristics of the antigenic proteins be well investigated.

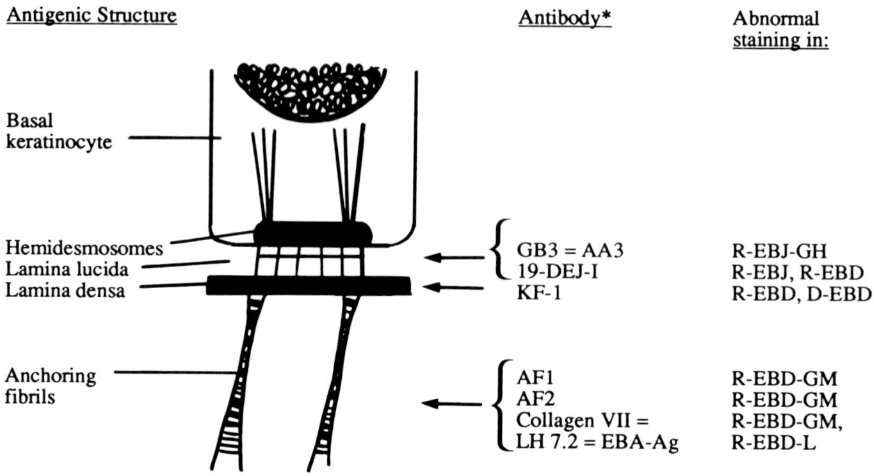

(a)

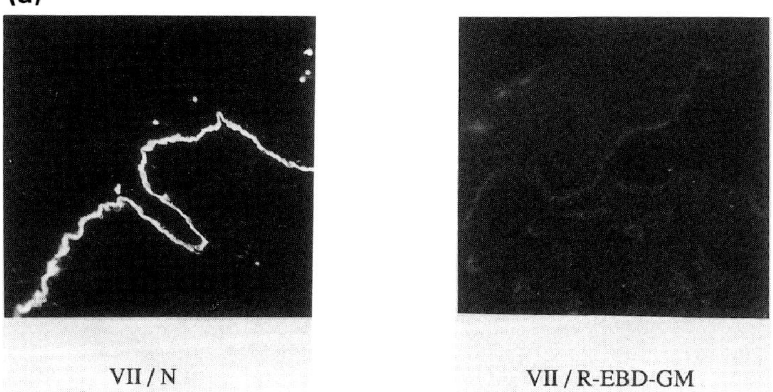

(b)

Figure 19.6 Antibodies with abnormal staining patterns in EB skin. (a) A schematic representation of the structures of the dermoepidermal junction zone. In center, the antibodies listed according to their respective level of binding and on the right the EB subsets in which abnormal staining was found.* The AA3 and GB3 antibodies recognize the same antigenic macromolecule. Both the LH 7.2 and EBA antibodies recognize the aminoterminal globular domain of collagen VII. (b) Lack of staining with antibodies to collagen VII in R-EBD-GM skin is shown on the right, a normal control on the left. Abbreviations: GH: gravis Herlitz; GM: generalized mutilating; L: localized.

No abnormal staining patterns have been observed with antibodies to well-characterized structural macromolecules of the basement membrane zone, such as collagen IV, laminin, nidogen, or heparans sulfate proteoglycan.

BIOCHEMICAL ABNORMALITIES

A number of abnormal biochemical reactions are associated with EB. However, studies on the involved reactions have often been performed with a small number of families or patients, and it seems that not all of these biochemical abnormalities are consistent enough to represent disease markers applicable to all cases. Not only clinical but also molecular heterogeneity is extensive. In Table 19.1 the abnormalities are summarily listed to give a better overview of defects reported as far. For reviews of original literature, see [1,3,6,8,9].

EB Simplex

It may be incongruous that the biochemical defects in an intraepidermal disease have been found in cultured fibroblasts. The activity of gelatinase, a collagen-degrading enzyme, was reduced to 15% of control levels in some patients with generalisata (EBS-G) and to about 30% in EBS localisata (EBS-L), whereas the activity was normal in other EB. Deficiency of an other enzyme, galactosyl-hydroxylysyl-transferase, was described in a single kindred. However, not all affected individuals displayed the defect. The relationship of these enzyme abnor-

Table 19.1 Biochemical Abnormalities in EB

EB subset	Abnormal findings
EBS	Reduced fibroblast gelatinase activity
	Reduced collagen galactosyl-hydroxylysyltransferase activity
	Defective epidermal cell membrane glycosylation
	Abnormal keratin filament expression
	Abnormal epidermal cell lectin-binding capacity
	Cellular immune defect
EBJ	Defective GB3 protein
	Abnormal 19-DEJ-1 antigen expression
EBD	Increased mutant collagenase activity
	Defective collagen VII
	Abnormal KF-1, AF1, AF2, 19-DEJ-1 antigen expression
	Abnormal chondroitin-6-sulfate proteoglycan expression
	Altered fibroblast behavior in collagen matrix
	Increased collagen synthesis
	Increased chondroitin sulfate in skin and urine
	Accumulation of glycosaminoglycans in vitro

malities to the pathogenesis of blistering is not clear, and the possibility of genetic linkage of two defects is not excluded.

Further abnormalities, (e.g., defective epidermal cell membrane structure or function, or abnormal keratin filament expression in vitro) have been suggested to be relevant to the etiopathogenesis of EBS.

EB Junctionalis

No biochemically defined abnormality has been reported (see section on immunochemical abnormalities).

EB Dystrophica

Dominant Subtypes

An accumulation of chondroitin-6-sulfate-proteoglycan in skin and urine, and increased proteoglycan synthesis by fibroblasts was found in EB dystrophica generalisata (D-EBD-G). The relationship of the findings and blistering in vivo remains unclear; interference of collagen matrix formation in skin has been hypothesized.

Recessive Subtypes

An excess of mutant collagenase was demonstrated in skin and fibroblasts of patients with different subsets of R-EBD. First, the overproduction of the structurally altered but catalytically equal enzyme was believed to represent a marker for about 80 % of R-EBD cases, but a later large study showed that only about 25 % of the patients demonstrated this abnormality.

New insight into the pathogenesis was gained by immunochemical experiments on R-EBD-GM skin that demonstrated absence of intact collagen VII. This finding provides a molecular basis for the absence of anchoring fibrils in this subtype. The pathologic mechanisms leading to lack of collagen VII are not yet solved, but several working hypothesis can be given: first, a gene mutation leads to synthesis of defective collagen VII that cannot build anchoring fibrils; second, an aberrant collagen VII is degraded by collagenase; third, normal collagen VII molecules are degraded by excessive mutant collagenase; fourth, some patients have mutant collagenase and others mutant collagen VII. Current and future research must determine which hypothesis applies to which subtype of R-EBD.

HOW TO DIAGNOSE EB

In Figure 19.7 a reasonable approach for diagnosis and classification of new patients with EB is described. For the genetic background a careful family history is obviously important. In evaluating the clinical presentation, onset and

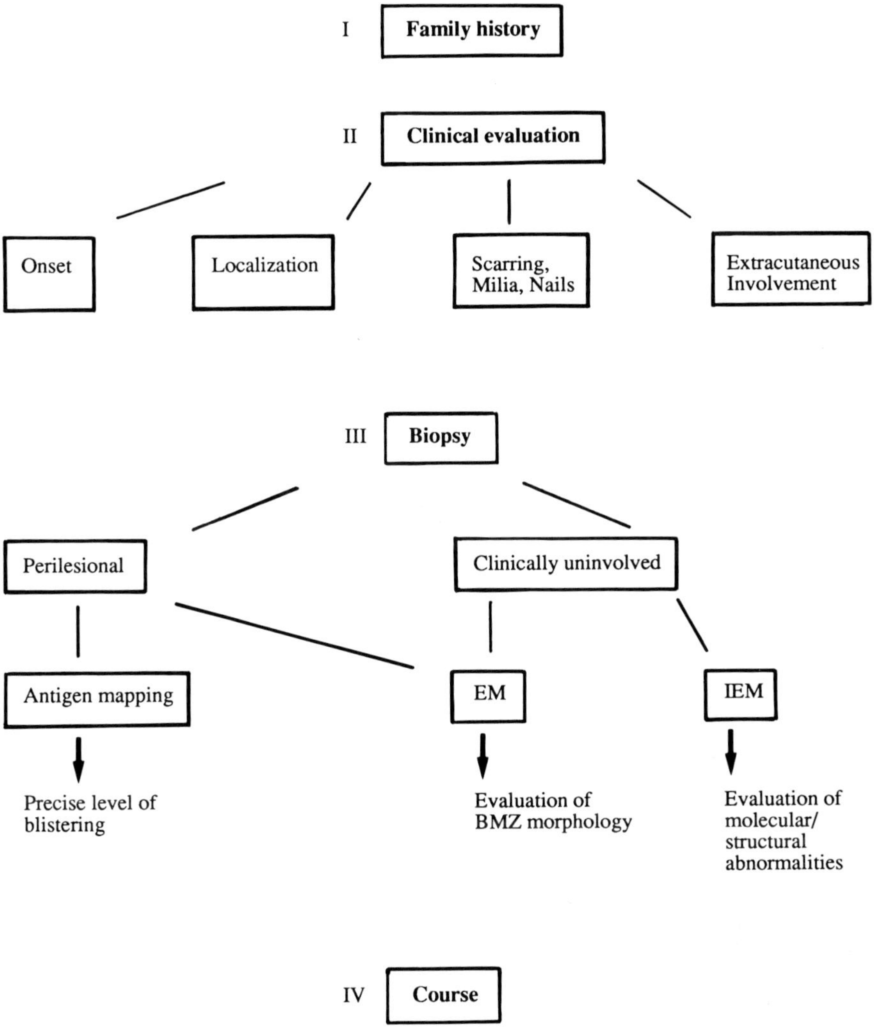

Figure 19.7 A flowchart of EB diagnosis.

localization of the blisters as well as scarring, milia formation, nail involvement, and involvement of extracutaneous tissues should be considered. A biopsy is essential. If possible, skin from the perilesional area, about 1 cm from the blister, as well as skin from a clinically normal looking uninvolved area should be obtained. A traditional light microscopic examination does not help in diagnosing EB, because the level of blistering in all three major categories is physically very close and cannot be differentiated on the light microscope without special markers. Instead, native biopsy material should be obtained for antigen mapping, electron microscopic examination and possibly immuno-electron microscopy. The potential of antigen mapping in determining the precise level of blistering is presented schematically in Figure 19.8. In addition, antibodies to collagen VII and GB3 protein can be used to diagnose R-EBD-GM and junctional (R-EBJ-GHEB), gravis, recessive respectively. In some cases it is not possible to diagnose EB in an early phase despite all the tests. The course of the disease, development, and final localization of the lesions will then help to establish the exact classification.

INVESTIGATION OF MOLECULAR MECHANISMS

Investigation of the molecular mechanisms leading to EB requires a multitude of biochemical methods. For screening of structural abnormalities, immunofluorescence and electron microscopic studies are useful. For a detailed analysis, more sophisticated methods, such as immuno-electron microscopy, immunoblotting, protein chemical analysis, DNA fragment analysis, and sequencing are required. Such methods are not routinely available in all clinics and laboratories, and international collaboration with specialized centers will be necessary for the investigation of as many patients as possible. In every case, it is advisable to save some native frozen skin and to establish and preserve fibroblast cultures (which is rather easy) from all patients for future analysis. Functional tests, such as enzyme activity measurements, are usually performed with fibroblasts established from patients' skin.

The investigation of the molecular mechanisms and defects is summarized in Figure 19.9.

CURRENT PROBLEMS AND PROSPECTS

Epidermolysis bullosa represents a growing group of genetic disorders of the dermoepidermal junction zone. New techniques have allowed a more precise characterization and further subdivision of clinically and genetically determined subsets: to date at least 23 subtypes can be identified. It is likely that while increased clinical research activity will reveal new entities, the laboratory researchers must dissect the known diseases to subtype further on the basis of molecular heterogeneity. In the future we may have to deal with a far more heterogeneous disease group than we now anticipate, and we may have to create a new classification based on molecular abnormalities.

For an optimal resolution of this complex set of disorders, biochemical characterization of the involved structural proteins and, subsequently, their molecular cloning, are imperative. With probes for normal and defective genes, questions about molecular defects and pathophysiological mechanisms underlying EB,

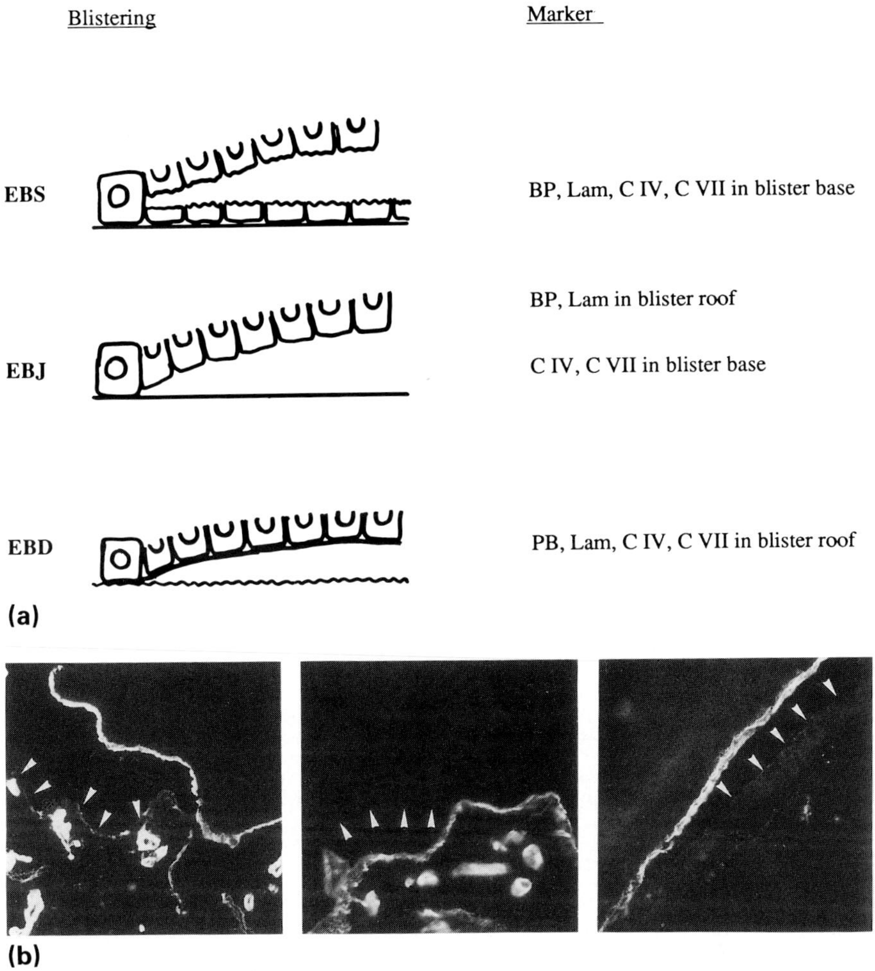

Figure 19.8 The principle of antigen mapping in the diagnosis of EB. (a) Antibodies to well-characterized antigens with known localization are selected as markers (e.g., bullous pemphigoid antigen on the lower pole of the basal cell, laminin in lamina lucida, collagen IV in lamina densa, and collagen VII in the anchoring fibrils). Clinically uninvolved skin should be gently rubbed prior to biopsy to induce splitting. (a) Immunofluorescent staining with the marker antibodies will be performed on frozen sections. The above fluorescence patterns are characteristic for the respective EB categories. BP, bullous pemphigoid antigen; Lam, laminin; C IV, collagen IV; C VII, collagen VII. (b) Laminin in blister roof in EBD (left), collagen IV in blister base in EBJ (center), and collagen VII in blister roof in D-EBD (right). The blister roof or base, respectively, is marked with arrows.

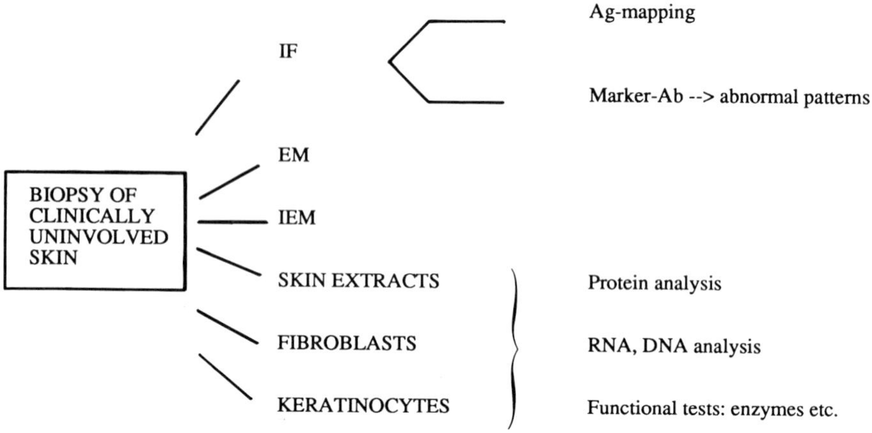

Figure 19.9 Investigation of defects in EB skin. To seek a structural or molecular defect, clinically uninvolved skin without secondary changes is required. A large biopsy should be divided into several portions for different investigations. See [5-10] for original literature describing the methods in detail.

molecular basis for gene linkage, or identification of carriers of the disease can be efficiently approached.

NOTE ADDED IN PROOF

Since the manuscript for this chapter was written more than a year ago, remarkable progress on the molecular biology and pathology of EB has been made. New structural proteins of the dermoepidermal junction and molecular abnormalities of some of the components have been defined, and recently, mutations of keratins 5 and 14 have been discovered in EBS and a mutation of collagen VII in EBD. The reader is referred to current literature data bases for original references.

REFERENCES

1. Gedde-Dahl T, Anton-Lamprecht I. Epidermolysis bullosa. In: Every AEH, ed. Principles and practice of medical genetics, vol I. 1990; 855–876.
2. Pearson RW. Clinicopathologic types of epidermolysis bullosa and their nondermatological complications. Arch Dermatol 1988; 124: 718–25.
3. Lin AN, Carter MD. Epidermolysis bullosa: when the skin falls apart. J Pediatr 1989; 114: 349–55.
4. Holbrook KA. Extracutaneous epithelial involvement in inherited epidermolysis bullosa. Arch Dermatol 1988; 124: 726–31.

5. Anton-Lamprecht I. Prenatal diagnosis of genetic disorders of the skin by means of electron microscopy. Hum Genet 1981; 59: 392–405.
6. Eady RAJ. Babes, blisters and basement membranes: from sticky molecules to epidermolysis bullosa. Clin Exp Dermatol 1987; 12: 159–70.
7. Bruckner-Tuderman L, Vogel A, Rüegger S, Odermatt B, Tönz O, Schnyder UW. Epidermolysis bullosa simplex with mottled pigmentation. J Am Acad Dermatol 1989; 21: 425–32.
8. Bruckner-Tuderman L, Mitsuhashi Y, Schnyder UW, Bruckner P. Anchoring fibrils and type VII collagen are absent from skin in severe recessive dystrophic epidermolysis bullosa. J Invest Dermatol 1989; 93: 3–9.
9. Fine JD. Changing clinical and laboratory concepts in inherited epidermolysis bullosa. Arch Dermatol 1988; 124: 523–6.
10. Verrando P, Pisani A, Ortonne JP. The new basement membrane antigen recognized by the monoclonal antibody GB3 in a large-size glycoprotein: modulation of its expression by retinoic acid. Biochem Biophys Acta 1988; 942: 45–56.

20

Acquired Bullous Diseases

Fenella Wojnarowska
The Churchill Hospital, Oxford, England

The acquired bullous diseases are autoimmune diseases in which circulating autoantibodies react with target antigens in the skin. This interaction sets off a cascade of mediators of inflammation that ultimately results in the formation of a blister. The site of the blister is chiefly determined by the ultrastructural localization of the antigen (Fig. 20.1). The intraepidermal bullous diseases, pemphigus vulgaris and pemphigus foliaceus, do not involve the connective tissues and will not be discussed further. The subepidermal bullous diseases are defined by their clinical picture and characteristic immunofluorescence findings. Recently there has been a move to define them in terms of their target antigens, using the techniques of immunoblotting and immunoprecipitation; however, these methods have revealed both overlap and heterogeneity among the diseases. These diseases comprise bullous pemphigoid (BP), pemphigoid gestationis (PG), cicatricial pemphigoid (CP), chronic bullous disease of childhood (CBDC), linear IgA disease of adults (LAD), epidermolysis bullosa acquisita (EBA), bullous lupus erythematosus (bullous LE), and dermatitis herpetiformis (DH). All of these are identified by the presence of tense vesicles or blisters or mucosal erosions, and they are all to some degree steroid- or dapsone-responsive. All, except DH, are associated with linear deposition of immunoreactants at the basement membrane zone (BMZ) and circulating antibodies to that region.

The involvement of the connective tissues in these disorders is of three kinds: in EBA and bullous LE the target antigen is type VII collagen [1], and it may

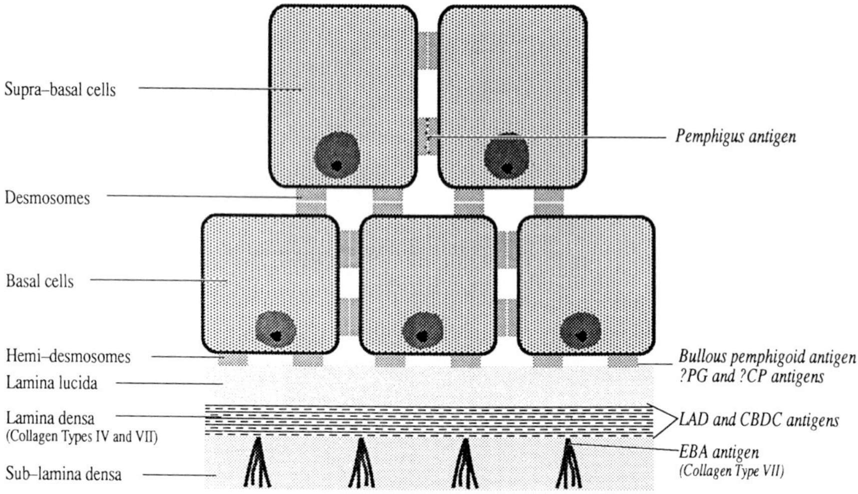

Figure 20.1 The BMZ and target antigens of the acquired bullous diseases. PG, pemphigoid gestationis; CP, cicatricial pemphigoid; CBDC, chronic bullous disease of childhood; LAD linear IgA disease of adults; EBA, epidermolysis bullosa acquisita.

also be anticipated, from the site of the deposition of the immunoreactants in DH, that the IgA is bound to connective tissue components; in all those diseases so far studied there is, during blister formation, activation of proteases including collagenase and elastase, which contribute to the formation of the lesions by destruction of connective tissue components of the BMZ and the dermis [2] The third mechanism is observed in CP, CBDC, LAD, EBA in which repeated blistering of mucosal epithelium, and also of skin in CP and EBA, results in scarring and fibrosis. The scarring in EBA is thought to result from the direct immunologic attack on type VII collagen.

BULLOUS PEMPHIGOID

This is the most common of the acquired subepidermal bullous diseases, and one of the best understood.

BP is a disease of the elderly, being rare in patients before the age of 60. The characteristic clinical presentation is of tense blisters arising either from normal skin or from red urticated plaques (Fig. 20.2). They are often although not invariably, flexural in distribution. Mucosae (e.g., the mouth, nasopharynx, and genitalia) may also be involved. The lesions heal without scarring. There is usually intense pruritus, which may precede the eruption.

Histopathologic examination shows a subepidermal blister containing eosino-

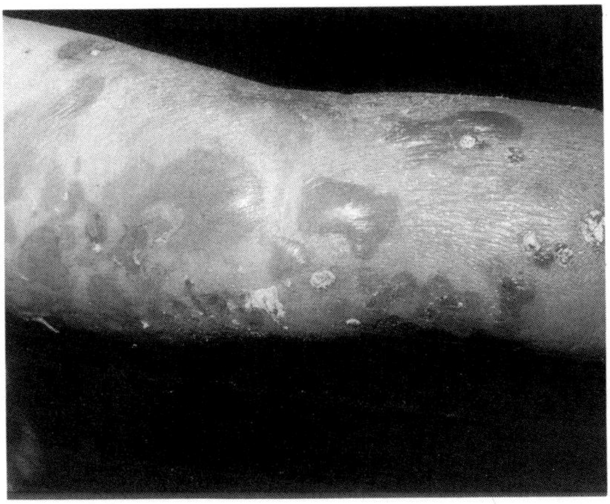

Figure 20.2 Bullous pemphigoid: tense blisters on the arm.

phils and sometimes neutrophils. Electron microscopic examination demonstrates that the split is through the lamina lucida. Immunofluorescent examination reveals linear deposition of IgG or C3 at the BMZ, and a circulating anti-BMZ antibody can be detected using normal skin or mucosa as substrate. The use of skin that has been artificially blistered through the lamina lucida using suction or prolonged incubation with 1M sodium chloride as substrate shows binding of the antibody to the epidermal aspect of the blister (Fig. 20.3) [3,4]. This suggests a close association of the antigen with keratinocytes. The BP antigen has an intracellular and extracellular component and is associated with the hemidesmosomes [5]. The immunoreactants deposited *in vivo* are found in the lamina lucida. The antigen has been identified in epidermal extracts and cultures by immunoblotting and immunoprecipitation as a glycoprotein of molecular weight 230 kD (220–240 kD)[6], although other antigens particularly, one of 180 kD, have been identified.

The mechanism by which reaction of the antibody with the target antigen triggers the inflammatory cascade leading to blister formation is not well understood. The demonstration in BP blister fluid of collagenase and elastase suggests that destruction of connective tissue constituents of the BMZ and the dermis is an essential step in lesion formation [2]. Recruitment of neutrophils and eosinophils is also involved.

Treatment is with steroids, both topical and systemic in moderate dosages (e.g., prednisolone 30–60 mg), and often azathioprine as a steroid-sparing agent. There is a substantial rate of mortality and morbidity from both disease and treatment. Most patients go into remission; the time taken to achieve this varies from a few months to many years.

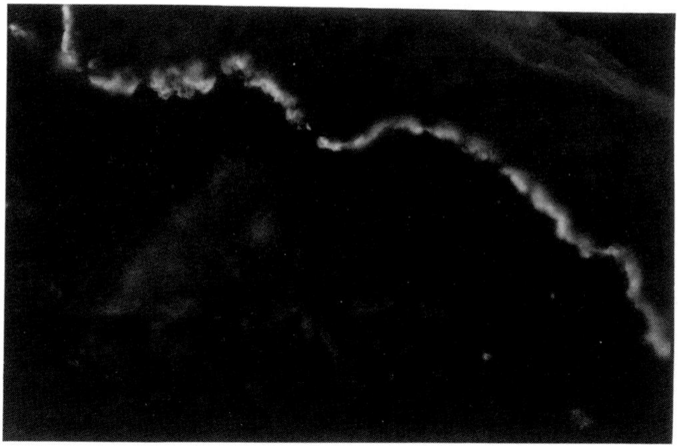

Figure 20.3 Bullous pemphigoid: binding of the BMZ antibody to the roof (epidermal) side of NaCl split skin.

PEMPHIGOID GESTATIONIS

This disease is one of the rarest of the bullous diseases, occurring in 1:50,000 pregnancies. It commences in the second or third trimester and even postpartum. It has also occurred in response to chorion carcinoma and injections of placental extracts.

The eruption begins around the umbilicus with urticated plaques that are often annular. The lesions spread to the rest of the abdomen (Fig. 20.4) and may become generalized. Blisters arise both from urticated lesions and from normal skin. Mucosal involvement, both oral and vaginal, does occur but rarely causes symptoms.

Occasionally there is transplacental transmission of the disease to the neonate, which develops urticated lesions and blisters within a few days of birth. These resolve spontaneously in a week or so.

The blister is subepidermal and contains eosinophils. Electron microscopic examination shows the split to be in the lamina lucida, but there may also be damage to the basal keratinocytes. There is deposition of C3 at the BMZ of both maternal and neonatal skin, and amnion placentae. IgG may sometimes be found. A circulating factor binds C3 to the BMZ of normal skin; this is an IgG1 antibody that avidly binds complement. The antigen is present in BMZ of skin, mucosae, and amnion placentae from the second trimester on [7]. It has been shown, using split-skin techniques, to be associated with the epidermal side of the split [7]. The antigen has been shown by immunoblotting to have a molecular weight of

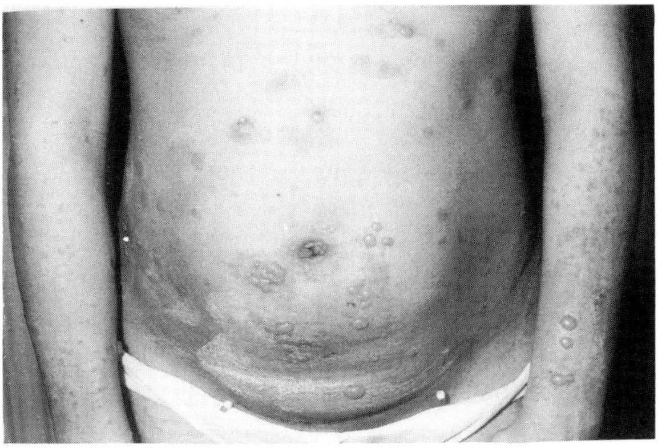

Figure 20.4 Pemphigoid gestationis: blisters on the abdomen (from Wojnarowska F, Briggaman RA, eds. Management of the blistering diseases. London: Chapman and Hall, 1990).

180 kD and there is sometimes also a 220 kD antigen (identical to the BP antigen) [8]. Thus the target antigens seem to be shared with BP

The mechanism of blistering has not been studied but may be assumed to be similar to that in BP.

The disease resolves postpartum but can take several months. It is very itchy and so treatment is required, usually with systemic steroids. The disease recurs in subsequent pregnancies unless the mother and fetus are human leukocyte antigen-(HLA) compatible. The mothers are usually HLA-DR3, DR4 [9].

CICATRICIAL PEMPHIGOID

This disease is much less common than BP. It affects middle-aged and elderly patients, but does also occur in young adults. The brunt of the disease is borne by the mucous membranes, but skin involvement is present in one-third of patients.

The usual presentation is with mucosal involvement; initially a single site or several may be affected. With time further sites are often involved, although there is wide variation in the extent of involvement at the different sites. The mouth and eyes are the most commonly affected. Oral lesions comprise blisters and erosions, and desquamative gingivitis in which the gums are painful, eroded, red, and inflamed. Ocular lesions include blisters and ulcers that may result in devastating scarring with symblepharon formation (i.e., adhesions between the eyelids and the globe) and also distortion of the eyelids and obstruction of the lacrimal ducts causing dry eyes. The most serious complication is involvement of the cornea, with ulceration and subsequent opacification due to epithelialization and vascularization, causing blindness (Fig. 20.5). Laryngeal lesions present with hoarseness and may progress to scarring with narrowing of the larynx, stridor, and asphyxia. The esophagus, rectum, vagina, and urethra may all be affected with erosions that can heal with stricture formation. The skin may manifest generalized blistering or there may be recurrent blistering and subsequent scarring at a localized site.

Histopathologic examination demonstrates a subepidermal blister with fibrosis of the underlying dermis. Electron microscopic examination shows the split to be within the lamina lucida. Immunofluorescence of perilesional tissue and of uninvolved skin or mucosa may show linear deposition of immunoreactants, IgG, C3, and sometimes IgA or IgM, at the BMZ. Suction blister studies show both epidermal and dermal binding [4,10]. Indirect immunofluorescence is positive in a minority of cases. Using split skin, unlike in BP, may show binding to either the roof or floor of the artificial blister, suggesting that the antigens are heterogeneous [4,10]. Immunoblotting studies have demonstrated that the circulating antibodies react with the BP antigen and with other epidermal proteins.

Studies of blister formation have not shown activation of proteases in the single case studied [2]. The mechanism by which the fibrosis and scarring occurs is unknown; however, unlike BP the inflammatory process at the BMZ stimulates proliferation and disorganization of the underlying collagen fibers.

This disease is resistant to treatment and often the scarring proceeds inexorably despite some periods of inactivity. Many patients obtain some symptomatic relief from topical and systemic steroids, immunosupressive drugs, or dapsone. Remission is rare.

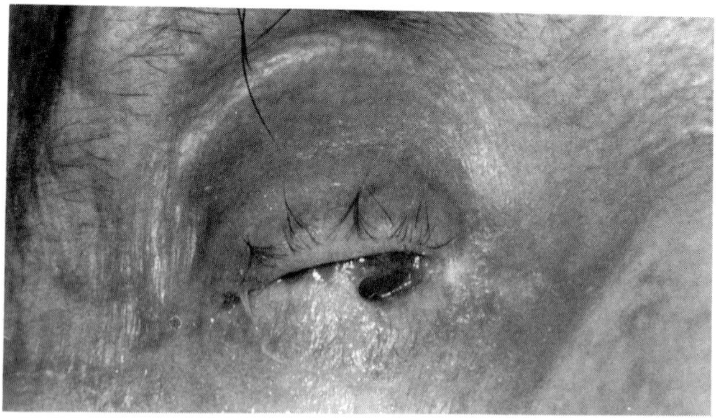

Figure 20.5 Cicatricial pemphigoid: severe ocular scarring.

CHRONIC BULLOUS DISEASE OF CHILDHOOD AND LINEAR IgA DISEASE OF ADULTS

These two diseases are now regarded as the same disease. They differ in the age of onset, cutaneous distribution, and immunogenetic basis. CBDC is associated with HLA-B8. They are both rare; LAD is more common than CBDC in the West; however the reverse is true in Asia and Africa. CBDC arises in early childhood (<5 years) and LAD in young adults or older persons.

The diseases present with tense blisters arising from normal or urticarial skin; the lesions are characteristically annular. In CBDC there is particular involvement of the perineum and face (Fig. 20.6). Mucosal involvement is common and may lead to scarring [11,12].

The blister is subepidermal and contains either eosinophils or neutrophils. There is linear deposition of IgA at the BMZ and a circulating IgA antibody in the majority of children and a minority of adults. The site of the antigen has been studied using split-skin and immunoelectron microscopy. An epidermal and a dermal site of antibody binding have been identified. The LAD antigen has only been found in dermal extracts. It may be heterogeneous, since preliminary reports have found its molecular weight to be 285 kD and 97 kD and in 3 cases the

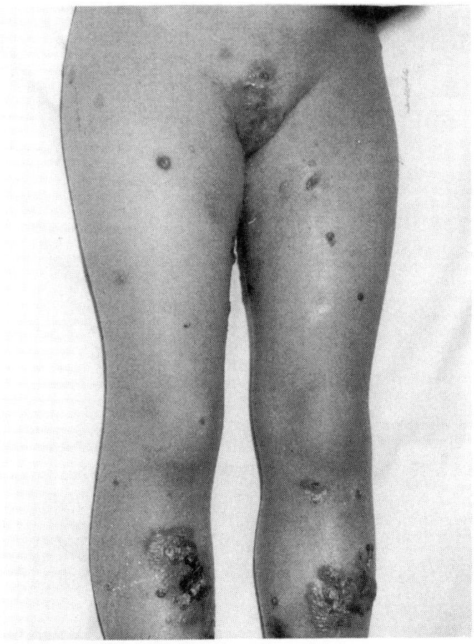

Figure 20.6 Chronic bullous disease of childhood: blisters, some in an annular pattern, on the perineum and legs.

antigen was identical to the EBA antigen (i.e., type VII collagen; see below). The CBDC antigen is indistinguishable from the 285 kD LAD antigen.

Serum from patients with LAD will cause blistering of normal skin in culture; this was prevented by protease inhibitors. Elastase and collagenase are present in the blisters of patients with CBDC [2]. These findings suggest that proteolytic destruction of BMZ and dermal components including collagens and elastin is part of the blistering process. Stimulation of fibrosis must occur when there is mucosal scarring.

These diseases respond to treatment with dapsone and sulfonamides. The majority attain remission within 5 years; however, a few do not remit. Some patients are left with mucosal scarring.

EPIDERMOLYSIS BULLOSA ACQUISITA AND BULLOUS LUPUS ERYTHEMATOSUS

These two diseases are very rare. Only a handful of cases of bullous LE have been reported in the world literature. EBA can occur at any age and is most common in black Americans. It is associated with HLA-DR2 [13] and with inflammatory bowel disease and other autoimmune diseases. Bullous LE affects young black patients with systemic LE; the immunogenetic basis is the same as EBA [13]. Their clinical features differ markedly, but the target antigen is the same in both diseases and is type VII collagen [1].

EBA is classically a mechanobullous disease: blisters are induced by trauma to the skin and thus are common on the hands and feet (Fig. 20.7). However, lesions are often present elsewhere and are often prominent on light-exposed areas. In some patients there is no relation to trauma and the presentation is indistinguishable from BP, but often becomes more typical with time. The lesions heal with scarring and milia formation. The skin is fragile, tearing in response to minor damage. Mucosal involvement occurs and may lead to scarring. The clinical picture is similar to epidermolysis bullosa dystrophica (Chapter 18), and hence the name.

Bullous LE manifests tense blisters or vesicles arising from normal or urticated skin; they may be annular. There is no skin fragility, no mechanobullous features, and scarring does not occur.

Histopathologic examination in both cases shows a subepidermal blister, but often in EBA there are very few inflammatory cells. In contrast, the blisters in patients with bullous LE usually contain many neutrophils. The BMZ can sometimes be demonstrated in the roof of a blister showing that the blister is dermal. This has been confirmed by electron microscopic examination, which also shows amorphous deposits below the lamina densa and reduction in anchoring fibrils. Direct immunofluorescence shows IgG and C3 and, rarely, IgA at the BMZ. Indirect immunofluorescence may demonstrate circulating BMZ antibodies in patients with EBA; this is less common in bullous LE. The use of NaCl split

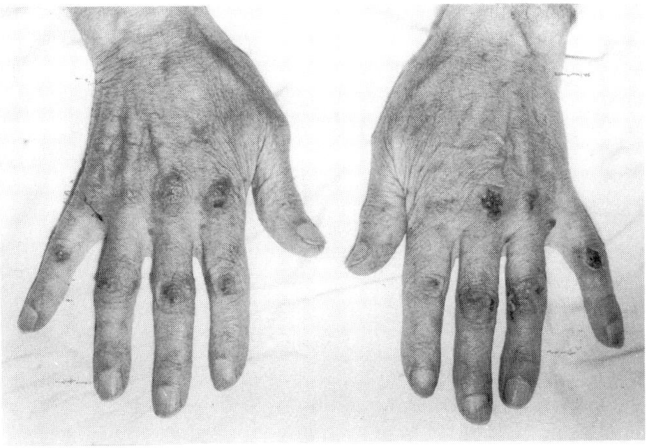

Figure 20.7 Epidermolysis bullosa acquisita: blisters at sites of trauma on the hands.

skin increases the detection of BMZ antibodies and shows dermal binding in all cases (Fig 20.8) [3]. Immunoelectron microscopic examination shows the immunoreactants deposited below the lamina densa and associated with anchoring fibrils. Immunoblotting has demonstrated that the antigen is collagen type VII, and that the antibodies are to the noncollagenous carboxy terminal globular domain [1] (see Chapters 1, 4).

The blisters result from the direct immunologic attack on the antigen, which recruits inflammatory cells and causes dermoepidermal separation. The mechanism by which attack on the anchoring fibrils results in weakening of the adhesion between the dermis and epidermis with the consequent skin fragility and trauma-induced blistering is still the subject of speculation. However, there is loss of anchoring fibrils and this may be associated with impaired function. It is a mystery why this does not occur in patients with bullous LE. The skin and mucosal scarring in EBA implies proliferation of dermal collagen and elastic fibers.

EBA runs a prolonged course and although steroids, immunosuppressive drugs, and dapsone have all been used often the response is poor. Bullous LE may have a short course and usually responds to treatment with dapsone.

DERMATITIS HERPETIFORMIS

DH is most common in Ireland and Scandinavia. It can present from childhood to old age, but does so most commonly in young adults. There is an absolute association with gluten-sensitive enteropathy. Although the immunogenetics of celiac disease and DH are similar relative to HLA B8, there are differences in the class 2 antigens.

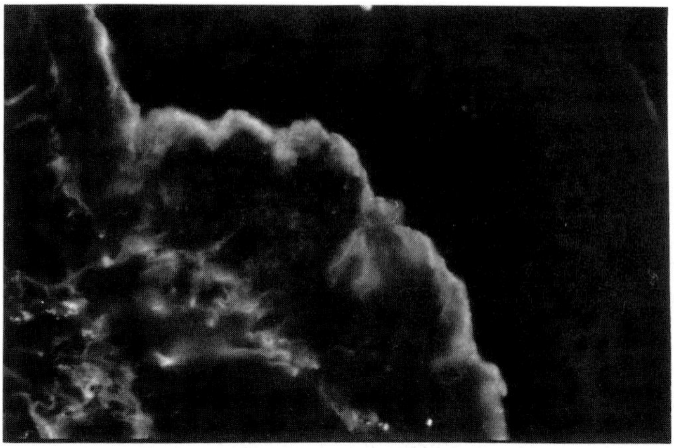

Figure 20.8 Epidermolysis bullosa acquisita: binding of the BMZ antibody to the floor (dermal) side of NaCl split skin.

The eruption is symmetrical and affects the extensor surfaces of the knees and elbows (Fig. 20.9), the nasal cleft, and often the shoulders, chin, and scalp. Other areas may be involved and oral lesions do occur. The lesions are extremely itchy and comprise small red, urticated papules that vesiculate and are usually excoriated.

Histopathologic examination reveals a papillary microabscess in the dermal papilla with marked edema and numerous neutrophils. Direct immunofluorescence is diagnostic and shows deposition of IgA in a granular fashion in the dermal papillae (Fig. 20.10). Immunoelectron microscopic examination shows the IgA to be associated with the microfibrillar–elastic fiber system. There are no circulating antibodies. The target antigen has not has been identified; it seems likely that it will be a protein component or fibril in the dermal papillae.

The production of a blister is a complex process. Although the edema is initially observed in the dermal papillae, there is separation in the lamina lucida. High levels of elastase are found in the blister fluid and in the inflammatory cells in the blister; collagenase levels are also elevated [2]. These findings suggest that destruction of the dermal connective tissue by proteases is a crucial step in the formation of lesions in DH.

DH responds dramatically to treatment with dapsone or sulphonamides, the eruption being controlled within 48 hr. Removal of gluten from the diet will, after many months (average, 2 years), also result in remission of the eruption. Reintroduction of gluten causes relapse, and treatment is lifelong. The IgA usually persists in the skin despite absence of lesions. Spontaneous remission is rare and usually temporary. The mechanism by which gluten causes the skin

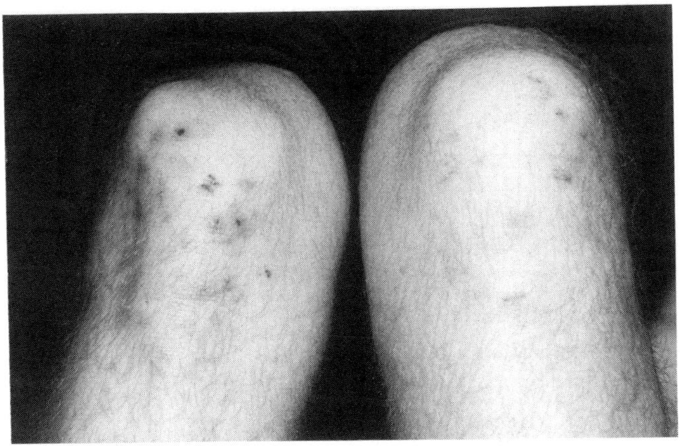

Figure 20.9 Dermatitis herpetiformis: excoriated papulovesicles on the knees.

Figure 20.10 Dermatitis herpetiformis: deposits of IgA in the dermal papillae of the skin.

lesions is unknown; both cross-reactivity with a dermal component and binding of a substance in wheat to a dermal component have been postulated. There is an increase in lymphomas in these patients, and it is hoped that this may be reduced by a gluten-free diet.

REFERENCES

1. Woodley DT, Burgeson RE, Lunstrum G, et al. Epidermolysis bullosa acquisita antigen is the globular carboxyl terminus of Type VII procollagen. J Clin Invest 1988; 81: 683–7.
2. Oikarinen AI, Zone JJ, Razzaque Ahmed A, et al. Demonstration of collagenase and elastase activities in the blister fluids from bullous skin diseases. Comparison between dermatitis herpetiformis and bullous pemphigoid. J Invest Dermatol 1983; 81: 261–6.
3. Gammon WR, Briggaman RA, Inman AO, et al. Differentiating anti-lamina lucida and anti-sublamina densa anti-BMZ antibodies by indirect immunofluorescence on 1.0 M sodium chloride-separated skin. J Invest Dermatol 1984; 82: 139–44.
4. Venning VA, Allen J, Millard PR, et al. The localization of the bullous pemphigoid and cicatricial pemphigoid antigens: direct and indirect immunofluorescence of suction blisters. Br J Dermatol 1989; 121: 305–15.
5. Mutasim DF, Morrison LH, Takahashi Y, et al. Definition of bullous pemphigoid antibody binding to intracellular and extracellular antigen associated with hemidesmosomes. J Invest Dermatol 1988; 92: 225–30.
6. Mueller S, Klaus-Kovtun V, Stanley JR. A 230-kD basic protein is the major bullous pemphigoid antigen. J Invest Dermatol 1989; 92: 33–8.
7. Kelly SE, Bhogal BS, Wojnarowska F, et al. Expression of a pemphigoid gestationis—related antigen by human placenta. Br J Dermatol 1988; 118: 605–11.
8. Kelly SE, Bhogal BS, Wojnarowska F, et al. Western blot analysis of epidermal extract in the characterisation of the antigen in pemphigoid gestationis. J Invest Dermatol 1988; 91: 397 (abst).
9. Shornick JK, Stastny P, Gilliam JN. Paternal histocompatibility (HLA) antigens and maternal anti-HLA antibodies in herpes gestationis. J Invest Dermatol 1983; 81: 407–9.
10. Fine J-D, Neises G, Katz SI. Immunofluorescence and immunoelectron microscopic studies in cicatricial pemphigoid. J Invest Dermatol 1984; 82: 39–43.
11. Leonard JN, Wright P, Williams DM, et al. The relationship between linear IgA disease and benign mucous membrane pemphigoid. Br J Dermatol 1984; 110: 307–14.
12. Wojnarowska F, Marsden RA, Bhogal B, et al. Chronic bullous disease of childhood, childhood cicatricial pemphigoid, and linear IgA disease of adults. J Am Acad Dermatol 1988; 19: 792–805.
13. Gammon WR, Heise ER, Burke WA, et al. Increased frequency of HLA-DR2 in patients with autoantibodies to epidermolysis bullosa acquisita antigen: evidence that the expression of autoimmunity to Type VII collagen is HLA class II allele associated. J Invest Dermatol 1988; 91: 228–32.

21

Localized and Systemic Scleroderma

Raul Fleischmajer

Mount Sinai School of Medicine, New York, New York

Scleroderma or systemic sclerosis is a disease that affects the connective tissue of various organ systems. Although the disease may be restricted to the skin, it may also affect the lungs, gastrointestinal tract, cardiovascular system, and kidneys. The cause of scleroderma remains unknown, although three hypotheses have been proposed suggesting an autoimmune process, a vascular disease affecting primarily capillaries and small arteries, and a metabolic abnormality in the regulation of collagen synthesis [1]. However, it is not possible to rule out the possibility that this disease may be an unusual reaction to some toxic chemical agent in susceptible individuals. More recently, several antinuclear antibodies have been described in patients with systemic sclerosis, although the role of humoral immunity remains speculative.

This chapter reviews the classification of scleroderma, discusses recent advances in the clinical and laboratory diagnosis, and the pathophysiology, and briefly evaluates the current management of this disease.

CLASSIFICATION

The classification of scleroderma remains unsatisfactory since there are no accurate clinical features or laboratory tests to identify distinct clinical subsets. However, more recently some attempts have been made to correlate some clinical forms with circulating antinuclear antibodies (ANA). Table 21.1 includes a classification of scleroderma, which, although simple, may be useful. There

Table 21.1 Classification of Scleroderma

Systemic
CREST
Diffuse
Localized
Morphea
Generalized morphea
Linear
Overlap Syndrome
Mixed connective tissue disease
Diffuse fasciitis with eosinophilia
Chronic graft-versus-host disease
Chemically induced scleroderma

are 3 basic groups: systemic sclerosis, localized scleroderma, and the overlap syndromes. Systemic sclerosis includes the calcinosis, Raynaud's phenomenon, esophageal involvement, sclerodactyly, and telangiectasis (CREST) and diffuse form; localized scleroderma is classified into morphea, linear scleroderma, and generalized morphea. The overlap syndromes include mixed connective tissue disease, chronic graft-versus-host disease, eosinophilic fasciitis, and chemically induced scleroderma.

CLINICAL PICTURE

The CREST syndrome appears to identify a relatively benign subset of systemic sclerosis. It is estimated that about 90% of patients with the CREST syndrome have a positive centromere antibody. The disease has a predilection for women, 30–40 years old, and runs a slow course with mild to moderate lung involvement and low incidence of kidney disease. However, this is not an entirely benign disease since serious complications, such as pulmonary hypertension and biliary cirrhosis, have been reported. The diffuse form of systemic sclerosis is characterized by widespread skin involvement, rapidly progressive disease with high incidence of lung and kidney involvement, usually accompanied by a positive Scl-70 (topoisomerase) antibody.

Skin Lesions

The skin is affected in 90% of patients with systemic sclerosis. Initially, there is a period of edema that affects the face and hands and lasts for about 3 months.

This is followed by sclerodactyly (sclerosis only restricted to fingers) or acrosclerosis: the skin induration extends to the face, upper chest, hands, and forearms. In the diffuse form, the sclerosis affects the trunk, upper, and lower extremities. In some patients, the skin induration may be initially accompanied by a passive erythema. Other skin manifestations include telangiectasis (macular or linear) that may involve face, hands, and oral mucosa, calcinosis cutis, ulcerations and gangrene of digits, symmetrical depigmentation, usually affecting the forehead and chest, and, less frequently, hyperpigmentation (Fig. 21.1). Raynaud's phenomenon is present in about 90 % of patients, and affects hands and feet, although it may be seen on the nose and knees and may precede the onset of systemic sclerosis by many years. An unusual feature of systemic sclerosis is the presence of multiple indurated nodules, 5–10 mm in diameter, dome-shaped, skin-colored or hyperpigmented, usually seen on the trunk and arms (nodular scleroderma) (Fig. 21.2).

Internal Involvement

The clinical picture of scleroderma has been well documented [2,3]. Lungs are affected in about 90% of patients with systemic sclerosis. The most common clinical symptom is dyspnea, although chest and pleuritic pain, congestion and sputum production, and even hemoptysis may occur. Pulmonary function studies usually reveal restricted disease and reduction in gas exchange. The severity of gas exchange reduction may be correlated with the incidence of mortality secondary to pulmonary involvement. Roentgenograms usually show linear or nodular densities to diffuse mottling and honeycombing. Pulmonary arterial hypertension is the most serious lung complication and can be diagnosed when a reduction in gas-diffusing capacity of 43% below the predictive value is combined with alterations in chest x-rays and electrocardiogram. Esophageal involvement is very common (90%) and is characterized clinically by dysphagia, dyspepsia, and reflux esophagitis. The best techniques for detecting esophageal hypomotility are the cine-esophagram and esophageal manometry, although barium swallow under fluoroscopic examination may be helpful. Some patients may develop malabsorption and steatorrhea, secondary to bacterial overgrowth that responds well to oral tetracyclines. Other gastrointestinal symptoms are constipation, ileus, and colonic diverticula.

Kidney disease may occur, particularly in the diffuse form, and has important prognostic implications. It is characterized by headaches, visual difficulties, hypertension, seizures, and sudden left ventricular failure. Persistent proteinuria is later followed by increase in serum creatinine, oliguria or anuria, azotemia, and high plasma renin levels. Recent studies showed that the heart is frequently involved in systemic sclerosis. Heart involvement is usually secondary to myocar-

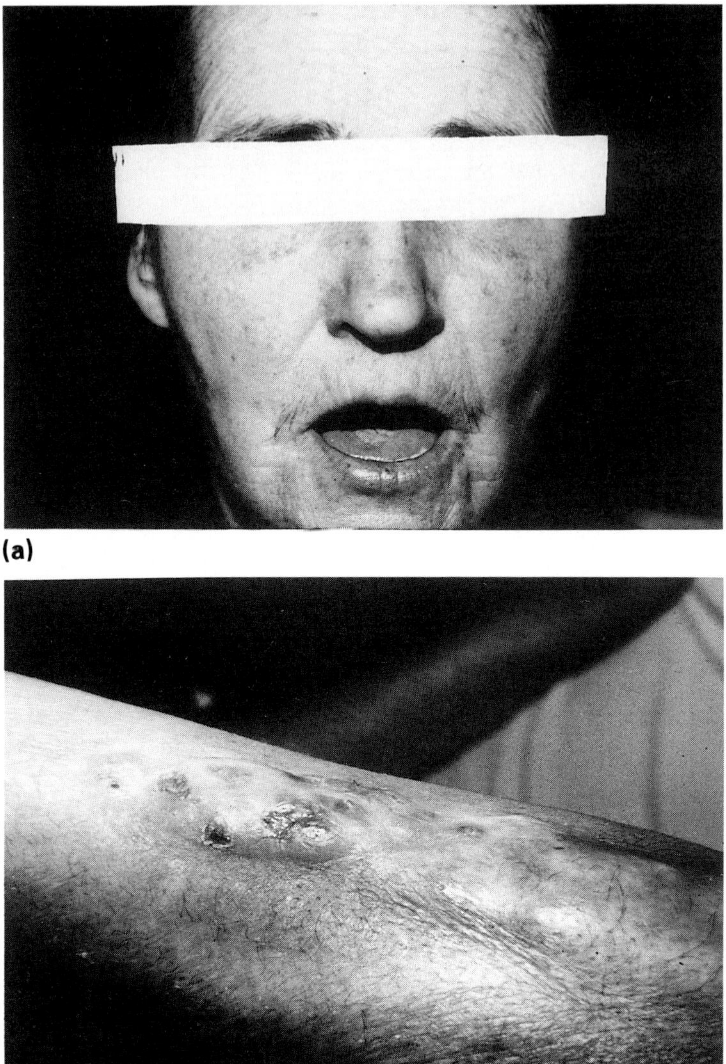

(a)

(b)

Figure 21.1 Findings in Systemic sclerosis include (a) radical furrowing around the mouth and telangiectasis (b), calcinosis cutis, (c) acroscelerosis and digital gangrene, and (d) symmetrical hypopigmentation.

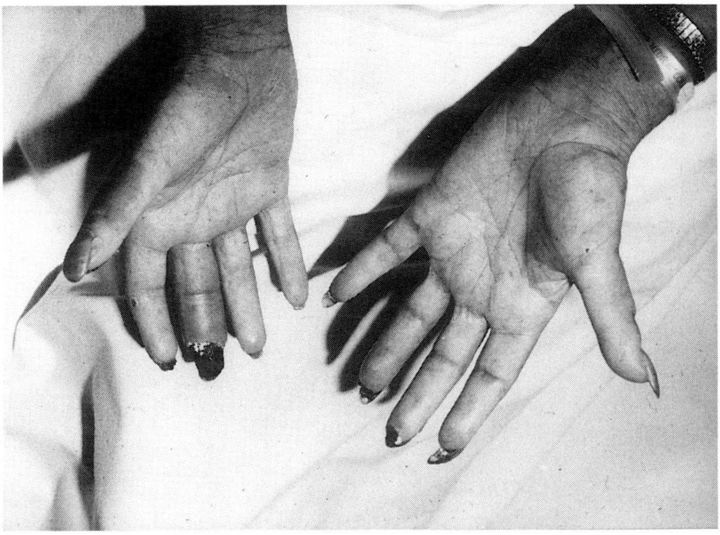

(c)

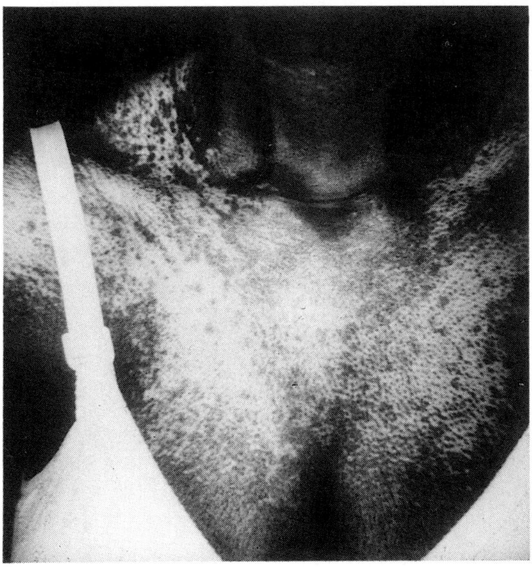

(d)

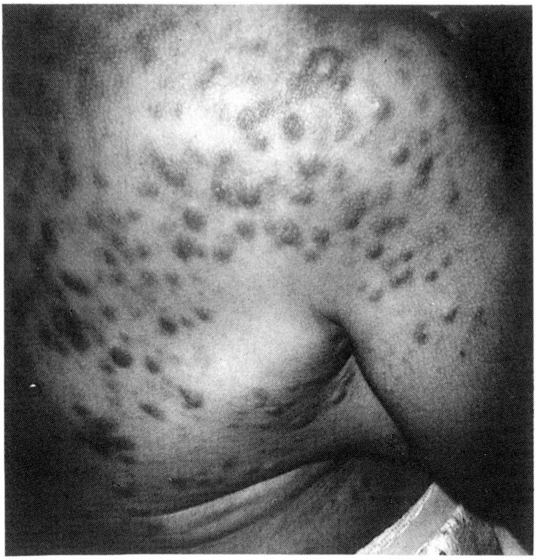

Figure 21.2 Patient with acrosclerosis and multiple nodular lesions on the back, abdomen, neck, and arms.

dial fibrosis or pulmonary involvement. Atherosclerosis and myocardial infarction are not common. Clinical findings are nonspecific and consist of atrial fibrillation, partial or complete atrioventricular block, atrial flutter, and other signs.

Sjogren's or sicca syndrome is not uncommon and consists of dry eyes, dry mouth, parotid enlargement, and an abnormal Schirmer's test. Acute myositis and symmetrical polyarthritis, although not common, may be seen in patients with systemic sclerosis.

Localized Scleroderma

Localized scleroderma is frequently seen in children, although it may affect persons of all ages. It has no sex predilection and usually undergoes spontaneous resolution in about 2–5 years, although occasionally it may persist for 10 or more years. This disease may cause severe atrophy involving skin, subcutaneous tissue, and even muscle and bone. These patients do not have Raynaud's phenomenon, sclerodactyly, or internal involvement. Conversion of localized forms to systemic sclerosis is rare, if it occurs at all. However, occasionally there are patients with systemic sclerosis who show bands of sclerosis resembling linear scleroderma. About 50% of patients with localized scleroderma have a positive ANA, usually with a homogeneous or nucleolar pattern at low titers. However, centromere, Scl-70, and RNP antibodies are usually not present.

Morphea

This clinical form is characterized by single or multiple, well-circumscribed indurated plaques, 5–10 cm, ivory-white, which may be surrounded by an inflammatory halo known as the ''lilac ring'' (Fig. 21.3). The lesions usually affect the trunk and extremities and resolve leaving areas of atrophy and hypopigmentation. Atrophoderma may accompany morphea and consists of soft, slightly depressed patches that are hyperpigmented. The superficial veins become prominent due to the dermal atrophy. In the author's experience, atrophoderma is an atrophic process from the onset and not a residual form of a morphea plaque.

Generalized Morphea

This is actually a widespread form of morphea that affects the trunk and extremities. The lesions may have a symmetrical distribution and consist of large, indurated, confluent plaques. The lesions may be 10–20 cm in diameter and show a ''lilac ring.'' Skin induration is severe enough to cause muscle atrophy, particularly when the lower extremities are affected. The breasts are frequently affected, although the periareolar area is not involved, and, thus, becomes prominent (Fig. 21.4). Some lesions show superficial erosions that become crusted and numerous telangiectasis. Involution starts at the periphery and slowly extends to the center of the lesion. Calcinosis, although rare, may occur.

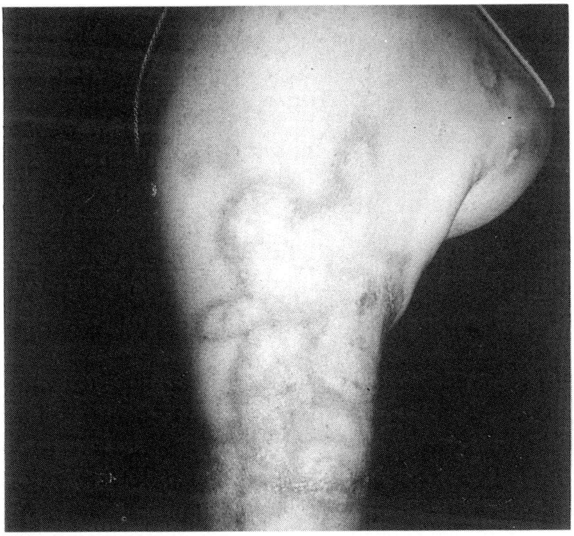

Figure 21.3 Coalescence of multiple morphea plaques surrounded by inflammation (lilac ring) in a patient with localized scleroderma.

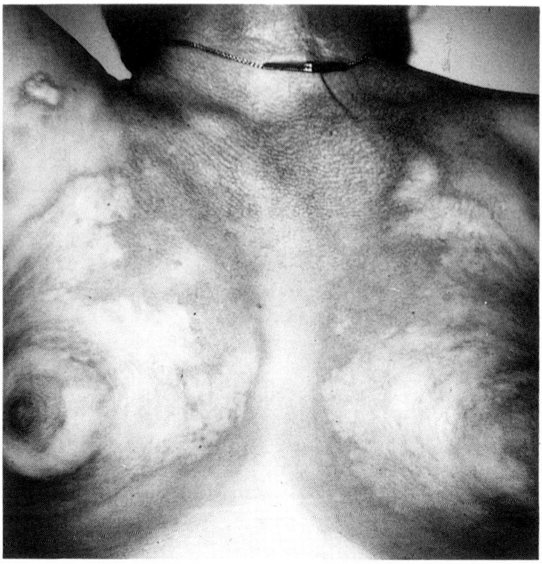

Figure 21.4 Severe sclerosis of the chest spares the periareolar area in a patient with generalized morphea. Note protruding nipples.

Linear Scleroderma

This clinical form affects primarily children and consists of indurated, bandlike, unilateral lesions involving the scalp, half of the face, arms, and legs. Although the disease has a self-limited course, it may cause severe disfiguration of the face. On the hands, it may cause flexion contractures, with severe functional impairment. There is no high association with spina bifida, as previously thought.

Overlap Syndromes

Mixed Connective Tissue Disease

This syndrome shows overlapping clinical features of lupus erythematosus, polymyositis, scleroderma, and occasionally, rheumatoid arthritis. Although some regard this syndrome as a distinct entity, others believe that it represents a mild form of lupus erythematosus with a low incidence of kidney disease. The clinical picture consists of Raynaud's phenomenon, swollen hands rather than acrosclerosis, polyarthralgia, esophageal hypomobility, myositis and pulmonary disease. Mixed connective tissue disease (MCTD) shows high titers of antibodies against ribonuclear protein (RNP), which are usually absent in scleroderma.

Eosinophilic Fasciitis

It is not clear whether eosinophilic fasciitis represents a new entity or may be part of the scleroderma spectrum [4]. This syndrome may resemble localized or systemic scleroderma and results in severe flexion contractures, carpal tunnel syndrome related to tenosynovitis, and occasionally synovitis. The involved skin may be tender and show a puckered or ''peau d'orange'' appearance. The blood reveals a severe eosinophilia ranging from 10 to 50%, high erythrocyte sedimentation rate, and transient hypergammaglobulinemia. Histopathologic examination reveals an inflammatory reaction in the deep fascia and sometimes lower dermis, consisting of lymphocytes, plasma cells, and eosinophils [5]. It has also been reported that patients with eosinophilic fasciitis may develop hematologic abnormalities including aplastic anemia, myeloproliferative disorders, Hodgkin's disease, and leukemia. A similar syndrome was also described following the ingestion of tryptophan.

Chronic Graft-versus-Host Disease

Following allogeneic bone marrow transplantation, patients may develop acute graft-versus-host disease (GVH) consisting of a morbiliform or scarlatiniform eruption, hepatitis, diarrhea, and lymphopenia [6]. In addition, those patients who survive 3 or more months may develop chronic GVHD. This syndrome consists of Sjogren's syndrome, lesions resembling lichen planus with oral involvement, chronic discoid lupus erythematosus, a maculopapular rash, cholestatic liver disease, and eventually a striking form of scleroderma. These lesions consist of severe acrosclerosis of hands and feet and flexion contractures. They also show large telangiectasis with hypo-and hyperpigmentation and atrophy resembling poikiloderma.

Chemically Induced Scleroderma

Workers exposed to polyvinyl chloride prior to its polymerization and to silica (miners, stone-masons) may develop a syndrome indistinguishable from systemic sclerosis. The clinical picture consists of acrosclerosis, Raynaud's phenomenon, dysphagia, arthralgia, calcinosis, kidney disease, and lung fibrosis. Lesions resembling scleroderma have been noted following the administration of bleomycin, pentazocine, after injections of paraffin or silicones, and following the ingestion of adulterated cooking oil that contained denatured rapeseed oil (toxic oil syndrome) [7].

LABORATORY DATA

Routine laboratory data are nonspecific and of little help to confirm the diagnosis or to ascertain the severity of the disease. There may be anemia, usually secondary to iron deficiency, although renal failure, malabsorption, and esophageal bleeding should be ruled out. Microangiopathic hemolytic anemia is usually seen in association with renal disease. White cell counts are usually normal, except for a mild transient eosinophilia [5]. About 50% of patients reveal a hypergammaglobulinemia usually due to an increase in IgG, less often IgM or IgA. Rheumatoid factor and anti-smooth-muscle antibodies may be present. Circulating immune complexes may be present and some were reported in the kidneys, although their significance is not clear. HLA-A and HLA-B histocompatibility antigens did not reveal specific patterns for scleroderma. Albuminuria may be present for many years and may precede kidney disease.

Antinuclear Antibodies

It is estimated that 70–95% patients with systemic sclerosis have ANA if the right substrate is used for the test [8–10]. In this regard, the highest positive rate was obtained with Hep-2 cells. Immunofluorescent microscopic examination revealed various patterns including fine or large speckles, homogeneous, or nucleolar. Centromere antibodies are usually seen in patients with the CREST syndrome and reveal a discrete speckled pattern on fluorescence [11, 12]. The anticentromere antibody can be seen in Sjogren's syndrome, diffuse scleroderma (about 12%), and in association with idiopathic Raynaud's disease (20%) [11]. Although the anticentromere antibody appears to carry a better prognosis, with less severity in pulmonary fibrosis and absence in renal disease, one has to be aware that this antibody has been found in association with two serious complications of the CREST syndrome, namely, pulmonary hypertension and primary biliary cirrhosis.

The scleroderma-70 antibody appears to be a marker for systemic sclerosis and is most often seen with the diffuse form. This antibody is directed against the nuclear enzyme DNA topoisomerase I, which controls chromosomal supercoiling during the cell cycle [10]. It is present in about 20% of patients with systemic sclerosis and gives a fine speckled pattern with or without nucleolar staining. Although specific for systemic scleroderma, it was also noted in idiopathic Raynaud's phenomenon.

Nucleolar antibodies are seen in 50–60% of patients with systemic sclerosis, sometimes at very high titers although the significance of these antibodies is yet to be determined. Nucleolar antibodies may have a wide range of antigen specifity including 4–6 S nucleolar RNA, anti-RNA polymerase I, fibrillarin, and nucleolar organizer. In addition, there is another antinucleolar antibody seen in some patients with scleroderma and polymyositis, known as PM-Scl previously known as PM-1 [13].

Histopathologic Characteristics

The histopathologic examination of localized and systemic scleroderma is similar and reveals three distinct features: mononuclear cell infiltrates, vascular changes, and fibrosis [14–16]. Cellular infiltrates, consisting of lymphocytes, plasma cells, and histiocytic type cells, were noted in 85% of patients with localized scleroderma and 50% of those with systemic sclerosis. These cellular infiltrates may be perviascular perivascular and frequently invade the subcutaneous tissue (Fig. 21.5). Electron microscopic examination of cellular infiltrates revealed lymphocytes with enlarged cytoplasm suggesting blast-transformation, immature and mature plasma cells, macrophages, and active fibroblasts (Fig. 21.6) [17]. Vascular changes refer to reduction in capillaries, development of ectatic vessels, and subintimal fibrosis of small arteries [18]. Arterioles may show thickening of their wall and narrowing of their lumen. Damage to endothelial cells was noted by electron microscopic examination [19]. The dermis and subcutaneous tissue reveals reveal marked deposition of collagen and glycosaminoglycans (Fig. 21.7). Electron microscopic examination reveals disorganization of collagen fibrils and great variety in fibril diameter (Fig. 21.8) and also an increase in microfibrils usually associated with elastin.

Pathophysiological Basis

The cause of scleroderma remains unknown, although it has been suggested that it may represent an autoimmune process. However, the evidence for an autoimmune process in scleroderma is not as well documented as in systemic lupus erythematosus. Circulating autoantibodies are common in scleroderma including those against centromere, topoisomerase, nucleolus, smooth muscle

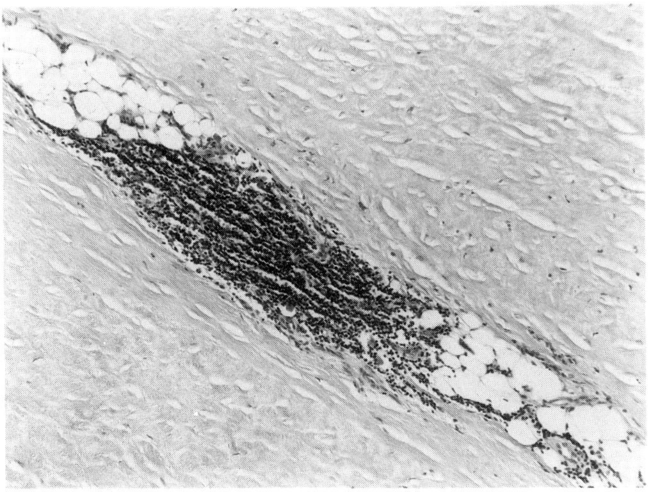

Figure 21.5 Celllular infiltrates within an area of adipose tissue in a patient with systemic sclerosis (hematoxylin and eosin, × 270; from [16]).

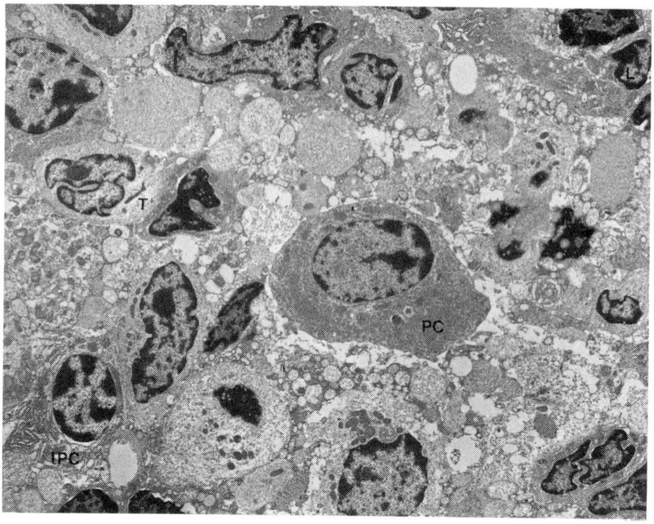

Figure 21.6 Cellular infiltration shows plasma cell (PC), immature plasma cell (IPC), blast lymphocyte (BL), and mature lymphocyte (L) (uranyl acetate–lead citrate [17]).

cells, and others. The role of these antibodies, however, is uncertain since some patients may show typical scleroderma without circulating autoantibodies. Furthermore, there is no good correlation between autoantibodies titers and severity of the disease. Autoantibodies against type I collagen, type IV collagen, and laminin have been reported, although they may represent a secondary phenomenon [20]. Furthermore, there are no consistent HLA-phenotypes to support an autoimmune process. Perhaps the most convincing evidence for an autoimmune process in scleroderma is its clinical similarity to chronic graft-versus-host disease. On the other hand, many diseases may show clinical features resembling scleroderma secondary to fibrosis and are probably unrelated to the pathogenesis of scleroderma.

Vascular changes are well documented in scleroderma. This disease affects capillaries and small arteries, as demonstrated by regular histologic examination, immunofluorescence microscopy with antibodies against blood vessels (laminin, type IV collagen) [21], and by electron microscopy [19]. There is a marked reduction in capillaries, probably secondary to endothelial cell injury. Small arteries show subintimal and perivascular fibrosis. Vascular damage is substantiated by an increase in von Willebrand's factor activity and factor VIII–von Willebrand's factor antigen [22]. In addition, there is also an increase in circulating platelet aggregates and plasma beta thromboglobulin [23]. Vascular ectasia has been reported and is characterized by an increase in endothelial cell prolifera-

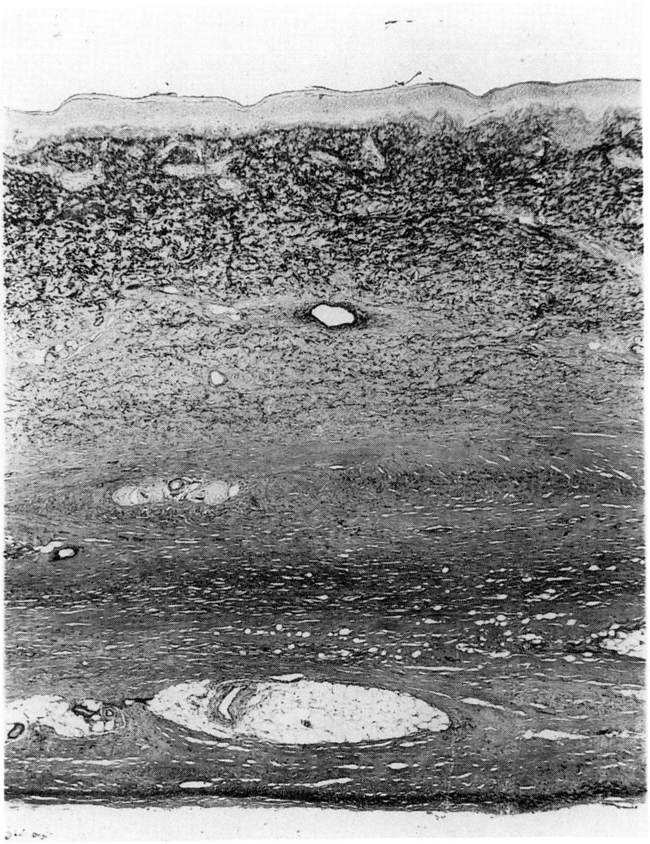

Figure 21.7 Massive fibrosis involving the dermis and subcutaneous tissue. Upper dermis reveals a heavy network of elastic fibrils, while the lower level shows an increase in glycosaminoglycans (aldehyde fuchsin, × 210 [16]).

tion [24]. This may represent a compensatory mechanism to counterbalance endothelial cell destruction.

The inflammatory reaction, triggered by the vascular damage or some unknown antigen, results in the recruitment of lymphocytes (T and B cells), macrophages, and fibroblasts. An increase in the T-helper population may explain the increase in B-cell activity with formation of autoantibodies and an expansion of reactive T-cell clones [25]. These activated T-cell clones may release lymphokines that are chemotactic for fibroblasts and may stimulate fibroblast proliferation as well as collagen and glycosaminoglycan synthesis. Monocytes could also be stimulated to release monokines and fibronectin, which is chemotactic for fibroblasts. Interleukin-1 may stimulate cell proliferation, collagen, collagenase,

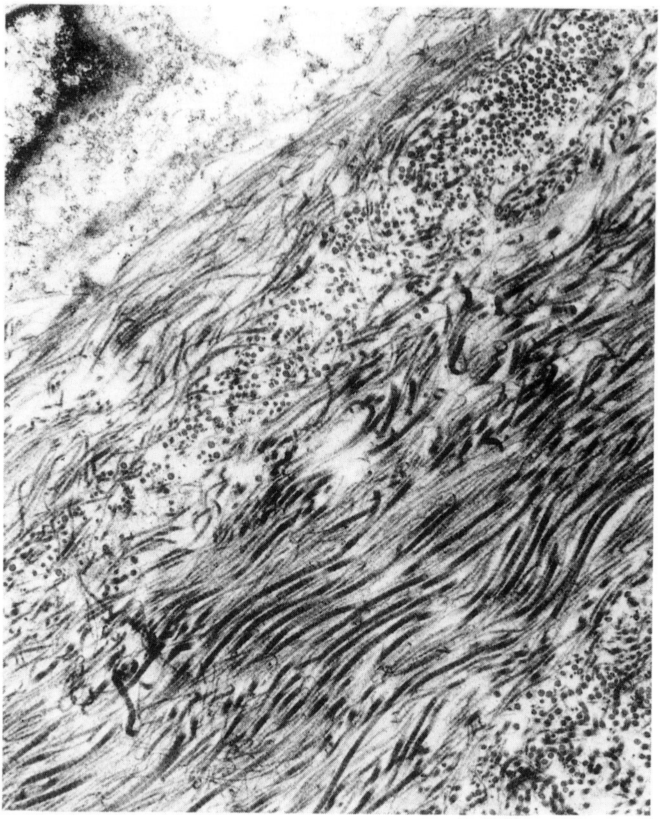

Figure 21.8 Lower dermis shows disorganization of collagen bundles and diversity of fibril diameter. (Uranyl acetate–lead citrate.)

and hyaluronate production by fibroblasts [25]. In addition, some lymphokines released by T cells may also be responsible for endothelial cell damage.

The fibrosis is likely to represent the end stage of the disease. There is an increase in collagen synthesis by scleroderma fibroblasts [26]. It appears that only selective populations of dermal fibroblast are activated, usually at the lower levels of the dermis [27, 8]. These is an increase in type I and type III collagen, although the ratio of these collagens remains normal. The increase in collagen synthesis is also expressed at the level of transcription [29,30]. It has recently been shown that the aminopropeptide of type I procollagen regulates collagen synthesis by negative feedback. This mechanism may be faulty in scleroderma fibroblasts that are high collagen producers [31]. Furthermore, an increase in type III collagen fibrils that retained the aminopropeptide was also demonstrated in scleroderma skin [32]. There have been recent reports showing an increase in mast cells in scleroderma skin [33]. However, at present it is not known how mast cells could influence the production of collagen [34].

TREATMENT

The treatment of scleroderma remains a great challenge to the clinician. Although there is no cure for scleroderma, certain therapeutic approaches may be helpful to patients.

General Measures

Patients are to avoid cold exposure, trauma, cigarette smoking, and emotional stress. Physiotherapy, in the form of exercises, massage, and hot water or paraffin baths, are of relative help.

Raynaud's Phenomenon

Raynaud's phenomenon and ischemia have been treated with sympatholytic drugs (phenoxybenzamine, reserpine, methyldopa). These drugs may improve peripheral blood flow and enhance wound healing of ulcers, but have little effect on the frequency and severity of Raynaud's phenomenon. More recently, calcium channel blockers (nifedipine) in dosages of 30–90 mg daily, have been found useful in some patients with Raynaud's phenomenon. These drugs inhibit the contraction of smooth muscle cells by reducing the uptake of calcium. Side effects consist of headaches, hot flashes, dizziness, palpitations, increased heart rate, nausea, drowsiness, and swelling of feet and ankles. Aspirin, 325 mg every other day, or dipyridamole, 225 mg daily, can be used for the antiplatelet aggregation effect. Prostaglandin E and prostacyclin are peripheral vasodilators and also inhibit platelet aggregation. They have been used in patients with systemic sclerosis with some benefits, although further controlled clinical trials are needed [35].

Arthralgia, Myalgia

Arthralgia and myalgia can be treated with short courses of prednisone, 40–60 mg daily, or with nonsteroidal anti-inflammatory agents, such as ibuprofen, 1200–1600 mg daily.

Fibrosis

Purine antimetabolites (6-thioguanine, azathioprine) and alkylating agents (chlorambucil, cylophosphamide) have been used in patients with scleroderma with variable results. Since the benefits have been questionable and side effects can be serious, the use of cytotoxic drugs is seldom justified.

Penicillamine interferes with intermolecular and intramolecular cross-linkages of collagen, but also has an immunosuppressive effect [36]. It has been suggested that penicillamine may soften the skin, improve pulmonary function, and prolong survival. The daily starting dosage is 250 mg for 4 weeks, increased progressively to 750 mg daily. Side effects include nephrotoxicity, bone marrow depression, gastrointestinal distress, and skin reactions, including atrophy. Complete blood cells counts and urinalysis should be performed every 2 weeks for the first 6 months of therapy and monthly thereafter. Colchicine has been used to treat the fibrosis in patients with scleroderma and biliary cirrhosis. This drug appears to interfere with the synthesis and excretion of collagen and in vitro it appears to enhance collagenase activity. The therapeutic efficacy of colchicine in patients with scleroderma has not been determined. However, there is a rationale for its use and the drug is very safe. The dosage is 0.6 mg twice or three times a day. The main side effect is diarrhea.

Ulcers

Ulcerations in scleroderma usually develop on digits and ankles, can be very painful, and have a tendency to heal slowly. Treatment consists of lukewarm compresses, followed by topical antibiotics such as bacitracin–polymyxin B, gentamycin, or benzoyl peroxide (10–20%). If there is a severe infection, systemic antibiotics, erythromycin, or dichloxacillin, should be used. Necrotic ulcers should be treated with enzymatic debridement, using collagenase, papain, fibrinolysin, or deoxyribonuclease. It is possible to control the pain by topical applications of 5–10% lidocaine ointment, every 4 hr alone or in combination with oral analgesics. The healing of ulcers can be enhanced with methlydopa, 250 mg twice daily, or reserpine, 0.25 mg twice daily.

Hypertension, Dysphagia

Hypertension crises have been well controlled with captopril, combination of diuretics and methyldopa, or guanethidine. Severe renal hypertension may require nephrectomy followed by kidney dialysis. Renal transplantation has not been useful. Reflux esophagitis responds to a treatment regimen for peptic ulcer, namely, head elevation, antacids, and, if necessary, H_2-blockers. Dysphagia requires the use of soft, well-chewed meals and antacids. Esophageal strictures can be improved by dilation and surgical procedures.

Experimental New Treatments

Photopheresis

This consists of extracorporeal photoactivation of 8-methoxypsoralen by ultraviolet A energy to a form that covalently cross-links to DNA. The patient receives oral methoxypsoralen followed by a centrifugation step to enrich blood lymphocytes. The lymphocytes are then exposed to an elaborate ultraviolet A system. It appears that the patient develops an immunologic response to the reinfused photodamaged lymphocytes. This treatment has been used with some success in the treatment of cutaneous T-cell lymphomas [37]. Since T cells may play a role in systemic sclerosis, a clinical trial is presently been conducted in various centers.

Cyclosporin-A

This strong immunosuppressant blocks antigen-specific T-cell proliferation. Its exact mode of action is not entirely known although it appears to inhibit the expression of interleukin-1 and interleukin-2 receptors on T cells. This drug is markedly nephrotoxic and should not be used in the treatment of systemic sclerosis unless a rigid experimental protocol can be instituted with all the necessary precautions.

Interferons

Interferons obtained from human cells or by a genetic engineering process have been used for the treatment of viral and neoplastic diseases. Mononuclear cells may be important mediators in the regulation of the fibrotic response. In this regard, these is evidence that gamma-interferon produced by activated macrophages inhibits collagen synthesis by scleroderma fibroblasts [38]. This drug has been suggested for the treatment of systemic sclerosis. Although interferon is considered safe, there are dose-dependent side effects including fever, chills, anorexia, malaise, fatigue, and leukopenia.

ACKNOWLEDGMENT

This work was supported by the National Institutes of Health grant AR27608 and by the Scleroderma Society, Inc.

REFERENCES

1. Fleischmajer R. Scleroderma, a model for fibrosis. Arch Dermatol 1983; 119: 957–62.
2. Kinder R, Fleischmajer R. Systemic scleroderma: a review of organ systems. Int J Dermatol 1974; 13: 382–95.
3. Jayson MIV, Black C M (eds). Systemic sclerosis: scleroderma. John Wiley and Sons 1988.
4. Shulman LE. Diffuse fasciitis with eosinophilia: a new syndrome. Trans Assoc Am Physicians 1975; 88: 70–86.
5. Fleischmajer R, Jacotot AB, Shore S, Binnick SA. Scleroderma, eosinophilia and diffuse fasciitis. Arch Dermat 1978; 114: 1320.

6. Lawley TJ, Peck GL, Moutsopoulos HM, Gratwohl AA, Deisseroth AB. Scleroderma, Sjogren-like syndrome and chronic graft-versus-host disease. Ann Intern Med 1977; 87: 707–9.
7. Phelps RG, Fleischmajer R. Clinical, pathological and immunopathological manifestations of the toxic oil syndrome. J Am Acad Dermatol 1988; 18: 313–24.
8. Tan EM. Antinuclear antibodies in scleroderma. Int J Dermatol 1981; 20: 569–73.
9. Catoggio LJ, Bernstein RM, Black CM, Hughes GRV, Maddison PJ. Serological markers in progressive systemic sclerosis: clinical correlations. Ann Rheum Dis 1983; 42: 23–7.
10. Douvas AS, Achten M, Tan EM. Identification of a nuclear protein (Scl-70) as a unique target of human antinuclear antibodies in scleroderma. J. Biol Chem 1979; 254: 10514–21.
11. Fritzler MJ, Kinsella TD, Garbutte E. The CREST syndrome: a distinct serologic entity with anticentromere antibodies. Am J Med 1976; 69: 520–6.
12. Moroi Y, Peebles C, Fritzler MJ, Steigerwald J, Tan EM. Autoantibody to centromere (Kinetochore) in scleroderma sera. Proc Natl Acad Sci 1980; 77: 1627–31.
13. Reimer G, Scheer U, Peters JM, Tan EM. Immunolocalization and partial molecular characterization of a nucleolar antoantigen (PM-Scl) associated with polymyositis scleroderma overlap syndromes. J Immunol 1987; 137: 3802–8.
14. Fleischmajer R, Perlish JS, Reeves JR, Cellular infiltrates in scleroderma skin. Arthritis Rheum 1977; 20: 975–84.
15. Fleischmajer R, Nedwich A. Generalized morphea. I Histology of the dermis and subcutaneous tissue. Arch Dermatol 1972 106: 509–14.
16. Fleischmajer R, Damiano V, Nedwich A. Alteration of the subcutaneous tissue in systemic scleroderma. Arch Dermatol 1972; 105: 59–66.
17. Fleischmajer R, Perlish JS, West WP. Ultrastructure of cutaneous cellular infiltrates in scleroderma. Arch Dermatol 1977; 113: 1661–6.
18. D'Angelo WA, Fries JF, Masi AT, Shulman LE.Pathologic observations in systemic sclerosis (scleroderma). Am J Med 1969; 46: 428–40.
19. Fleischmajer R, Perlish JS. Capillary alterations in scleroderma. J Am Acad Dermatol 1980; 2: 161–70.
20. Mackel AM, De Lustro F, Harper FE, Leroy EC. Antibodies to collagen in scleroderma. Arthritis Rheum 1982; 25: 522–31.
21. Fleischmajer R, Dessau W, Timpl R, Krieg T, Luder-Schmidt C, Wiestner M. Immunofluorescence analysis of collagen, fibronectin and basement protein in scleroderma skin. J Invest Dermatol 1980; 75: 270–5.
22. Kahaleh MB, Osborn I, LeRoy EC. Increased factor VIII–von Willebrand factor antigen and von Willebrand factor activity in scleroderma and in Raynaud's phenomenon. Ann Intern Med 1981; 94: 482–4.
23. Kahaleh MB, Osborn I, Leroy EC. Elevated levels of circulating platelet aggregates and beta-thromboglobulin in scleroderma. Ann Intern Med 1982; 96: 610–3.
24. Fleischmajer R, Persh JS. ^{3}H-Thymidine labeling of dermal endothelial cells in scleroderma. J Invest Dermatol 1977; 69: 379–82.
25. Postlethwaite AE, Kang AH. Cellular immunity in systemic sclerosis: scleroderma. In: Janson MIV, Black CM, eds. John Wiley and Sons, 1988: 61.

26. LeRoy EC. Connective tissue systhesis by scleroderma skin fibroblasts in cell culture. J Exp Med 1972; 135: 1351–62.
27. Fleischmajer R, Perlish JS, Krieg T, Timp R. Variability in collagen and fibronectin synthesis by scleroderma fibroblasts in primary culture. J Invest Dermatol 1981; 76: 400–3.
28. Scharffetter K, Lankat-Buttgereit B, Krieg T. Localization of collagen mRNA in normal and scleroderma skin by in-situ hybridization Eur J Clin Invest 1988; 18: 9–17.
29. Graves PN, Weiss IK, Perlish JS, Fleischmajer R. Increased procollagen mRNA levels in scleroderma skin fibroblasts. J Invest Dermatol 1983; 80: 130–2.
30. Uitto J, Bauer EA, Eisen AZ. Scleroderma: increase in biosynthesis of triple helical type I and type III procollagens associated with unaltered expression of collagenase by skin fibroblasts in culture. J Clin Invest 1979; 64: 921–30.
31. Perlish JS, Timpl R, Fleischmajer R. Collagen synthesis regulation by the aminopropeptide of procollagen I in normal and scleroderma fibroblasts. Arthritis Rheum 1985; 28: 647–51.
32. Perlish JS, Lemlich G, Fleischmajer R. Identification of collagen fibrils in scleroderma skin. J Invest Dermatol 1988; 90: 48–53.
33. Hawkins RA, Claman HN, Clark RAF, Steigerwald JC Increased dermal mast cell populations in progressive systemic sclerosis: a link in chronic fibrosis. Ann Intern Med 1985; 102: 182–6.
34. Pearson ME, Huff JC, Giorno RC, Panicheewa S, Claman HN, Steigerwald JC. Immunologic dysfunction in scleroderma: evidence for increased mast cell releasability and HLA-DR positivity in the dermis. Arthritis Rheum 1988; 31: 672–7.
35. Belch JJF, Newman P, Drury JK, McKenzie F, Capell H, Lieberman P, Forbes CD, Prentice CRM. Intermittent epoprosterol (prostalyclin) infusion in patients with Raynaud's syndrome. Lancet 1983; 1: 313–5.
36. Steen VD, Medsger TA, Rodnan GP. D-Penicillamine therapy in progressive systemic sclerosis (scleroderma). Ann Intern Med 1982; 97: 652–9.
37. Edelson R, Berger C, Gasparro F, et al. Treatment of cutaneous T-cell lymphoma by extracorporeal photochemotherapy. Engl J Med 1987; 316: 297–303.
38. Jimenez SA, Freundlich B, Rosenbloom J. Selective inhibition of human diploid fibroblasts collagen synthesis by interferons. J Clin Invest 1984; 74:1112–6.

22

Pseudoscleroderma: Clinical, Morphological, and Biochemical Aspects

Stefania Jablonska
Warsaw School of Medicine, Warsaw, Poland

Several conditions mimic both systemic scleroderma (SSc) and localized cutaneous scleroderma (LS). These diseases, both atrophic and indurative, of various causes and different pathomechanisms [1], are important because they need to be differentiated from scleroderma. Comparison of their clinical and pathologic features as well as of changes in collagen with those in scleroderma may help to delineate the basic differences and to allow us to understand better the pathogenesis of scleroderma.

This chapter discusses eosinophilic fasciitis (EF), regarded as a nosologic pseudosclerodermatous entity, which appears to be in essence an unusual form of symmetrical LS, and the newly described inborn pseudoscleroderma syndromes: congenital fascial dystrophy and restrictive dermopathy.

EOSINOPHILIC FASCIITIS vs. SYMMETRICAL MORPHEA

Eosinophilic fasciitis (EF) has been recognized as a separate entity since it differs from all other forms of scleroderma by clinical and histologic features, and usually benign course with full recovery [2,3]. However, sporadic cases with coexistent symptoms of systemic scleroderma and/or transitional into scleroderma [4–6] were reported by several authors.

We have observed four cases of typical EF transformed within several months to a few years into symmetrical morphea. The onset was sudden after physical exertion and/or trauma, there were symmetrical indurations of the limbs with no cutaneous changes, peripheral eosinophilia and hypergammaglobulinemia, as well as a characteristically enlarged fascia with profuse inflammatory infiltrations containing abundunt eosinophils. The progressively developing sclerotic changes were generalized; however, they were most pronounced on the trunk, and somewhat on the limbs. In two persons (a 9-year-old boy and a 57-year-old woman) the morphea-type lesions regressed spontaneously within 2–3 years, with full restoration of movement and full regression of cutaneous changes. In one 28-year-old man the symmetrical morphea became widespread, almost generalized, and persisted for almost 10 years, with no involvement of the internal organs, muscle, or bones. In those cases, peripheral and tissue eosinophilia and gammaglobulinemia disappeared first and the clinical picture acquired all the characteristic features of an ordinary, although symmetrical, widespread morphea.

In a 12 year-old girl, whom we followed up for 15 years (Fig. 22.1-3),

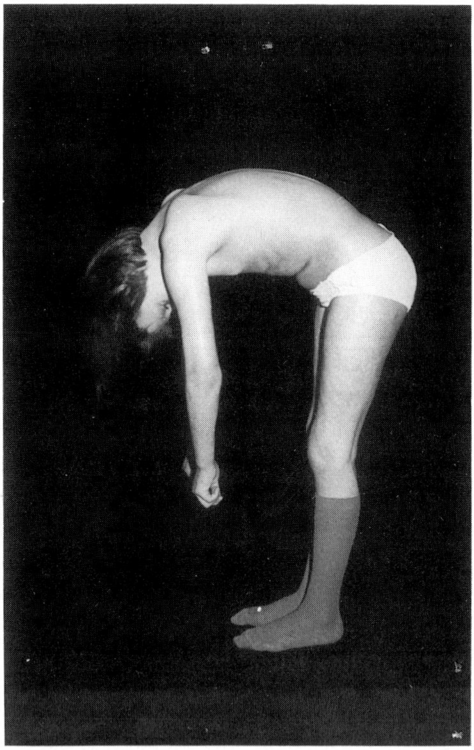

Figure 22.1 Patient with early eosinophilic fasciitis with indurations of the extremities not preventing normal activity.

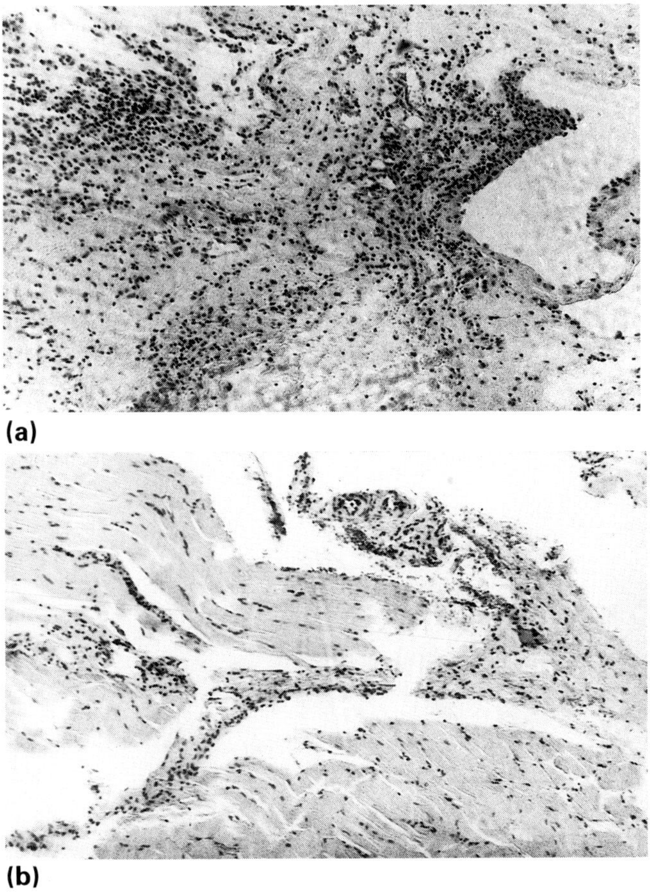

Figure 22.2 (a) Enlarged fascia with pronounced inflammatory infiltrates (hematoxylin and eosin [H&E], × 100). (b) Fascia with some inflammatory infiltrates in the later stage (H&E, × 180).

symmetrical indurative lesions on the trunk developed progressively, sparing nipples that were unusually enlarged, surrounded by sclerotic skin. This patient had no visceral involvement except for decreased respiration of the restrictive type due to tight thoracic skin. No immune abnormalities were disclosed, although at some times antinuclear antibody titers were 80–320. However, the results of repeated immunofluorescent examinations for almost the whole duration of the disease were negative. This girl developed pronounced sclerodactyly, with contractures of the hands and feet (Fig. 22.3). At this time the pattern of tryptophan metabolism changed from high kinurenine level characteristic of EF to that

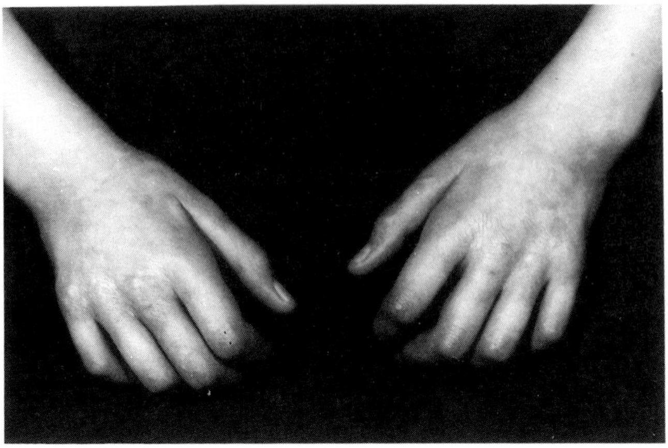

Figure 22.3 The same patient, 3 years later. Indurations and contractures of eosinophilic fasciitis are evident. Transformation of eosinophilic fasciitis into scleroderma, with fascia remaining as a target for inflammatory reaction.

of tryptamine and indolacetic acid characteristic of scleroderma [1]. A biopsy specimen of the skin and muscle at the onset of the disease showed pronounced inflammatory changes with numerous eosinophils in the considerably enlarged fascia, and no muscle involvement (Fig. 22.2a). In the later stage, the fascia was significantly less enlarged, with no eosinophils, but with some inflammatory infiltrates penetrating the fibrotic interstitial connective tissue of muscle (Fig. 22.2b). In this patient, the course of the disease was unusually severe, with fatal outcome due to secondary amyloidosis.

Thus, EF is not invariably a benign, self-regressing disease, although in a majority of the cases this scleroderma-like disease has a more favorable prognosis than other subsets of symmetrical morphea or deep linear scleroderma. The differing pattern of tryptophan metabolic pathways might be of diagnostic and prognostic significance.

The transformation of some typical cases of EF into widespread symmetrical morphea, with or without spontaneous regression, is suggestive of their close relationship.

CONGENITAL FASCIAL DYSTROPHY

In contrast to inflammatory fascial involvement in EF, the noninflammatory fibrosis of the body fascia, described under the name of congenital fascial dystrophy, does not appear to be a subset of scleroderma despite the stony-hard indurations of the skin and deeper tissues (Figs. 22.4 and 22.5) [8]. The disease is

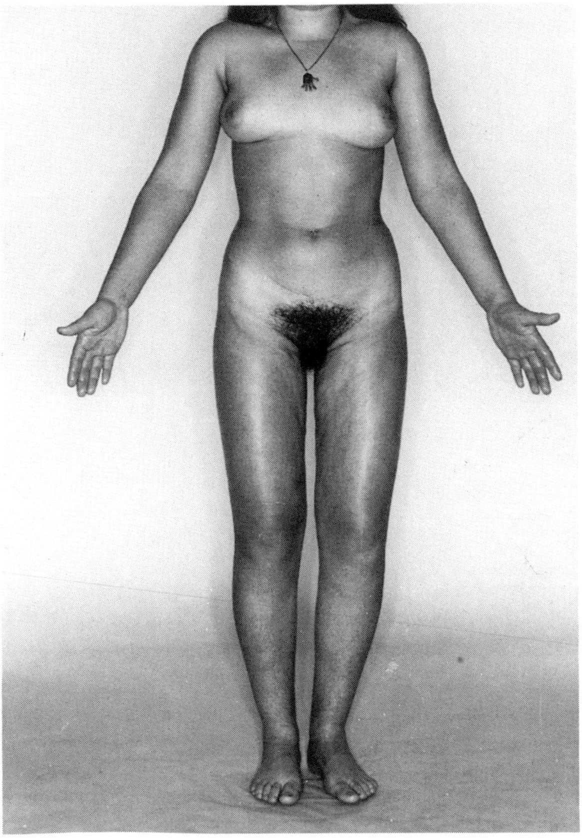

Figure 22.4 Congenital fascial dystrophy with stony-hard indurations of the extremities.

inheritable, since most of the described cases were either siblings or children of consanguinous marriages [8–11], but the mode of inheritance is not fully established. It differs from scleroderma by its genetic and congenital character, absence of inflammatory and vascular changes, absence of visceral involvement and immune abnormalities, as well as by a nonprogressive course. The only abnormality is a considerably (at least four times) enlarged fascia (Fig. 22.6), especially remarkable in areas of its abundance on the buttocks and thighs.

The bones and muscle are not involved due to the normal vascular and nerve supply, not impeded by the thickened fascia. The limitations of joint mobility and contractures in the lower limbs are responsible for a characteristic tiptoe posture and peculiar manner of walking (Fig. 22.5).

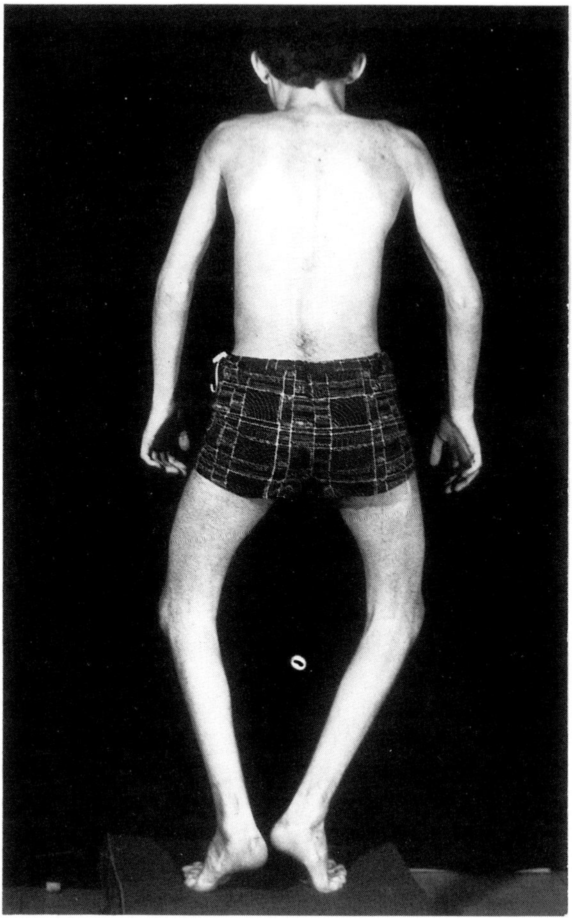

Figure 22.5 Congenital fascial dystrophy. Characteristic tip-toe posture, contractures of the lower extremities, small thorax, with well-developed shoulder muscles (van Gieson, × 180).

The disease is usually noticed in early infancy and is not progressive, except for the functional impairment of the lungs, probably due to thickened thoracic fascia. Despite limitations of movements and the bizarre posture, patients are well adjusted to their disability and do not require any management except for proper rehabilitation procedures. This disorder of supportive connective tissue described previously as a stiff skin syndrome [9,10], was suggested as being related to a defective local regulation of mucopolysaccharide synthesis by fibroblasts.

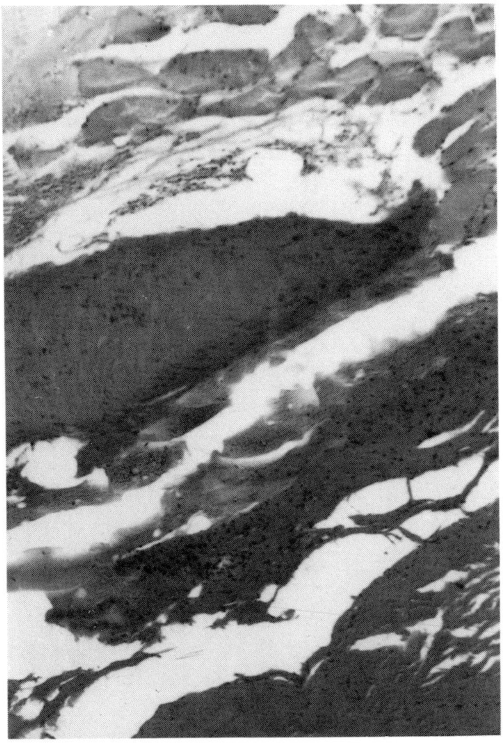

Figure 22.6 Enlarged fascia without inflammatory infiltrates; normal muscle (van Gieson, × 180).

We found an increased collagen synthesis by the fibroblasts derived from the deeper portions of the skin, without any abnormality of its pattern and normal production of mucopolysaccharides and fibronectin. However, electron microscopic studies disclosed abnormal amianthoid-like fibers in the fascia, 400 nm in diameter. We postulated that their appearance could be related to the disturbances of the structural glycoproteins and glycosaminoglycans (i.e., the noncollageneous glycoprotein component of the matrix) [8]. We also found a striking similarity to collagen alterations in the tight skin mouse, a dominant mutant of an inbred mouse strain characterized by scleroderma-like accumulation of collagen in the thickened skin, firmly bound to the underlying tissue [11]. This mouse presents a model for hereditary excessive collagen production, resulting in indurations of the skin and supportive tissues, with no inflammatory changes of immune abnormalities characteristic of scleroderma.

FATAL SCLERODERMALIKE GENETIC DISORDER OF NEWBORN INFANTS (RESTRICTIVE DERMATOPATHY)

This apparantly autosomal recessive disorder with invariably fatal outcome was reported under different names as aplasia cutis congenita [12, 13]; contractures, edema, hyperkeratosis, and intrauterine growth retardation [14]; and restrictive dermatopathy [15, 16]. A similar fatal case in a prematurely born 3-month-old infant [17] was reported as a case of scleroderma in an infant.

In this new syndrome, the entire skin is tight, except for the palms and soles, does not pit on pressure, and in some areas shows peeling of the superficial layers. The facies is characteristic with micrognathia, small open mouth, and beaklike nose. The hair is sparse or absent. In some infants with thick rigid facial skin, ectropion develops with secondary keratitis. All infants show flexion contractures due to the tight skin, and the restricted respiratory movements appear to be the cause of death.

The histologic study by Holbrook et al. [15] disclosed signs of arrested epidermal morphogenesis with hyperplastic, hyperkeratotic, and parakeratotic epidermis, and aberrant patterns of keratin. The connective tissue of the dermis appeared stretched resembling the tendon in its orientation, and collagen fibers were smaller in diameter. Skin appendages and sweat ducts showed arrested development, the hair follicles did not show evidence of hairs, and sweat ducts were thickened and coiled beneath the epidermis. The subcutaneous fat was preserved and twice the thickness of the thin dermis. These authors believe that the primary defect is an alteration in the mechanisms regulating dermal–epidermal interactions.

We have observed five cases of this genetic disorder (D. Rosinska et al., in press). Two were siblings, and three unrelated infants. In one of them, there was family history of similar disease in a sibling who died in the first week of life, and another was born to a mother in whose family several neonatal deaths had occurred. All infants were born prematuraly to apparently healthy parents. Two survived for more than 10 months.

The infants showed typical dysmorphic facial changes from the first week of life and sclerodermiform lesions from the third month of age. The boy died at the age of 20 months, and the girl survived up to the age of 3 years.

These two children were subjected to more detailed study. Both cases were very similar to that reported by Labeille et al. [18] as neonatal progeria with sclerodermiform lesions. The cutaneous involvement, the typical facies, and course of the disease were identical to our cases, but in their case there was also osteolysis of the outer part of the clavicule and terminal phalanges (i.e., features characteristic of progeria). However, there was an increased synthesis of collagen by the patient's fibroblasts, similar to that in patients with scleroderma [19], whereas progeria is associated with decreased collagen synthesis, characteristic of the aged skin [18].

In none of our cases did we succeed in maintaining the cultured fibroblasts, although the cultures were performed in three different laboratories.

In the child who survived to the age of 3, the clinical features became strikingly similar to progeria syndrome, with characteristic facial hypoplasia and micrognathia, beaked thin nose, and distorted ear lobes. Repeated cultures of skin fibroblasts were unsuccessful, and this is reported as characteristic of progeria, together with a markedly reduced life span of progeroid fibroblasts in vitro [20]. Progeria is, however, a disease of hypoplastic, atrophic, and degenerative changes occurring in initially fairly well developed tissue. This is probably the cause of its later appearance, usually after the first year of age [21], while the avarage life span of affected individuals is 12 years. Single sporadic neonatal cases of progeria with early fatal outcome [22–25], some presenting features of scleroderma in early infancy [18, 26], might have been, in reality, cases of restrictive dermatopathy.

The most important recent finding is the detection of the increased elastin gene expression in progeroid fibroblasts [27], believed to be a biochemical marker of the phenotype. The increased elastin production might be related to the accelerated aging, but proper fibrillogenesis and interactions with other connective tissue molecules appear to be of basic importance [28]. Although tropoelastin production by progeroid fibroblasts was found to be six-to ninefold increased at the protein and mRNA levels, the relative collagen synthesis was similar to control. Thus, there is presently available a marker for progeria that until now was recognized exclusively on the basis of a very characteristic appearance.

The difference between progeria and fatal restrictive dermatopathy consists of an onset in fetal life, early fatal outcome, and evident genetic character of the latter, while most cases of progeria are sporadic. However, the relationship between these two patterns of malformation in infants who die from the condition is not entirely clear.

EOSINOPHILIA MYALGIA SYNDROME

At the end of 1989 the first cases were reported of a new syndrome characterized by severe myalgia, peripheral eosinophilia, and various cutaneous manifestations: ill-defined rash, edema, and hard indurations, involving mostly extremities, sometimes also the trunk but characteristically sparing the digits, and not associated with Raynaud's phenomenon. Thus cutaneous changes were similar to deep indurations in eosinophilic fasciitis (EF), or to subcutaneous generalized and/or symmetrical morphea [29, 30]. However, this syndrome differs from EF due to the much more severe myalgia, intensive pruritus, maculopapular or urticarial rash, alopecia of systemic lupus erythematosus (SLE) type, visceral involvement (lung, heart), polyneuropathy, derangement of central nervous system, and fever. As in EF, the most characteristic pathologic findings are edematous and sclerodermalike skin changes, enlargement of fascia with abundant inflammatory infiltrates consisting of lymphocytes, plasma cells, mast cells, and usually numerous eosinophils. Peripheral eosinophilia is present in about 39% of the cases, with the median eosinophil count 5,296/mm^3, similar to or even more pronounced than in EF. Unlike in EF, there is usually no hypergammaglobulinemia, and the platelet count is elevated, which may result in thromboembolism. It should be stressed that despite severe muscle involvement, the creatine phosphokinase level is in most cases normal, whereas the aldolase level is usually elevated. Antinuclear antibodies are present in the majority of the patients, whereas they occur as the exception in patients with EF.

The clinical features and the course of the disease are variable, sometimes severe, even with fatal outcome (in 27 cases). From the first reported cases in October, 1989, to February, 1990, more than 1300 cases have been uncovered, and by August, 1990 the number was up to 1556 (L. Shulman, personal communication).

A clear association between this new syndrome and the intake of L-tryptophan (L-TRY) had been firmly established. All patients had ingested L-tryptophan, some for several or more than 10 years, in median dosages of 1.5 g daily, with a range of 0.5–16 g daily, for treatment of insomnia, depression, anxiety, or other neurologic complaints. Although the association of the syndrome with ingestion of L-tryptophan is generally recognized, the causal relationship and the reason for epidemic outbreak are poorly understood. One suggestion is that the toxic effects are related to some contaminants (bacterium amyloliquefaciens) introduced during the production by genetic engineering technique, since almost all of the American patients have used a Japanese product. High-performance liquid chromatographic (HPLC) analysis revealed one additional peak E (97) that could represent a novel amino acid linked with TRY [31], and responsible for the toxic effects.

However, new cases have been reported from Europe in patients treated with drug produced by other companies: in Germany by Biologische und Pharmazeutische Produkte [32, 33]. Ingested L-TRY is accumulated in the organism and, following discontinuation of supplementation, there is only a slow improvement. Corticosteroids are usually not effective. After a prolonged ingestion, if a chronic disease develops, the course may be steadily progressive [34].

The relationship of scleroderma and scleroderma like chages with tryptophan metabolism was studied by several authors [35, 36]. For EF the characteristic feature was found to be the deranged kynurenine pathway of L-TRY metabolism [37]. The excretion of kynurenine was high during the whole active period of the disease, and 1.0 g L-TRY induced in patients with EF a very pronounced increase; three times higher than in scleroderma and four times more than in controls. The first case of scleroderma-like changes induced by therapy with L-5-hydroxytryptophan and carbidopa had features of EF and EMS, with pronounced increase of plasma kynurenine concentration [38]. The abnormal TRY metabolism could explain appearance of sclerodermalike changes in patients with eosinophilia myalgra syndrome (EMS) [30, 39–41]. Silver et al. [42] also found high levels of kynurenine and its further metabolite, quinolinic acid. These authors presented an interesting suggestion concerning the role of interferon-gamma, which might induce indoleamine -2,3-dioxygenase, associated with abnormalities of kynurenine pathway. Varga et al. [43] stressed a causal relation between the effect of TRY metabolites and the stimulation of collagen expression resulting in dermal and fascial fibrosis. Elevated expression of the genes for TGF_B and type VI collagen in the affected fascia could suggest a role for TGF_B in the induction of sclerodermalike changes [44].

The explosive epidemic of EMS has evident similarity to the toxic oil syndrome [TOS], attributed to the ingestion of industrial-grade denaturated cooking oil sold in 1981 in Spain [45]. In 1982, there were 19,828 cases reported, with 315 deaths [29]. There were several systemic manifestations: fever, headache, pulmonary edema, severe muscle pain, thromboembolism, and peripheral eosinophilia. The cutaneous rashes, edema followed by induration of the extremities, and hematologic and serologic abnormalities were similar to the findings in EMS, and the histologic changes of the skin and fascia were comparable to both EMS and EF. The systemic symptoms (neurologic, pulmonary, cardiac) in TOS were more severe than in EMS, and the patients with EMS have higher levels of pulmonary, cardiac, neurologic, myopathic, and gastrointestinal involvement than patients with EF, but these differences appear to be quantitative.

No contaminant was isolated from the oil but some samples contained high levels of aniline, which is a known toxin, closely releated to the anthranilic acid, a product of the kynurenine pathway [46]. Most important, is that both kynurenine and quinolinic acid levels were found to be increased in patients with TSO, like in EMS [42], thus providing the first evidence of the biochemical linkage of EMS and TOS.

There is a marked female preponderance of patients with chronic stages of both EMS and TOS, while EF appears with equal frequency in both genders.

Despite the differences, there is a remarkable similarity in the sclerodermalike type of fasciitis in all these three diseases. In EMS there is an evident causal relation to ingestion of large amounts of L-TRY, and the abnormal kynurenine metabolism has been well established [30, 42, 47], similar to the kynurenine pathway of TRY metabolism in EF [37, 48]. In TOS, although the offending agent remains unknown, TRY metabolism was also found to be involved.

It is assumed that the incidence of EMS will be declining since L-TRY as a drug has been removed from the market; however, new cases might be due to ingestion over a long period of low doses contained in various amino acid compositions.

The outbreak of EMS has raised great interest in a possible toxic causes of scleroderma and sclerodermalike diseases. However, various sclerodermatous changes were reported to be induced also by several other environmental factors, both occupational (e.g., vinyl chloride, trichlorethylene, epoxy resin, and especially exposure to silica dust in miners) [48, 49], and iatrogenic (e.g., after augmentation mammoplasty with silicone implants) [50]. A proportion of the cases showed features of true scleroderma. Thus, induced disease might be either scleroderma or pseudoscleroderma.

Recognition of these pseudosclerodermatous syndromes and detection of diverse causative factors should allow a better understanding of the pathogenesis of scleroderma and provide a basis for rational prophylaxis and therapy.

REFERENCES

1. Jablonska S. Scleroderma and pseudoscleroderma. Warsaw: Polish Medical Publishers, 1975.
2. Shulmann LE. Diffuse fasciitis with eosinophilia: a new syndrome? Trans Assoc Am Physicians 1975; 88: 70–86.
3. Rodnan GP, DiBartolomeo AG, Medsger TA, Barnes LE. Eosinophilic fasciitis: report of seven cases of a newly recognized scleroderma-like syndrome. Arthritis Rheum 1975; 18: 422–3.
4. Torres VM, George WM. Diffuse eosinophilic fasciitis. A new syndrome or variant of scleroderma? Arch Dermatol 1977; 113: 1591–3.
5. Jarrat M, Bybee JL, Ramsdell W. Eosinophilic fasciitis: an early variant of scleroderma. J Am Acad Dermatol 1979; 1: 221–6.
6. Jablonska S, Hamm G, Kencka D, Sieminska S. Fasciitis eosinophilica—Übergang in eine eigenartige Sklerodermie (Sklerodermie-Fasciitis). Z Hautkr 1984; 59: 711–21.
7. Jablonska S, Rodnan GP. Localized forms of scleroderma. Clin Rheum Dis 1979; 5: 215–41.
8. Jablonska S, Groniowski J, Krieg T, Nerlich A, Peltonen L, Oikarinen A, Dabrowski J, Pietrow D. Congenital fascial dystrophy—a noninflammatory disease of fascia: the stiff skin syndrome. Pediatr Dermatol 1984; 2: 87–97.
9. Esterly NB, Mc Kusick VA. Stiff skin syndrome. Pediatrics 1971; 47: 360–9.
10. Kikuchi I, Inoue S, Hamada K, Ando H. Stiff skin syndrome. Pediatr Dermatol 1985; 3: 48–53.
11. Jablonska S, Schubert H, Kikuchi I. Congenital fascial dystrophy—stiff skin syndrome: a human counterpart of the tight skin mouse. J Am Acad Dermatol 1989; 21: 943–50.
12. Garmi R, Sofer S, Karplus M, Ben-Yaker Y, Madler D, Bar-ziv J. Aplasia cutis congenita in two sibs discordant for pyloric atresia. Am J Hum Genet 1982; 11: 319–28.
13. Toriello HV, Higgins JV, Waterman DF. Autosomal-recessive aplasia cutis congenita—report of two affected sibs. Am J Hum Genet 1983; 15: 153–6.

14. Lowry RB, Machin GA, Norgan K, Mayock D, Marx L. Congenital contractures, edema, hyperkeratosis and intrauterine growth retardation: a fatal syndrome in Hutterite and Mennonite kindreds. Am J Med Genet 1985; 22: 531–43.
15. Witt DR, Hayden MR, Holbrook KA, Dale BA, Baldwin VJ, Taylor GP. Restrictive dermatopathy: a newly recognized autosomal recessive skin dysplasia. Am J Med Genet 1986; 24: 631–48.
16. Holbrook KA, Beverly AD, Witt DR, Hayden MR, Toriello HV. Arrested epidermal morphogenesis in three newborn infants with a fatal genetic disorder (restrictive dermatopathy). J Invest Dermatol 1987; 88: 330–9.
17. Heilbron B, Saxe N. Scleroderma in an infant. Arch Dermatol 1986; 122: 1417–9.
18. Labeille B, Dupuy P, Frey-Follezou, Larrégue M, Maquart FX, Borel JP, Gallet M, Rosbourg B, Denceux JP. Progeria de Hutchinson-Gilford néonatale avec atteinte cutanée sclérodermiforme. Ann Dermatol Venereol 1987; 114: 233–42.
19. Fleischmajer R, Nedwich A. Progeria (Hutchinson-Gilford). Arch Dermatol 1973; 107: 253–8.
20. Goldstein S. Studies on age-related diseases in cultured skin fibroblasts. J Invest Dermatol 1979; 73: 19–23.
21. De Busk FL. The Hutchinson-Gilford progeria syndrome. Report of 4 cases and review of the literature. J Pediatr 1972; 80: 697–724.
22. Wiedemann HR. An unidentified neonatal progeroid syndrome: follow-up report. Eur J Pediatr 1979; 130: 65–70.
23. De Martinville B, Sorin M, Briand ML, Frezal J. Progerie de Gilford-Hutchinson à début néonatal chez des jumeaux monozygotes. Arch Fr Pediatr 1980; 37: 679–81.
24. Snigula F, Rautenstrauch T. A new neonatal progeroid syndrome. Eur J Pediatr 1981; 136: 325.
25. Devos EA, Leroy JG, Frijns JP, Van Den Berghe H. The Wiedemann-Rautenstrauch or neonatal progeroid syndrome. Report of a patient with consanguinous parents. Eur J Pediatr 1981; 136: 245–8.
26. Moynahan EJ. Progeria (Hasting-Gilford) presenting as scleroderma in early infancy. Proc R Soc Med 1962; 55: 233–4.
27. Sephel GC, Sturrock A, Giro MG, Davidson JM. Increased elastin production by progeria skin fibroblast is controlled by the steady-state levels of elastin mRNA. J Invest Dermatol 1988; 90: 643–7.
28. Kornberg RL, Hendler SS, Oikarinen AI, Matsouka LY, Uitto J. Elastoderma—disease of elastin accumulation within the skin. N Engl J Med 1985; 312: 771–4.
29. Shulman LE. The eosinophilia-myalgia syndrome associated with ingestion of L-tryptophan. Arthritis Rheum 1990; 33: 913–7.
30. Silver RS, Heyes MP, Maize JC, Quearry B, Vionnet-Fuasset M, Sternberg EM. Scleroderma, fasciitis and eosinophilia associated with the ingestion of tryptophan. N Engl J Med 1990; 332: 874–81.
31. Mayeno AN, Lin F, Foote ChS, Loegaring DA, Ames MM, Hedberg CW, Gleich GJ. Characterization of "peak E," a novel amino acid associated with eosinophilia–myalgia syndrome. Science 1990; 250: 1707–8.
32. Zillikens D, Bammel A, Lurz Ch, Elsner P, Burg G. Eosinophilie-Myalgia-Syndrom nach Einnahme von L-Tryptophan. Hautarzt 1991; 42: 154–7.

33. Von Gizycki-Nienhaus B, Meurer M, Krieg T, Braun-Falco O. EMS und L-Tryptophaneinahme. Hautarzt 1991; 42: 179–82.
34. Bulpitt KJ, Verity MA, Clements PJ, Paulus HE. Association of L-tryptophan and an illness resembling eosinophilic fasciitis. Arthritis Rheum 1990; 33: 918–29.
35. Price JM, Yess N, Brown RR, Johnson AM. Tryptophan metabolism: a hitherto unreported abnormality occurring in a family. Arch Dermatol 1967; 9: 462–72.
36. Stachow A, Jablonska S, Skiendzielewska A. 5-Hydro-xytryptamine and tryptamine pathway in scleroderma. Br J Dermatol 1977; 97: 147–54.
37. Stachów A, Jablonska S, Kencka D. Tryptophan metabolism in scleroderma and eosinophilic fasciitis. In: Black CM, Myers AR eds. Current topics in rheumatology: systemic sclerosis. (scleroderma). New York: Gower Medical, 1985: 13–4.
38. Sternberg EM, van Woert MH, Young SN, Magnussen I, Baker H, Gauthier S, Osterland CK. Development of a scleroderma-like illness during therapy with L-5-hydroxytryptophan and carbidopa. N Engl J Med 1980; 303: 782–7.
39. Connolly SM, Quimby SR, Griffin WL, Winkelmann RK. Scleroderma and L-tryptophan: a possible explanation of the eosinophilia-myalgia syndrome. J Am Acad Dermatol 1990; 23: 541–7.
40. Gordon ML, Lebwohl MG, Phelps RG, Cohen SR, Fleischmajer R. Eosinophilic fasciitis associated with tryptophan ingestion. Arch Dermatol 1991; 127: 217–20.
41. Walz-Leblanc BAE, Inman RD. Eosinophilia myalgia syndrome-old questions for a new syndrome. J Rheumatol 1990; 17: 1435–8.
42. Silver RM, Sutherland SE, Carreira PE, Heyes MP. Alteration of tryptophan metabolism in the toxic oil syndrome and in the eosinophilia–myalgia syndrome. Presented at the conference on scleroderma, Swievadow, June 1991.
43. Varga J, Griffin R, Newman JH, Jimenez SA. Eosinophilic fasciitis is clinically distinguishable from the eosinophilia–myalgia syndrome and is not associated with L-tryptophan use. J Rheumatol 1991; 18:259–63.
44. Peltonen J, Varga J, Sollberg S, Uitto J, Jimenez SA. Elevated expression of the genes for transforming growth factor-B_1 and type VI collagen in diffuse fasciitis associated with the eosinophilia–myalgia syndrome. J Invest Dermatol 1991; 96: 20–5.
45. Kilbourne EM, Rigau-Perez LA, Heath CW JR, Zack MM, Falk H, Martin-Marcos M, de Carlos A. Clinical epidemiology of toxic oil syndrome: manifestations of a new illness. N Engl J Med 1983; 309: 1408–14.
46. Roubenoff R, Cote T, Watson R, Levin ML, Hochberg MC. Eosinophilia–myalgia syndrome due to L-tryptophan ingestion: report of four cases and review of the Maryland experience. Arthritis Rheum 1990; 33: 930–8.
47. Mainetti C, Fathi M, Saurat JH. L-tryptophan-induced eosinophilia-myalgia syndrome. II Partial correction of abnormal tryptophan metabolism by pyridoxine. Dermatologica 1991; 18(3): 62–5.
48. Owens GR, Medsger T AJ. Systemic sclerosis secondary to occupational exposure. Am J Med 1988; 85: 114–6.
49. Haustein UF, Ziegler V: Environmentally induced systemic sclerosis disorders. Int J Dermatol, 1985; 24: 147–51.
50. Varga J, Schumacher HR, Jimenez SA. Systemic sclerosis after augmentation mammoplasty with silicone implants. Ann Intern Med 1989; 111: 377–83.

23

Healing, Ulcers, and Keloids

Charles M. Lapière

University of Liège, Sart Tilman, Belgium

Healing is required for the survival of all multicellular organisms in contact with an aggressive, toxic, or infectious environment responsible for trauma and tissue necrosis. It is a homeostatic function operated by the cells of the connective tissue that allows for the recovery of mechanical properties required for the organization of epithelial, endothelial, and parenchymal cells.

Although the pathogenic mechanisms that will trigger the repair reaction are multiple, they are all related to cell death and share a common feature: the release of a variety of cytokines and other mediators (Table 23.1). Healing is a sequence of integrated cellular reactions initiated and regulated by chemical and physical mediators. These informational molecules and mediators are similar throughout the organism. However, the time sequence, the nature, and the concentration of these molecules operating during the healing process can vary between organs.

Tissue repair can be arbitrarily classified into its connective tissue phase and its organ-specific phase (i.e., repair of epithelial, endothelial, or parenchymal tissue). In several steps of the process, interaction between these phases will occur. The common aspect of the healing reaction in all organs occurs within the connective tissue. Various resident cells of the connective tissue, fibrocytes, smooth muscle cells, pericytes, endothelial cells, and others, interacting with cells from the blood, participate in the process. Their involvement can be schematically organized into three overlapping mechanisms: inflammation, granulation tissue formation, and scar organization.

Table 23.1 Mediators Active in Healing

Growth factors and cytokines
Interleukins
Endothelins, interferons, TIMPs, transferrin
Serotonin, acetylcholine, epinephrine, prostaglandins, nitric oxide
Complement, coagulation factors
Hormones

TIME COURSE OF SKIN HEALING

The injury, whether physical, chemical, bacteriologic, or immunologic, results in blood vessel destruction, extravasation of blood, and/or its coagulation. Coagulation and platelet aggregation release an array of biologically active substances that trigger a sequence of events [1] listed in Table 23.2 for a skin wound. Within a few hours after the injury and the accumulation of macrophages and leukocytes, cells surrounding the traumatized area undergo changes that witness their activation [2]. Endothelial cells, activated monocytes, and fibroblasts rapidly colonize the wound space, supported in their migration by the loose network of polymeric fibrin–fibronectin in the blood clot. This initial scaffold is progressively replaced by polymeric collagen, offering a differentiated support to the cell. Cell multiplication and neovascularization result in the formation of the granulation tissue. The contractile activity of the cells induces the migration of the edges of the wound toward its center. The progressive organization of the granulation tissue by differentiation of the cell and reduction of their number results in a scar with increasing mechanical strength that will, however, remain lower than the initial structure. The process of cell differentiation and tissue remodeling extends to the neighboring connective tissue and persists for a long time.

Table 23.2 Healing of a Full-Thickness Skin Wound

Timing	Event
Minutes	Formation of the blood clot
Hours	Migration of blood cells
Days	Multiplication of neighboring cells
Days	Formation of the granulation tissue
Week	Wound contraction
Week	Migration of epithelial cells
Month	Organization of the scar and neighboring tissues
Year	Maturation of the scar

CYTOKINES, GROWTH FACTORS, AND CELL–MATRIX INTERACTION DURING TISSUE REPAIR

Blood coagulation triggered by the activation of thrombin, complement, and the kinin system as well as aggregation and degranulation of platelets upon contact with nonendothelial surfaces such as collagen and the death of all types of cells result in the release of growth factors that act specifically on the various connective tissue cells that participate in the healing reaction (Table 23.3). The basic cellular mechanisms required for healing are similar to those involved in development, growth, and aging. They are chemokinesis, multiplication, and differentiation.

A population of cells that has been recruited into the wound space by chemotaxis undergoes several modifications in shape and phenotype [3]. Their endoplasmic reticulum develops and filaments of contractile proteins migrate to a peripheral location and form in the cytoplasm large bundles oriented parallel to the long axis of the cell. These so-called myofibroblasts display obvious contractile capacities and defined biosynthetic activities. Mediators of this transformation include the growth factors released by platelets and by several other types of cells in the injured tissue.

The complex regulation of the myofibroblast (MF) during the formation of the scar is shown in Figure 23.1. The progressive modeling of the extracellular matrix (ECM) to form a granulation tissue depends on controlled chemotaxis (CHEM), multiplication (X), synthesis (SYN), and degradative (DEG) activity. Growth factors (GFs) and cytokines (CYTs) produced by migrating cells (macrophage and lymphocytes, for example) act on myofibroblasts by a paracrine pathway and their activity is concentration-dependent and nature-specific [4]. The type and the density of the membrane receptors (GCRs) on the recipient cell also condition their activity. The production of collagen (COLLs), fibronectin

Table 23.3 Activity of Growth Factors in Vitro

	EC	F	SMC	K
PDGF	X	X, T, S, C	X, S, C	—
FGF	X, T, D	X	X, S, C	X, T, S
EGF	X, T	X, D	X, C	X, T
TGFB	X–, S	X–, T, S, C	X–, T, S	X–, T, D
TNF	X–, T	X, S, D	X–, S	X

T, chemotaxis; X, multiplication or X-reduced proliferation; S, synthesis; D, degradation; C, contraction; EC, endothelial cells; F, fibroblasts; SMC, smooth muscle cells; K, keratinocytes.

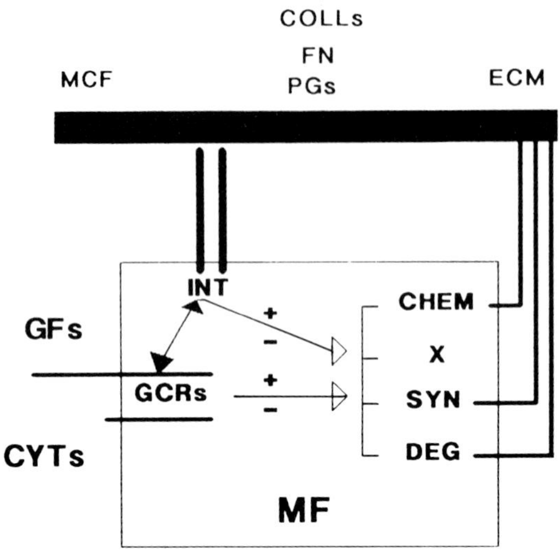

Figure 23.1 Sketch of the multiple interactions (indicated by arrows) involved in the control of cell function during maturation of the granulation tissue and scar. The abbreviations are defined in the text.

(FN), and proteoglycans (PGs) is modulated by cytokines and growth factors (see Chapter 12) and also by the chemical composition of the extracellular matrix and the density and type of integrins (INT) in the cell membrane (see Chapters 11, 7). Information received by integrins will modulate the receptors for growth factors and cytokines and vice versa. Mechanical forces (MCF) transferred to the cells by the network of connective tissue macromolecules also interact in this complex regulation of the cells of the granulation tissue in their evolution to form the scar [5].

Growth factors, cytokines, and extracellular matrix components are also responsible for the controlled proliferation and differentiation of endothelial cells. After migration into the wound bed by chemotaxis, the endothelial cells differentiate into capillaries. Cell multiplication is triggered by a set of growth factors of the FGF family, while differentiation into capillaries and the formation of the new network is under the control of growth factors and polymeric collagen [6].

The granulation tissue is capable of contraction, and wound retraction is a significant mechanism in the closure of a full-thickness skin wound. Two mechanisms should be considered for this process. The first relies on the contractile activity of the granulation tissue inside the wound pulling on the edges. The other depends on the directional migration of myofibroblasts of the edge of the wound toward its center. The second mechanism is supported by the persistence of contraction even when the granulation tissue filling the wound has been removed.

SCAR FORMATION AND REMODELING

The initial network present shortly after trauma is the blood clot made of blood cells entrapped in polymeric fibrin and fibronectin stabilized by FXIIIa. It is progressively removed under the activity of macrophages and replaced by polymers of collagen. This process is related to continuous differentiation of the cells. Their initial phenotype leads to the deposition of fibronectin and type III collagen. Type I collagen forming larger fibrils will progressively replace the thin polymers of collagen type III and increase the resistance of the scar. Additional types of collagen (type V and type VI) will also be deposited and participate in the restructuring of the tissue and acquisition of mechanical resistance.

Mechanical forces are again significant mediators involved in modeling the scar. Tension within the repair tissue is maintained by the cells as do fibroblasts in vitro in a collagen gel. Forces transmitted to the cells by the framework of polymers regulate their phenotype.

Hyaluronic acid present in the early granulation tissue will be later removed and replaced by sulfated proteoglycans. Proteoheparan sulfate will serve in the organization of the tissue and the relationship between the cells and their support. Elastin and fibrillin are also synthesized during the formation of the granulation tissue and the remodeling of the scar. The amount and the organization of the elastic fibers will, however, never attain that in the surrounding nonwounded tissue [7].

Early during the process of healing in skin, a layer of epithelial cells will migrate over the granulation tissue. The interface between epidermal cells and the granulation tissue will host the formation of a new basement membrane [8]. Collagen type IV and the basement membrane glycoproteins and collagen type VII will be progressively deposited in the basement membrane zone. Epithelial–connective tissue interaction mediated by cytokines and secretion products of the cells from the two compartments are known to participate in the modeling of the scar.

It is interesting to note that fetal skin heals without formation of a visible scar [9]. It has been claimed to depend on its large and persistent concentration of hyaluronic acid [10]. A similar scarless healing has been attained in adult animals by suppressing the activity of TGF beta using a specific antibody [11]. Grafting wounded fetal human skin onto the nude mice either exposed to air or subcutaneously results in healing without scar only in the latter conditions. A multifactorial control is probably involved in scarless healing.

PATHOLOGIC HEALING

Physiological healing (i.e., tissue repair occurring in an otherwise noncompromised organism) will proceed at an optimal rate. Delayed or suppressed healing resulting in chronic wounds, also called ulcers, depends on a variety of alterations impairing the function of some of the cells required for the repair process. Disturbed tissue functions related to healing may also be encountered in all organs in the form of retraction, as in the burn patient and in the stenosis of the hollow organs, the esophagus, intestine, heart valves, blood vessels, and urinary tract.

Ulcers

Ulcers are wounds, spontaneous or induced, that do not heal for a specific reason related to a disturbed relationship of the wounded tissue and the rest of the organism (see Table 23.4).

Most skin ulcers in the human are located on the lower legs and result from defective blood supply. Impaired sensation of pain, peripheral or central, is responsible for various types of pressure sores. Altered functions of the cells participating in the various aspects of the healing process resulting from metabolic, immunologic, or iatrogenic causes, are also responsible for delayed healing. Defective cross-linking of fibrin in FXIII deficiency, altered protein metabolism in prolidase deficiency, reduced multiplication of cells by antimitotic agents, and defective function of inflammatory cells, macrophages, lymphocytes, and polymorphonuclear leukocytes in immunodeficiency and corticotherapy are also known causes of ulcers.

Animal models of vascular ulcers can be created, as in the spontaneous necrosis of the tip of a long pedunculated graft in the rat. Chemically induced diabetes in the rat also induces a retardation of skin wound healing. Delayed healing of experimental wounds can be obtained by administration of drugs such

Table 23.4 Causes of Ulcers

Arterial	Immunodeficiency
Arteriolal	Iatrogenic
Venous	Antimetabolites
Lymphatic	Corticosteroids
Neurologic	
Metabolic	
Sickle cell anemia	
Prolidase deficiency	
Factor XIII deficiency	

as corticosteroids or antimetabolites or by application of ionizing radiation. In the experimental animal but also in humans, application of various growth factors has demonstrated a benefical effect in such delayed healing processes [12].

Keloids and Hypertrophic Scars

During the process of their formation, scars can be transiently hypertrophic (i.e., present an excessive volume compared to the neighboring surface). Most often this hypertrophy will regress (skin, bone, hollow organ) and the scar will finally become atrophic. The hypertrophic state of a scar can persist for a long time. One year is considered the longest limit. Keloids are somewhat similar excesses of scar tissue that extend outside of the initial wound [13]. There is no consensus on the pathologic basis of keloids, although a few facts are worth mentioning. Black and Asian persons are more prone to hypertrophic scarring and keloids than white persons, which introduces the notion of a potential genetic control of the healing reaction. Keloids and hypertrophic scars are more vascularized, contain more connective tissue, and endothelial cells and are covered by a thicker epidermis than usual scars. The connective tissue cells in keloids are hyperactive in terms of protein and collagen synthesis. Hypoxia and increased lactate production might be one of the causative mechanisms explaining some of the above-mentioned modifications. Continuous external pressure in excess of the inherent capillary pressure has been shown beneficial in reducing and preventing hypertrophic scars and even keloids.

Healing and its pathologic basis represent fields of high interest ranging from basic biology to applied medicine. The future of the discipline is very promising.

REFERENCES

1. Clark RA. Cutaneous tissue repair: basic biologic considerations I. J Am Acad Dermatol 1985; 13: 701–24.
2. Scharffetter K, Kulozik M, Stolz W, Lankatbuttgereit, B, Hatamochi A, Sohnchen R, Krieg T. Localization of collagen alpha 1 (I) gene expression during wound healing by in situ hybridization J Invest Dermatol 1989; 93: 405–12.
3. Sappino AP, Schürch W, Gabbiani G. Biology of disease. Differentiation repertoire of fibroblastic cells: expression of cytoskeletal proteins as marker of phenotypic modulations. 1990; Lab Invest 63: 144–61.
4. Adelmann-Grill BC, Wach F, Cully Z, Hein R, Krieg T. Chemotactic migration of normal dermal fibroblasts towards epidermal growth factor and its modulation by platelet-derived growth factor and transforming growth factor-beta. Eur J Cell Biol 1990; 51: 322–6.
5. Lambert CA, Soudant EP, Nusgens BV, Lapière CM.Pretranslational regulation of extracellular matrix macromolecules and collagenase expression in fibroblasts by mechanical forces. Lab Invest 1992; 66: 444–51.

6. Montesano R, Vassalli JD, Baird A, Guillemin R, Orci L. Basic fibroblast growth factor induces angiogenesis in vitro. Proc Nat Acad Sci USA 1986; 83: 7297–302.
7. Quaglino D, Nanney LB, Kennedy R, Davidson JM. Transforming growth factor beta stimulates wound healing and modulates extracellular matrix gene expression in pig skin. 1. Excisional wound model. Lab Invest 1990; 63: 307–19.
8. Rigal C, Pieraggi MT, Vincent C, Prost C, Bouissou H, Serre G. Healing of full-thickness cutaneous wounds in the pig. 1. Immunohistochemical study of epidermodermal junction regeneration. J Invest Dermatol 1991; 96: 777–85.
9. Krummel TM, Nelson JM, Diegelmann RF, Lindblad WJ, Salzberg AM, Greenfield J, Cohen IK. Fetal response to injury in the rabbit. J Pediatr Surg 1987; 22: 640–4.
10. Siebert JW, Burd DAR, McCarthy JG, Weinzweig J, Ehrlich HP. Fetal wound healing: a biochemical study of scarless healing. Plast Reconstr Surg 1990; 85: 495–502.
11. Shah M, Foreman DM, Ferguson MWJ. Control of scarring in adult wounds by neutralizing antibody to transforming growth factor beta. Lancet 1992; 339: 213–4.
12. Kingsnorth AN, Slavin J. Peptide growth factors and wound healing. Br J Surg 1991; 78: 1286–90.
13. Rockwell WB, Cohen IK, Ehrlich HP. Keloids and hypertrophic scars: a comprehensive review. Plastic Reconst Surg 1989; 84: 827–37

24

Collagen in Dermatological Applications

Frank DeLustro
Collagen Corporation, Palo Alto, California

Samuel J. Stegman
University of California, San Francisco, California

Xenogeneic dermal collagen has long enjoyed a valuable place in biomedical applications, especially as a resorbable suture and a hemostatic agent. Its applicability has been enhanced by its biocompatibility and weak immunogenicity. Since type I collagen provides the major structural support for connective tissue and thus all organ systems, it has inherent properties of fibrillar structure, protease resistance, and malleability that contribute to a multitude of formulations and highly diverse applications. These physical/chemical attributes are combined with biological properties that promote interactions with a wide variety of cell types including fibroblasts, epidermal cells, endothelial cells, platelets, and others. These cell–matrix combinations can result in directed tissue replacement, repair, and regeneration. This biological, physical, and chemical flexibility has led to the resurgence and expansion of the roles of collagen devices in medicine [1,2].

Although numerous genetically distinct collagen types have been identified (I–XII), the availability and characteristics of type I collagen have contributed to its leading role in dermatologic applications. In addition to its use in surgery as resorbable suture material and to obtain hemostasis, the dermatologic practitioners have utilized these biomaterials for soft tissue augmentation in the form of injectable collagen and, more recently, in dressings for the promotion of wound healing. These specific applications are detailed below.

INJECTABLE COLLAGEN IN DERMATOLOGY

The dermatologist faces numerous types of soft tissue contour defects due to aging, scars, trauma, and congenital deformity. The search for a safe and effective material to augment these irregularities has gone on for many years with limited success. Since collagen is the major structural protein of the dermis, it was a logical extension of its biomedical application to explore injectable collagen for the correction of dermal contour defects. The advent of a highly purified form of injectable xenogeneic dermal collagen has provided the dermatologist and plastic surgeon with a valuable tool in the treatment of these medical problems [3].

The severe inflammation and granuloma formation associated with alloplastic materials have been overcome by the use of injectable collagens, which have become highly biocompatible implants for dermal augmentation. Collagen provided a biologically natural substance consistent with surrounding dermal structure and is compatible to infiltration of host connective tissue cells. The clinical utility of these biomaterials has rapidly expanded since their first introduction for soft tissue augmentation.

In clinical dermatology, treatment of aging changes is extremely popular at present. Those physical changes attributed to aging include the effects of gravity, sun, or facial movement, and the loss of subcutaneous support tissue including fat, cartilage, and muscle. Injectable collagen is helpful in correcting some of the changes due to sun exposure, facial movement, and loss of support. (Figs. 24.1-3).

Facial movement (smiling, frowning, squinting, eating) causes skin to fold and crease. The effect on the skin is passive in that there is no direct muscle pull on the facial skin, but rather the muscles of expression and mastication below the skin contract, resulting in a relative skin redundancy. The skin then mounds up (a fold); bends down (a furrow); or is compressed (a crease). For example, when the corrugator muscles contract during knitting of the brow, the glabellar skin forms vertical, linear creases or folds (Fig. 24.2A). When the perioral area is pulled into to broad smile, several creases, folds, or furrows are formed around the mouth. It is these lines that collagen treats so well (Fig. 24.1B, 2B)

The lines from facial expression are soft and develop in normal skin; (Fig. 24.3A), that is, skin with normal composition and thickness of dermis. Injectable collagen placed into the dermis by needle is laid evenly along the crease or furrow and elevates the overlying skin (Fig. 24.3B) back to its pre-expression height [4]. Thus the line is eradicated. There are several areas on the face where the lines are successfully corrected by collagen; for example, the pucker lines that radiate around the lips, the smile lines on the cheeks and chin, the vertical (and sometimes horizontal) lines on the forehead, and the crow's feet lines radiating from the eyes (Fig. 24.1).

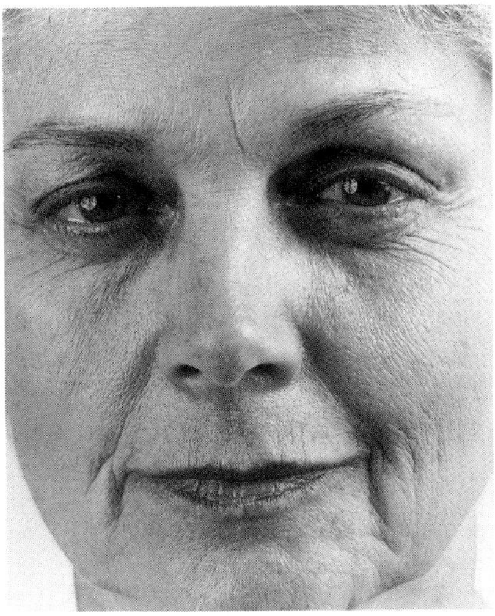

(a)

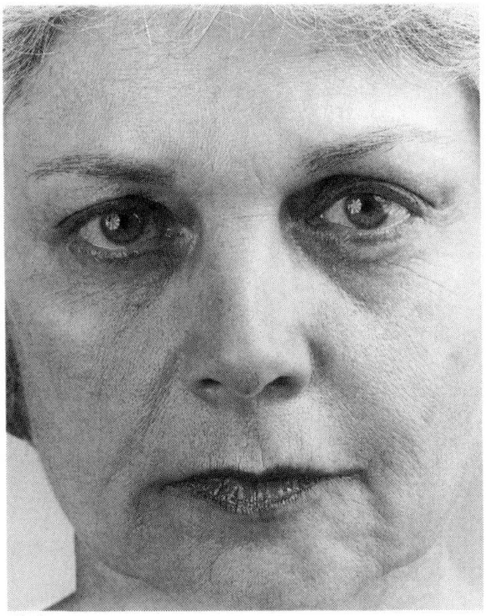

(b)

Figure 24.1 Photograph of a 60-year-old female (a) before treatment with injectable collagen and (b) after treatment with 3.75 ml Zyplast implant in nasolabial, glabellar, and oral commissure lines.

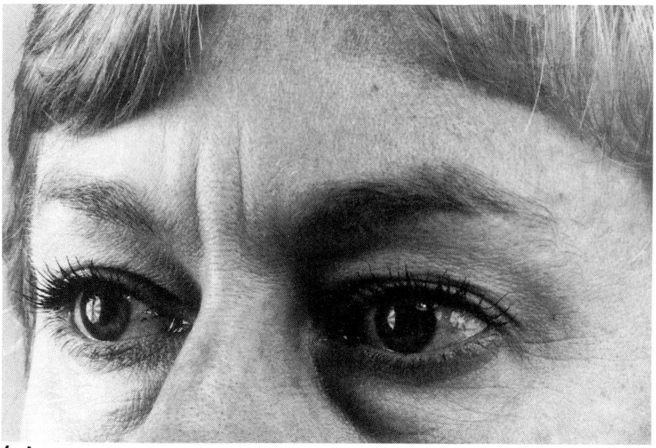

(a)

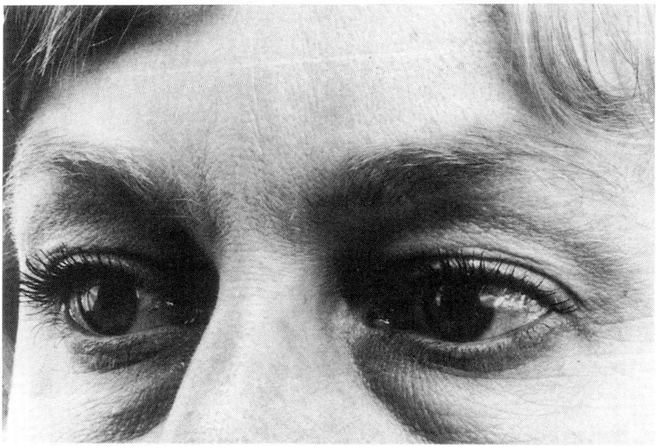

(b)

Figure 24.2 A 35-year-old woman (a) before treatment and (b) after two treatment sessions with a total of 1.35 ml Zyplast implant to correct glabellar frown lines.

Another aging change helped by collagen injection is the loss of subcutaneous support. Sometimes as early as age 40, the fat in the cheeks will begin to flatten; the same is true for the temples and zygomatic area. These areas can be augmented with collagen to restore partially the youthful roundness.

Scarring, both postdisease (e.g., acne or varicella) and posttrauma (either accident or surgical), is amenable to collagen injections that elevate depressions [5]. When the patient has soft, saucer-shaped scars from acne (Figs. 24.4A, 5A)

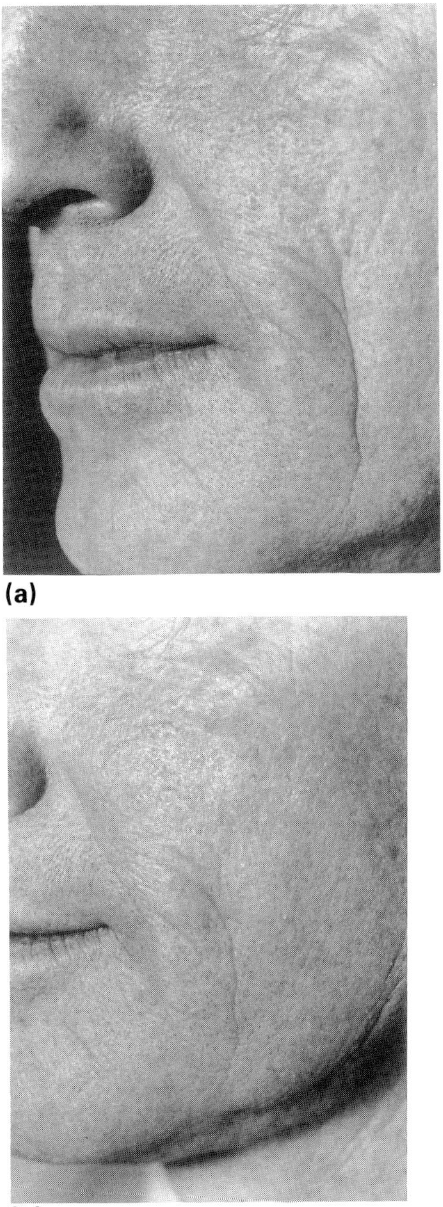

(a)

(b)

Figure 24.3 An expression line on the cheek of this 44-year-old man (a) before treatment and (b) 4 weeks after injection with 0.75 ml Zyplast implant.

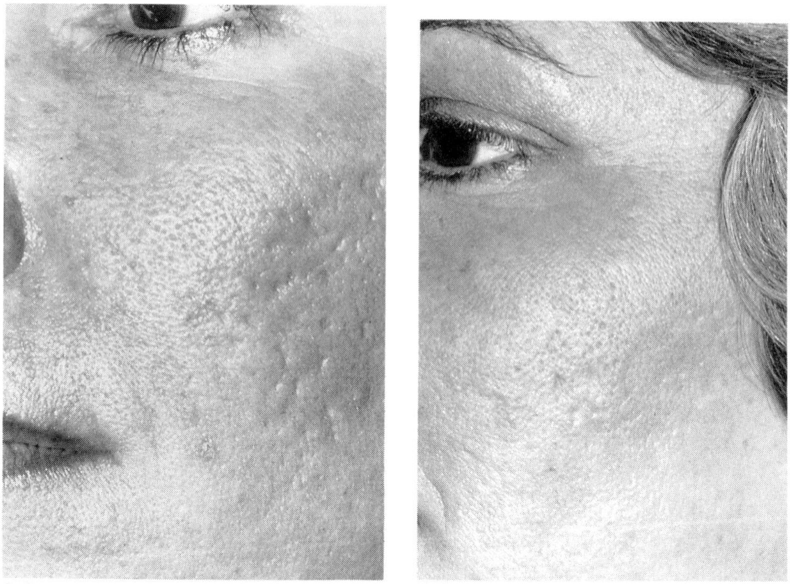

(a) (b)

Figure 24.4 A 28-year-old subject with soft, depressed postacne scars on the cheeks (a) before and (b) 4 weeks after treatment with 1.5 ml Zyderm II collagen.

or soft, depressed linear scars from trauma, the implant will rebuild the normal flat contour and greatly improve the cosmetic appearance. The material does not alter the scar but fills and elevates the irregularities (Figs. 4B, 24.5B)

When scars are firm and fibrotic, either there is no response from collagen injections or the entire scar may raise up. This phenomenon has been seen when collagen was injected into and under so-called ''ice-pick'' acne scars. These narrow (1–2 mm) diameter scars are relatively deep and fibrotic. The physician attempts to place the implant just under the base of the scar. But the base is so small and the walls so firm that the whole scar is elevated en mass. The ice pick scar is therefore converted to a mound with a hole in the center. Thus it is called ''the donut.'' The same problem is experienced with larger surgical or traumatic scars; if they are firm and fibrotic, there is no response or the whole scar raises up. If collagen can be injected into a firm scar (a difficult task) there may be some softening of the scar. Repeated injections become easier and some clinical improvement may become evident.

Collagen is delivered to the physician in 1 ml syringes filled with 0.5, 0.75,

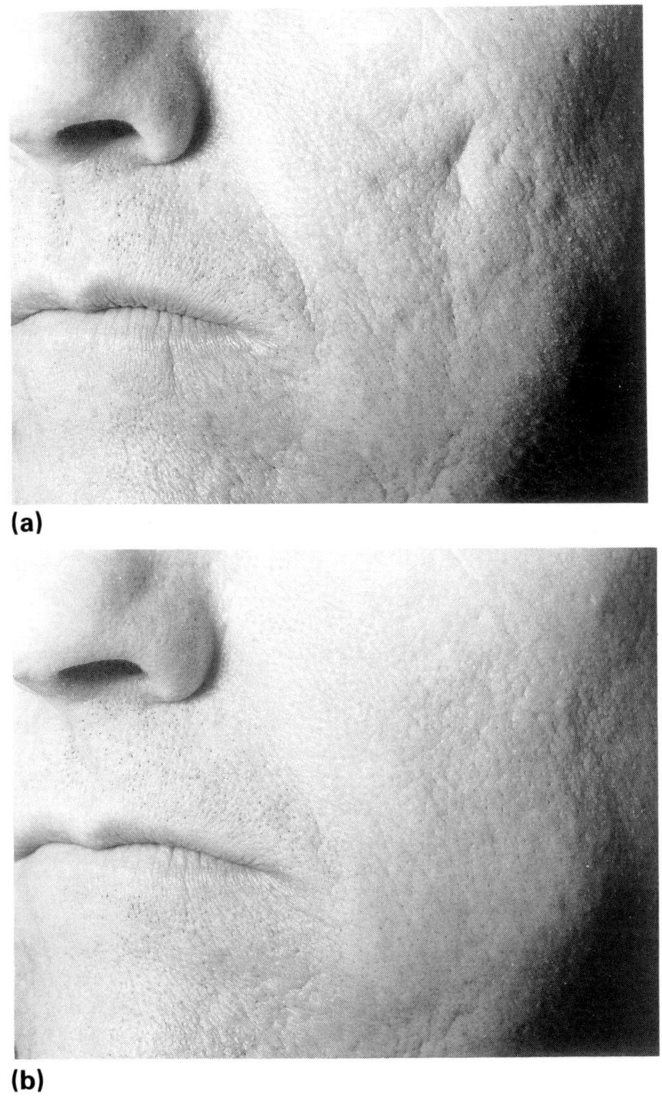

Figure 24.5 Prominent acne scarring of the cheek (a) before treatment and (b) 2 weeks after the last of three treatments with a total volume of 2 ml Zyderm I collagen and 1 ml Zyderm II collagen.

or 1.0 ml of material. There are three preparations available now: Zyderm I collagen, Zyderm II collagen, and Zyplast implant. The difference between Zyderm I and II collagens is concentration; the latter has approximately twice as much as collagen per milliliter as the former (65 vs. 35 mg/ml). Zyplast implant is the same product as Zyderm collagen except that it has been lightly cross-linked with glutaraldehyde, making it a firmer product that can be used for patients with deeper defects and thicker, heavier skin.

Over the 11 years since the product was introduced, physicians have learned empirically how best to inject the material. Placement is best in the dermis. If it is injected just under the epidermis, it will look bumpy and sometimes form little epidermal pockets much like milia. If it is placed below the dermis in the subcutaneous fat, it will require far greater amounts to effect a clinical improvement and the longevity of the correction is greatly shortened. Thus efforts have been directed toward techniques that deposit the implant evenly within the dermis. This is more difficult in patients with thin or scarred skin.

A very successful approach begins by stabilizing the skin with the operator's hand or help from assistants. The physician then injects tiny amounts of collagen through multiple punctures along the long axis of the line [4]. We have learned over the years that a 30 gauge needle with the bevel pointing upwards is effective. Often the needle is bent at the hub so that it approaches the skin at a very acute angle. Early on, injections were too often inadvertently placed too deeply; the bent, acute angled needle helped to prevent this problem.

All three products have been popular, with each physician acquiring his or her own favorite. Zyderm I collagen is usually used in patients with thin skin or in anatomical areas of thin skin [6]. The wrinkled cheeks of older women often have very thin skin; Zyderm I collagen corrects the wrinkles and is not visible in the skin, nor is it lumpy. Zyderm II collagen in that situation would appear visible through the thin skin as a creamy colored implant and may be a little elevated during the first 2 or 3 weeks postinjection. The same problems accompany treatment of the shallow lines around the eyes.

Zyderm II collagen and Zyplast implant are used interchangeably by many physicians for creases in normal or thick skin; they are injected into the middermis. Not as much overcorrection is required for Zyderm II collagen and none for Zyplast implant, since these products are more concentrated or robust.

Experience has also taught us to use magnification and back lighting, to have the patient sitting so the lines are under the full effect of gravity, and to massage the implant lightly after injection. Since approximately ⅔ of the volume of Zyderm I Collagen and ⅓ of the volume of Zyderm II Collagen will rapidly resorb during syneresis (loss of saline), overcorrection is the key. For best results a line or crease is overcorrected by 50–100%. Within the first 24–48 hr, the fluids are lost from the implant and the remaining bovine collagen exerts the correction. The patient looks bumpy only on the first day, and thereafter has the value of the treatment.

Two limitations occur often enough to discuss. The first is the longevity of the clinical correction. Animal and human studies have demonstrated that the implant itself has approximately a 2 year life. However, clinical corrections do not last nearly that long. Several clinical studies indicate that the improvement generally lasts 6–9 months for lines, and 9–18 months for scars.

The best explanation for this phenomenon is that the collagen implant "sinks" deeper into the skin and eventually works its way out of the dermis and "falls" into the subcutaneous space [7]. Once it is below the dermis it can no longer exert any effect to elevate the original defect, whether a scar or line. If the treated depression happens to be directly overlying a bony prominence, the implant "falls" into the subcutaneous space, exerts some upward pressure, and seems to provide longer-lasting correction.

The other problem is the predictable 3–5% incidence of hypersensitivity. Since this material's first usage, a consistent 3% of the population exhibit hypersensitivity to the intradermal skin challenge. Also since the beginning, an additional 1–2% become hypersensitive with one of the subsequent treatment exposures [3]. Hypersensitivity has always been only a localized reaction limited to the area of the implant. On histologic examination it is an allergic granulomatous reaction with varying numbers of infiltrating cells including lymphocytes, macrophages, leukocytes, and mast cells [8]. There is some indication that the timing of the biopsy may affect the number and type of cells detected; the earlier reactions are more cellular and the later ones more granulomatous. The reactions are self-limiting, with an average resolution in 4 months. Some reactions have taken more than 1 year to resolve and a very few have been so intense that they healed with small atrophic scars. Treatment is not indicated and of course the patient is not treated with collagen again.

The application of injectable collagen for soft tissue augmentation has expanded beyond the practice of dermatology and plastic surgery. Recent clinical studies have demonstrated that injectable collagen can be effectively utilized to augment the urinary sphincter in the treatment of urinary incontinence, to augment the lower esophageal sphincter in the treatment of gastroesophageal reflux, and to augment the larynx in the treatment of glottic insufficiency. In addition therapeutic embolization with injectable collagen has been used to treat a variety of inoperable tumors and has been found to be an effective vehicle for the local delivery of antineoplastic drugs along with the embolic result. It is apparent that augmentation of soft tissue with a natural matrix, collagen, is having an increasing benefit to patients and an expanding role in the physician's search for new, effective modalities in the treatment of disease. In the future, we will see the improvement of injectable collagens for soft tissue augmentation to achieve a reduced incidence of hypersensitivity, an increased duration of clinical correction, and improved handling properties.

COLLAGEN IN WOUND HEALING

As the outermost barrier to the outside world, the skin and its integrity are essential to the maintenance of homeostasis and the prevention of infection. In light of this, the repair of damage to this barrier system due to burns, acute wounds (e.g., surgical or traumatic), or chronic wounds (e.g., decubitus or venous stasis ulcers) is imperative for the safety of the individual, and is of key interest to dermatologists who specialize in the skin and its functions. The challenge to the body when the barrier of the skin has been violated is to repair the defect, with re-epithelialization and granulation tissue deposition (both connective tissue and vasculature) being of uppermost importance. However, the avoidance of scar or keloid formation is critical. While myriad complex cellular and matrix events take place during these wound healing responses, we focus here solely on the application of collagen as a biomaterial to these indications and refer the reader to recent reviews for more extensive discussions [9].

Being the major structural component of the skin, collagen's role in dermal wound repair is obviously a central one that has an impact on every phase of the process. Application of collagen-based biomedical devices is thus an obvious extension of the biology of the skin and the natural progression of wound healing. An exciting application of collagen matrices is as a major component of artificial skin in the treatment of severe burns. This bilayer system incorporates collagen and chondroitin sulfate as the inner layer that promotes fibroblast infiltration and new matrix formation, while an outer layer of silicone can be removed when epidermal grafting is desired. This artificial skin provides protection from infection and fluid loss, and stimulates dermal regeneration through its collagen components.

The arena of occlusive dressings in the treatment of acute and chronic wounds has expanded dramatically in the last decade [10]. Dermal collagen has recently been incorporated into several of these dressings. Data demonstrate that enhanced re-epithelialization and accelerated connective tissue regeneration can be achieved by the use of a collagen scaffolding in dressing design. It has been suggested that collagen peptides may be chemotactic for connective tissue cells, recruiting them to the site, and that the collagen matrix supplied by the dressing may regulate the quality of the healing response, reducing the degree of contraction. Collagen biomaterials have demonstrated that they can contribute to the key components of repair: promotion of wound re-epithelialization, deposition of granulation tissue, and reduction in wound contraction.

The future application of collagen-derived devices to wound care in dermatology will clearly involve the incorporation of growth factors known to regulate various steps in the wound repair process (e.g., transforming growth factor beta [TGF-β], platelet-derived growth factor [PDGF], etc.) and the creation of delivery systems that will optimize the local activity of these proteins [9]. These devices will make maximal utilization of the facilitative "bridge" provided by matrices of collagen and the inductive "promotional" signals provided by the naturally occurring proteins (growth factors) of wound repair. These matrix/growth factor combinations will closely mimic the natural process of wound repair that takes place in the normal biology of wound healing.

There are other volumes that review the biology, chemistry, and medical applicability of collagen [11]. In brief, it is apparent that there is a burgeoning of the uses of collagen-derived medical devices in the practice of dermatology. Following the original use of collagen in surgery, collagen in injectable form has been of great value in the treatment of soft tissue contour defects. Application to wound healing has just begun. It is apparent that we will see increasing use of collagen-based devices as dressings and matrices in wound care. This promotion of healing will no doubt be accompanied by the use of growth factors that naturally regulate the dermal healing process. The future will also see collagen as a drug delivery system for the treatment of multiple diseases, including those of the skin. This progression from present applications to future uses of collagen will accelerate very rapidly in the coming decade.

It should not be surprising that collagen, the major structural component of the skin, has been so well conserved during evolution and provides an effective environment for cell activity, a sturdy scaffolding for the tissues, and a resilient milieu for growth and repair. Collagen is providing a natural solution to elusive problems in dermatology and medicine in general.

REFERENCES

1. Simpson RL. Collagen as a biomaterial. In: Rubin LR, ed. Biomaterials in reconstructive surgery. St Louis: CV Mosby, 1983: 109–17.
2. Pachence JM, Berg RA, Silver FH. Collagen: its place in the medical device industry. MD DI 1987; 9: 49–55.
3. Kligman AM, Pharriss BB, eds. Symposium on injectable collagen implants. J Dermatol Surg Oncol 1988; 14, suppl. 1.
4. Stegman SJ. Zyderm. In: Roenigk H, Roenigk R, eds. Dermatologic surgery. New York: Marcel Dekker, 1988: 1313–37.
5. Bailin PL, Bailin MD. Correction of depressed scars following Mohs' surgery: the role of collagen implantation. J Dermatol Surg Oncol 1982; 8: 845–9.
6. Cooperman LS, Mackinnon V, Bechler G, Pharriss BB. Injectable collagen: a six-year clinical investigation. Aesth Plast Surg 1985; 9: 145–52.
7. Stegman SJ, Chu S, Bensch K, Armstrong RA. A Light and electron microscopic evaluation of Zyderm collagen and Zyplast implants in aging human facial skin. Arch Dermatol 1987; 123: 1644–9.

8. Stegman SJ, Chu S, Armstrong RC. Adverse reactions to bovine collagen implant: clinical and histologic features. J Dermatol Surg Oncol 1988; 14 (Suppl): 39–48.
9. Clark RAF, Henson PM, eds. The molecular and cellular biology of wound repair. New York: Plenum Publishing, 1988.
10. Falanga V. Occlusive wound dressings. Why, when, which? Arch Dermatol 1988; 124: 872–7.
11. Nimni ME, ed. Collagen, vol. I-III. Boca Raton, FL: CRC Press, 1988.

25

In Vitro Reconstructed Skin for Grafting in Humans

Bernard Coulomb
Hôpital Henri Mondor, Créteil, France

Louis Dubertret
Hôpital St. Louis, Paris, France

One of the major problems in the treatment of extensive skin defects (e.g., burns) is the small area of normal skin available for grafting. Rapid covering is increasingly indicated since the management of shock, infection, and metabolic disturbances in burn patients has improved substantially. Indeed, the lack of skin is now the limiting factor in survival. Despite the common use of autologous mesh grafts, with further grafts after healing of the donor site, the area of skin available often remains inadequate.

FROM TEMPORARY SKIN SUBSTITUTES TO LIVING SKIN EQUIVALENTS

Allogenic temporary skin substitutes, including xenografts, homografts, and cadaver skin, provide short-term relief but their availability is limited and they are eventually rejected. Synthetic dressings, such as silicone polymers, have the advantage of better availability but, again, covering is only temporary, despite the addition of biological components such as collagen.

The need for a permanent physiological dressing has engendered several research programs aimed at the development of permanent skin substitutes. Some have given rise to acellular biological products that are progressively colonized by mesenchymal cells and integrated by the host [1]. Nonetheless, such dressings still require completion by a living epidermis.

Most types of skin cell have been cultured during the past few years. In particular, a method for serial cultivation of normal human keratinocytes [2] permits the growth in vitro of an autologous epidermis from a small biopsy specimen, thus offering the surgeon coherent epidermal sheets for grafting. This technique, successfully used to engraft two extensively burned children [3], is now routinely employed in several burn centers worldwide, although the need for temporary skin substitutes during the weeks necessary for cell culture is not obviated. The main advantage of such keratinocyte cultures is that they provide large quantities of autologous epidermal sheets that restore the barrier function of the skin. Although the latter conditions are sufficient for patient survival, in the case of deep wounds (in which epidermal sheets do not survive after direct grafting on the fascia), part of the skin (i.e., the dermis) is missing. The presence of the dermis appears to be of prime importance for the mechanical quality of the skin graft.

The development of novel cell culture techniques has offered the opportunity to reconstitute not only an epidermis but also a living dermis, and to use them in association, as they are found in normal skin. The dermis is constructed by incorporating fibroblasts into a three-dimensional collagen matrix; the fibroblasts then reorganize the collagen fibrils, producing a tissue-like structure [4]. This living dermal equivalent, when covered by cultured keratinocytes, represents a living skin equivalent composed, as in vivo, of a dermis and an epidermis. When grafted in animals (rats and rabbits) this simplified autologous skin becomes vascularised, inhibits wound contraction and persists [11].

RECONSTRUCTION OF A HUMAN SKIN EQUIVALENT WITH DERMIS AND EPIDERMIS

In 1981, we started to evaluate the potential of this living skin equivalent for grafting in humans. We chose to start a preliminary clinical evaluation involving burned patients and also patients with giant nevi, since the need to provide large grafts from the small areas of skin available resembles the situation in burned patients. However, patients with giant nevi do not present the metabolic disorders and bacterial infection that occur in the latter context; work can thus take place in a nonemergency situation.

Fibroblast Cultures

Autologous Fibroblasts

For patients with giant nevi, fibroblasts were established from punch biopsies (1 mm diameter) obtained from the future graft recipient. Cells were propagated in Earle's modified Eagle culture medium (EMEM, Flow or Boehringer Labs) containing 10% fetal calf serum (FCS; Flow Labs), in the absence of antibiotics to avoid latent bacterial contamination. Depending on the size of the skin samples taken and the number of dermal equivalents required, fibroblast multiplication by successive passage in culture flasks took from 1 to 2 months.

Allogeneic Fibroblasts

Allogeneic fibroblasts were prepared for burned patients from biopsies of normal skin obtained during plastic surgery, usually from young women. The donor was subjected to the tests used for blood transfusion (Departmental Center of Blood Transfusion, Créteil, France) to avoid viral contamination of the graft recipient during engraftment.

Reconstruction of a Living Dermal Equivalent

Fibroblasts from subconfluent or just-confluent cultures were removed by trypsin treatment, then suspended at 4×10^5 fibroblasts/ml of EMEM with 10% of human AB serum instead of fetal calf serum (FCS) used for the preparation of the fibroblast monolayers.

Fibroblasts were then incorporated into a three-dimensional collagen matrix by mixing in cold glass flasks the following solutions in the following order: 80.5 ml concentrated EMEM (1.76×), 15.75 ml human AB serum, 52.5 ml of type I calf skin collagen solution (5 mg/ml) in 0.02M acetic acid (Bioetica, Lyon, France), 8.75 ml 0.1N NaOH, and 17.5 ml of fibroblast suspension (4×10^5 cells/ml) in EMEM (1×) with 10% of human AB serum.

This mixture (total volume, 175 ml) was then immediately poured into 25 × 25 cm plastic dishes (Costar) and placed at 37°C in a 95% air / 5% CO_2 atmosphere. The collagen rapidly polymerized, forming a gel in which the fibroblasts were uniformly distributed. The gel was then separated from the dish by gentle shaking and 50–100 ml of complete medium was added to avoid readhesion of the gel to the dish during contraction. During the next few days, by a process of active compaction of collagen fibrils by the fibroblasts, a tissue-like structure, the dermal equivalent, was formed, measuring 10×10 cm^2 after 1 week. The size and mechanical properties obtained in these conditions made the dermal equivalents easy to handle, and the thickness was compatible with rapid vascularization after grafting.

Epidermalization

The epidermis was reconstituted using epidermal cells of the future graft recipient, by means of small skin biopsies, as previously described [5]. Punch biopsies 1 or 2 mm in diameter were taken from areas of healthy skin either under local anesthesia with 1% lidocaine (without epinephrine), or from skin removed with a dermatome after general anesthesia. The latter method was mainly used for burned patients undergoing routine grafting and had the advantage of standardizing the depth of the biopsies.

The first method used for epidermalization was the implantation of the biopsies into the collagen gel before the contraction occurred, 1–3 hr after polymerization. The implantation was performed using a stereomicroscope to position the dermal–epidermal junction of the biopsy level with the surface of the collagen gel. Several biopsies were implanted no more than 4 cm apart, giving a separation of no more than 1 cm after contraction.

The second method involved the use of biopsies (as thin as possible) that were not implanted, but glued to the dermal equivalents following contraction. The dermal equivalent was then placed on a stainless-steel grid to avoid deformation and further contraction. The biopsies were placed every 1 cm, or less, on the dermal equivalent. A stereomicroscope was generally used to place the horny layer uppermost, although epidermal outgrowth was found to be similar regardless of the orientation. A mixture of fibrinogen and thrombin (Tissucol, Immuno France Labs.) was then sprayed over the biopsies, which, after a few minutes, became glued to the dermal equivalent by this fibrin sealant. Culture medium (EMEM containing 10% of human AB serum) was then added, submerging the culture. After 3–5 days and then twice a week, the medium was renewed and supplemented with 20 ng/ml epidermal growth factor (EGF; Collaborative Research). The time of culture after epidermalization varied from 12 to 20 days, according to the surgical schedule. For patients with giant nevi, cultures were performed without antibiotics, while those for burn patients were supplemented with 4 μg/ml pefloxacine and 10 μg/ml ceftazidime from epidermalization until the end of the culture period.

Cultures were rinsed several times in serum-free medium during the 24 hr before grafting. Pefloxacine and ceftazidime were added to the rinsing medium of cultures for burned patients.

GRAFTING OF THE LIVING SKIN EQUIVALENT

The area to be grafted was excised, with careful hemostasis to avoid bleeding under the graft. In the case of burned patients, excision was performed a few days before grafting to obtain a granulation tissue. The skin equivalent was gently placed on the graft bed and adjusted, taking care not to touch the epidermal surface or distend the collagen matrix, since this would shear the epidermis from the dermal equivalent. Air pockets were expelled before the graft was sutured along its edges. The skin equivalent was kept humid using culture medium throughout surgery. Only one $10 \times 10\ cm^2$ graft was used per patient during each intervention to facilitate conventional skin grafting in case of failure.

Implantation of the skin punch biopsies into the collagen gel just after polymerisation was found to give the shortest time (two weeks) between epidermalization and grafting, since epidermal growth occurred during the contraction of the dermal equivalent and mechanical properties were suitable for handling (Fig.25.1: protocol 1). However, the collagen matrix was apparently not sufficiently reticulated,

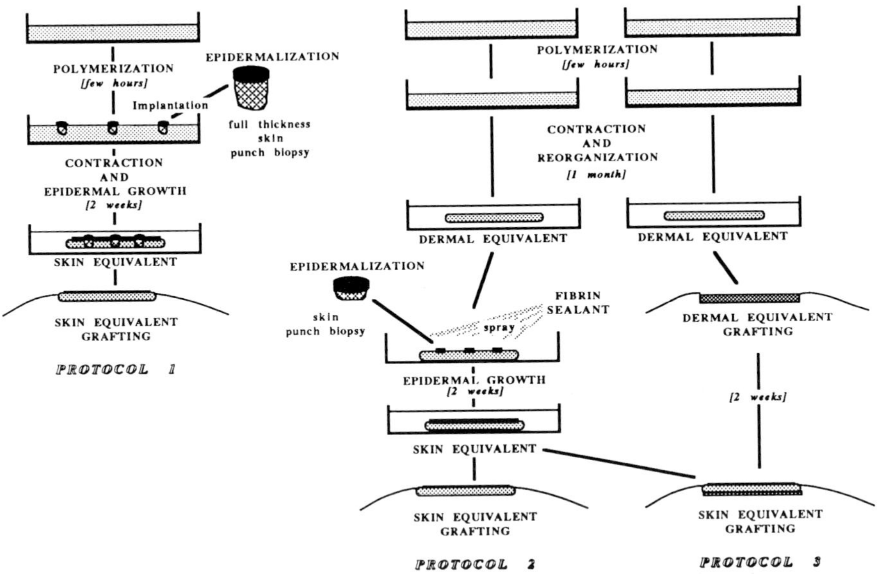

Figure 25.1 Human living skin equivalents were reconstructed and grafted according to three different protocols. **Protocol 1.** Human dermal fibroblasts incorporated into a three-dimensional collagen matrix that permitted the reconstruction of a dermal equivalent. Just after polymerization of the collagen, skin punch biopsies, used as a source of keratinocytes, were implanted before the contraction of the dermal equivalent. Epidermal growth on the dermal equivalent was concomitant with matrix organization by fibroblasts. The only advantage was the short time (2 weeks) between reconstruction and grafting. **Protocol 2.** Dermal equivalents constructed as above were cultured for at least 1 month. Skin biopsies were then glued onto the surface of the organized dermal equivalents and the epidermis grown for another 2 weeks. The main advantage was the resistance of the dermal equivalents to collagenases in vivo. **Protocol 3.** The same as protocol 2, but a dermal equivalent was grafted 2 weeks before the skin equivalent. This gave the further advantage of preparing the graft bed during the time necessary for the epidermalization in vitro of another dermal equivalent.

since the dermal equivalent was frequently found to be lysed at the time of the first dressing (the first observation after grafting). Nevertheless, localized areas of epidermis were still present, as shown either by the presence of a thin whitish film, or by the persistance of localised spots of epidermis during later observations of the graft. A further disadvantage of this method was the time required to place the biopsies on the dermal equivalent. The quality of epidermal growth was also highly dependent on the precise pattern of implantation.

In further experiments, to avoid the disorganization of the collagen matrix (which could lead to complete destruction of the graft), the dermal equivalent was cultured for at least 1 month before grafting. The increased cross-linking between collagen molecules enhanced not only mechanical resistance, but also resistance to bacterial collagenases, as previously observed in vitro [12]. This protocol improved the success of grafting and involved the use of thin skin punch biopsies glued to contracted dermal equivalents. The preparation of these grafts was longer but was compatible with the non-urgent grafting of patients with giant nevi. In addition, the reconstruction in advance of dermal equivalents containing allogenic fibroblasts made the dermal component ready for immediate use on burned patients (Fig. 25.1: protocol 2).

The grafted area was rapidly painless, became supple, and the cutaneous microrelief was visible 3 or 4 months after the graft. Histologic studies performed at this time showed a normal dermal architecture and normal epidermal differentiation. However, the most important observation was the reappearance of a normal undulating dermal–epidermal junction responsible for the normal microrelief of the graft (Fig. 25.2A). In addition, elastic fibers were present in the dermis, demonstrating rapid and extensive synthesis of this component of the extracellular matrix after grafting (Fig. 25.2B).

Since the preparation of the graft bed appeared to be of prime importance, a dermal equivalent (without an epidermal layer) was grafted 2 weeks before the complete skin equivalent. Two identical dermal equivalents were thus constructed. After 1 month of culture, one was grafted, while normal skin obtained during the same surgical intervention served to epidermalize the other dermal equivalent in vitro. After 2 further weeks required for epidermal culture, the skin equivalent (dermis and epidermis) was, in turn, grafted. In this way, the patient could be rapidly covered by a collagen dressing that was homeostatic and reduced pain. Vascularization was initiated by this biological dressing and improved the success of the complete skin equivalent graft (Fig. 25.1: protocol 3).

Several dressings were used in this work: fine mesh gauze coated with petroleum jelly, a nylon gauze associated with a silicon membrane and coated with collagen (Biobrane, Woodroof Laboratories Inc.), or a thin polyurethane film (Omiderm, Omikron Scientific Ltd.). Dressings were applied directly to the graft, with care taken not to displace them, to avoid cleavage of the epidermis and dermal equivalent. A compressive dressing was then applied. The dressings were renewed 5 days later without removal of the layer directly in contact with the cultured epidermis; the graft was closely inspected for infection at this time.

EVALUATION OF THE GRAFTED HUMAN LIVING SKIN EQUIVALENT

Apart from preliminary grafts, five patients with giant nevi and nine burned patients received 100 cm^2 skin equivalent grafts. Some patients received several grafts (during several interventions), mainly for the treatment of giant nevi. In

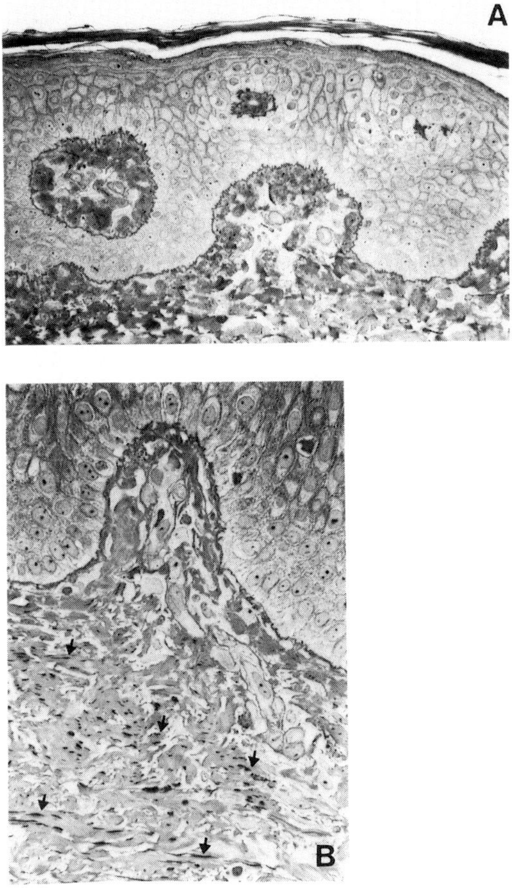

Figure 25.2 Histologic appearance of a living skin equivalent 4 months after grafting, in a patient with giant nevi. (A) In contrast to the flat dermal–epidermal junction usually found when a cultured epidermis is grafted alone, the presence of a dermal component in the graft permits a rapid reappearance of a normal undulated junction. This noncicatricial dermal–epidermal junction is responsible for the normal microrelief of the surface of the graft. (B) Concomitant with the reappearance of the normal cutaneous microrelief, elastic fibers are observed in the dermis (arrows), demonstrating a rapid synthesis of elastin when a living dermal equivalent is grafted.

particular, one of the first patients to be grafted with this technique, a young girl, received a total of five grafts. Two burned patients received a living dermal equivalent prior to the graft of a living skin equivalent.

Not all the grafts were successful, but sufficient data were collected to evaluate the potential and limits of this living skin equivalent for grafting in humans. In this preliminary clinical evaluation, three grafts were a partial success in burned patients and four grafts in patients with giant nevi were satisfactory. The technique was modified and improved as experience was gained.

Importance of the Dermis

After the graft of a simple epidermis reconstructed according to the Rheinwald and Green technique [2], rete ridge formation takes from 6 months to 1 year, and elastic fibers reappear only 3–5 years after grafting [6]. Compared to the time necessary for the reappearance of elastic components when a dermal equivalent is present (4 months), it is clear that a dermis at the time of engraftment improved the mechanical properties of the graft, and thus its success.

In addition, grafting a dermal equivalent alone prior to the graft of the skin equivalent greatly increased the success rate in burned patients. This could be because the living dermal equivalent permits early covering, even if the barrier function had to be provided temporarily by a complementary synthetic dressing; infection is thus reduced and the graft bed is more suitable.

Homogeneity of the Epidermis

Epidermalization is crucial for the persistance of the dermal equivalent in vivo and for the long-term quality of the graft itself. Confluency between the epidermal outgrowths (around each skin punch biopsy) has to be obtained in vitro, since the areas devoid of epidermis in vitro can be clearly recognized after grafting, and epidermal healing of these areas is very slow in vivo. Even when confluency is obtained, although the clinical result seems satisfactory just after grafting, the junctions between the different epidermal outgrowth areas lead to scar formation after a few months. In addition, the centers of the punch biopsies become pigmented with time; this technique of epidermalization thus gives poor cosmetic results. Clearly, the long-term quality of the grafts depends on the homogeneity of the epidermis obtained in vitro.

Tolerance of the Living Skin Equivalent

Collagen

The reorganization of collagen molecules into fibrils and the packing of the fibrils by fibroblasts, and thus the mechanical resistance of the dermal equivalents, requires the presence of the terminal telopeptides. However, these peptides (preserved during acidic extraction of collagen) are also responsible for antigenicity. Therefore, although the immunogenicity of collagen is low from one species to another, the presence of bovine collagen antibodies should be sought in the serum of graft recipients.

Culture Medium

The medium used for the culture of most living skin substitutes is very similar to that used in cell culture, and usually contains calf serum. In most cases, several rinses in serum-free medium before the graft are sufficient to eliminate animal proteins that could lead to rejection. However, in the case of the dermal equivalent, animal proteins are trapped in the collagen matrix and graft rejection can be observed even after several rinses in serum-free medium over 24 hr. We therefore use human serum at the time of incorporation of the fibroblasts into the collagen gel. In our experience, the use of human serum prior to this step does not, however, seem to be necessary. The development of defined culture media may avoid this type of rejection and allow the standardization of the manufacture of skin substitutes necessary for large-scale production.

Fibroblasts

Although the tolerance of allogeneic fibroblasts previously reported in animals [7] remains to be demonstrated in humans, no rejection phenomenon was observed when the dermal equivalents contained allogenic fibroblasts. Furthermore, although we have not studied their persistence in the host, a progressive replacement of donor fibroblasts would not affect the outcome of the graft. The use of allogenic fibroblasts allows dermal equivalents to be made in advance for use in emergency situations (e.g., burns), given that in vitro maturation of the collagen matrix takes several weeks. If necessary, compatibility between the donor fibroblasts and the host could be checked by DNA analysis. A "bank" of such living dermal substitutes could thus be prepared with a view to epidermalization or direct grafting to prepare the graft bed.

Epidermis

Autologous cells were always used here for the epidermalization of the dermal equivalents. In effect, even in the absence of observable Langerhans cells (responsible for allogenic antigen presentation) in this living skin equivalent in vitro [8], the use of allogenic epidermal cells was not justified in this preliminary clinical evaluation.

Dressing

Correct dressing is crucial to the success of living skin substitutes. In the context of burn injury, dressings are required for immediate covering while the living skin substitute is being prepared, and then for protecting the cultured epidermis during its differentiation in vivo.

None of the living skin substitutes available at present possesses in vitro the barrier function of the skin. Dressings are thus required during the time (> 1 week) required for full differentiation in situ. In our experience there is no ideal dressing. Tulle gras with petroleum jelly obscures the surface of the graft, making observation impossible. The collagen present in Biobrane (an advantage in classic use) leads to the colonization of the dressing by keratinocytes and subsequent damage to the cultured epidermis during removal. Of the dressings used during this work, Omiderm was found to be most suitable, despite the fact that it is excessively occlusive.

With progress in cell culture methods, in particular with the development of defined culture media, differentiation of cultured epidermis may eventually be obtained in vitro without diminishing the keratinocyte proliferation rate (although at present this would appear incompatible).

CONCLUSION

We have shown that this living skin equivalent, composed of a dermis and an epidermis, can be used in humans, even in the context of burn injury. The most important observation is that the living dermal substitute permits rapid neosynthesis of elastic tissue leading to the reappearance of cutaneous microrelief and to mechanical properties (e.g., elasticity) closer to those of normal skin than the cicatricial skin usually obtained with simple epidermal substitutes. The major improvement of this living skin equivalent is now the quality of the epidermis; other techniques of epidermalization currently used for epidermal sheet grafts [2] may provide the solution.

The need for a dermal substitute to avoid secondary scar contraction and to contribute to a good cosmetic result is now generally agreed. The question is now to define the type of dermis. Several permanent dermal substitutes devoid of cells are now in development [1, 9], although we consider that the presence of living fibroblasts improves biological function [10]. Nevertheless, this has to be balanced with the need for large-scale production in which cost, storage, and facility of use during surgery have to be taken into account.

In conclusion, in vitro skin reconstruction is still in its infancy. Further clinical studies comparing the various techniques forwarded will be required to identify advantages and disadvantages of each, with the view to extending the use of permanent skin substitutes to a large number of patients, in various clinical situations.

ACKNOWLEDGMENTS

The authors thank Drs. Baruch and Raulo (Service de Chirurgie Plastique et Reconstructive, Hôpital Henri Mondor, Créteil); Guilbaud, Perrot, and Garcin (Service des Brûlés, Hôpital Percy, Clamart); Richard, Marsol, Perrier, and Masquelet (Service des Brûlés, Hôpital Trousseau, Paris); Glicenstein (Hôpital Bretonneau, Paris); and Neveux (Centre de Recherche du Service de Santé des Armées) for their active participation that made this work possible.

This work was supported by grants from Direction des Recherches Études et Techniques (DRET 82/105, 82/1051, 84/125, and 88/211) and from Assistance Publique des Hôpitaux de Paris (Contrat de Recherche Clinique de l'AP, 1988 and 1989).

REFERENCES

1. Burke JF, Yannas IV, Quinby WC, Bondoc CC, Jung WK. Successful use of a physiologically acceptable artificial skin in the treatment of extensive burn injury. *Ann Surg* 1981; 194: 413–27.
2. Rheinwald JG, Green H. Serial cultivation of strains of human epidermal keratinocytes: the formation of keratinizing colonies from single cells. *Cell* 1975;6: 331–44.
3. Gallico GG, O'Connor NE, Compton CC, Kehinde O, Green H. Permanent coverage of large burn wounds with autologous cultured human epithelium. *N Engl J Med* 1984; 311: 448–51.
4. Bell E, Ivarsson B, Merrill C. Production of tissue-like structure by contraction of collagen lattices by human fibroblasts of different proliferative potential in vitro. *Proc Natl Acad Sci USA* 1979; 76: 1274–8.
5. Coulomb B, Saiag P, Bell E, Breitburd F, Lebreton C, Heslan M, Dubertret L. A new method for studying epidermalization in vitro. *Br J Dermatol* 1986; 114: 91–101.
6. Barrandon Y. Communication during EC workshop, Skin equivalents: problems of development and clinical usage in Europe. Lyon, March 13–15, 1989.
7. Sher SE, Hull BE, Rosen S, Church D, Friedman L, Bell E. Acceptance of allogeneic fibroblasts in skin equivalent transplant. *Transplantation* 1983; 36: 5052–7.
8. Bagot M, Bertaux B, Heslan M, Coulomb B, Dubertret L. Reconstructed human epidermis: absence of Langerhans cells and failure to stimulate allogeneic lymphocytes in vitro. *Clin Exp Immunol* 1988; 71: 138–43.
9. Echinard C, Dantzer E, Poinsignon F, Damour O, Vescovali C, David MF, Marchetti B, Adhoute H, Sahabeddin L, Collombel C. Mise au point d'un derme acellulaire, un pas vers la peau artificielle totale. *Ann Chir Plast Esthét* 1989; 34: 346–52.
10. Coulomb B, Lebreton C, Dubertret L. Influence of dermal fibroblasts on epidermalization. *J Invest Dermatol* 1989; 92: 122–5.

11. Bell E, Ehrlich P, Buttle D, Nakatsuji. Living tissue formed in vitro and accepted as skin-equivalent tissue of full thickness. *Science* 1981; 211: 1052–54.
12. Rowling PJE, Raxworthy MJ, Wood EJ, Kearney JN, Cunliffe WJ, Reorganization of collagen lattices in the presence of human dermal fibroblasts. *J Invest Dermatol* 1987; 89: 320.

26

Drugs Acting on Connective Tissue

Aarne Oikarinen
University of Oulu, Oulu, Finland

Several hormones and vitamins modulate the synthesis and degradation of macromolecules in connective tissue. Especially important in dermatology are glucocorticoids, which can cause atrophy of the skin and osteoporosis. During recent years mechanisms of glucocorticoid action have been revealed and these are discussed below in detail. Retinoids have also gained much interest due to studies in which they have been shown to improve photodamaged skin. For these reasons the mode of retinoid action on connective tissue is emphasized in this chapter.

The knowledge of the biosynthetic steps of collagen has already resulted in the identification of compounds that specifically modulate collagen biosynthesis (see Table 26.1). Especially interesting in the future will be compounds that inhibit prolyl hydroxylase, a key enzyme in collagen synthesis. In this chapter, the modes of action of the specific inhibitors of collagen synthesis now available and future compounds are summarized.

HORMONES AND HORMONE ANALOGS

Glucocorticosteroids

Short-term systemic glucocorticoid treatment is often used for acute clinical conditions such as allergic reactions and anaphylactic shock. Since treatment is usually brief, side effects on connective tissue are uncommon. Several diseases,

Table 26.1 Compounds Acting on Specific Steps in Collagen Synthesis and Degradation

Level of action	Compound acting	Direction of regulation
DNA		
↓	Bleomycin	↑
mRNA	Glucocorticoids	↓
	Retinoids	↓
	Interferons	↓
↓	TGFβ	↑
Translation	Vitamin C	↑
↓		
Hydroxylation of proline	Vitamin C	↑
↓	Inhibitors of prolyl hydroxylase	↓
Triple helix formation	Analogs of proline	↓
↓ Intracellular degradation	cAMP	↑
Secretion	Colchicine	↓
↓		
Removal of propeptides	Polyamines	↓
↓	Divalent cations	↓
Cross-link formation and fibrillogenesis	D-penicillamine	↓
	B-aminoproprionitrile	↓
↓	Colchicine	↑
Degradation	Glucocorticoids	↓
	Retinoids	↓
	TGFβ	↓

however, require long-term glucocorticoid therapy, including dermatologic conditions such as pemphigus vulgaris, bullous pemphigoid, systemic lupus erythematosus, and sarcoidosis. Most patients receiving prolonged steroid therapy will develop adverse effects manifested in the form of generalized connective tissue weakness (Table 26.2) [1–3].

A relatively common side effect is the development of varying degrees of osteoporosis. This detrimental action on bone tissue seems to be a result of two simultaneous events: a reduction in bone formation with an associated increase in detectable resorption sites. The latter is believed to be caused by a raised

Table 26.2 Connective Tissue Side Effects after Long-Term Glucocorticoid Treatment

Tissue	Symptoms	Mechanism of connective tissue pathologic change
Skin	Atrophy	Decrease in connective tissue components: decrease in water content
Skin	Striae	Loss of elastin
Skin	Telangiectasia	Expansion of abnormal blood vessels Loss of connective tissue
Skeleton and bones	Osteoporosis	Decrease in bone formation, osteoblast function is inhibited, changes in calcium metabolism
Skeleton and bones	Reduced skeletal growth in children	Inhibition or cessation of linear bone growth
Tendon	Fragility	Loss of connective tissue

level of parathyroid hormone, presumably secondary to a corticosteroid-mediated inhibition of calcium absorption from the gastrointestinal tract.

The glucocorticoid action on bone metabolism was investigated in a recent study. Systemic glucocorticoid treatment in patients with various dermatoses decreased markedly the serum markers of bone metabolism [4]. The levels of carboxyterminal propeptide of type I procollagen (PICP), which is mostly derived from bones, and osteocalcin, which reflects osteoblastic activity, were decreased in the serum by 38 and 49%, respectively, during steroid treatment (Fig. 26.1). In contrast, systemic glucocorticoid did not affect the degradation of bone collagen, which was monitored by measuring the cross-linked telopeptide of type I collagen (P. Autio et al, unpublished). These results indicate that glucocorticoids have mostly an antianabolic effect on collagen and osteocalcin of bones.

Glucocorticoids may cause growth retardation in children, although permanent arrest of growth is unusual, since in addition to inhibiting bone growth, the steroids also delay epiphyseal closure, thus allowing growth once steroid therapy is discontinued.

The most common cutaneous side effect of steroid treatment is thinning and atrophy of the skin, especially after use of potent glucocorticoids (Fig. 26.2). The affected skin is thin, shiny, and translucent, and is easily bruised. Topical or systemic application of glucocorticoids may also lead to the formation of striae, characterized histologically by loss of the elastic fibers. A relatively

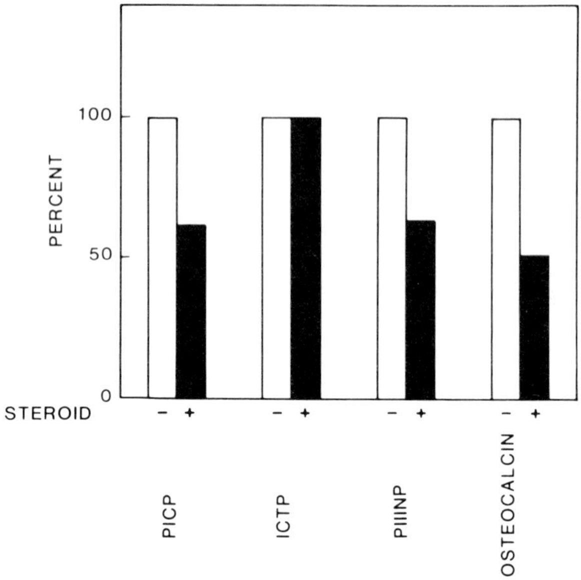

Figure 26.1 Effect of systemic glucocorticoid treatment on the serum levels of carboxyterminal propeptide of type I procollagen (PICP), cross-linked telopeptide of type I collagen (ICTP), aminoterminal propeptide of type III procollagen (PIIINP), and osteocalcin in dermatologic patients. PICP, PIIINP, and osteocalcin values are modified from the original study with permission (Ref. 4).

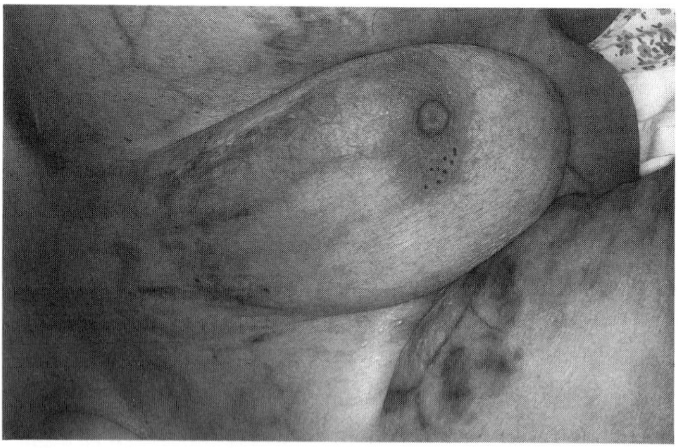

Figure 26.2 Marked skin atrophy in a 76-year-old woman who had used clobetasol-17-proprionate-cream for more than 2 months. Note prominent blood vessels and ecchymosis.

common side effect of the topical application of potent synthetic steroids is the development of telangiectasias resulting from altered properties of the blood vessel walls in tissues.

Several animal and cell culture studies have shown that glucocorticoids inhibit collagen synthesis [1–3]. Recent studies have revealed that glucocorticoids in human skin fibroblasts reduce the amount of collagen messenger RNA, leading to diminished synthesis of collagen (Table 1). The details of how glucocorticoids regulate the amount of collagen mRNA are not known. An especially interesting observation has been that glucocorticoids regulate type I collagen synthesis by decreasing the larger transcript of type I collagen messenger RNA, the decrease correlating significantly with the decrease of total collagen mRNA [3]. Increased degradation of collagen mRNA could partially explain reduced levels of mRNA after glucocorticoid treatment. In addition, glucocorticoids decrease the activity of enzymes needed for the intracellular biosynthesis of collagen [1, 2].

Only a few studies in humans demonstrate the decreased collagen synthesis after glucocorticoid administration. As discussed earlier, systemic glucocorticoid treatment decreased markedly the carboxyterminal propeptide of type I procollagen in serum [4]. Systemic glucocorticoid treatment likewise diminished the aminoterminal propeptide of type III procollagen (PIIINP) (Fig. 26.1). Since type I and III collagens are the major components of skin, this indicates that systemic glucocorticoid treatment may lead to skin atrophy.

The action of topical glucocorticoids on skin collagen synthesis in vivo has not been studied in detail due to lack of reliable methods. For these reasons a new assay was developed to follow changes in collagen synthesis in human skin in vivo. In the assay propeptides of type I and III collagen are measured from suction blisters. By this assay it was shown that topical glucocorticoids after a 2 day treatment markedly decreased both PICP and PIIINP in blister fluids (Fig. 26.3) [5]. It should be noted that even hydrocortisone diminished collagen propeptides markedly, suggesting that it may also cause skin atrophy in certain subjects.

The net amount of collagen in tissue is dependent not only on the synthesis but also on the degradation of collagen. Thus it is of special interest that glucocorticoids drastically inhibit the activity of collagenase, an enzyme able to degrade collagen [2, 3].

Glucocorticoids also modulate other components of the connective tissue. The synthesis of elastin and fibronectin is increased in the presence of glucocorticoids. In human skin fibroblasts, the ratio of fibronectin/collagen synthesis and the levels of mRNA were markedly increased in the presence of dexamethasone.

Glucocorticoids inhibit the synthesis of glycosaminoglycans (GAGs) in vitro. Also in vivo a decrease in ground substance consisting of GAGs was noted after glucocorticoid treatment, resulting in smaller interfibrillar spaces between the collagen and elastic fibers. This could partially explain the rapid thinning of the dermis after glucocorticoid treatment [2, 3].

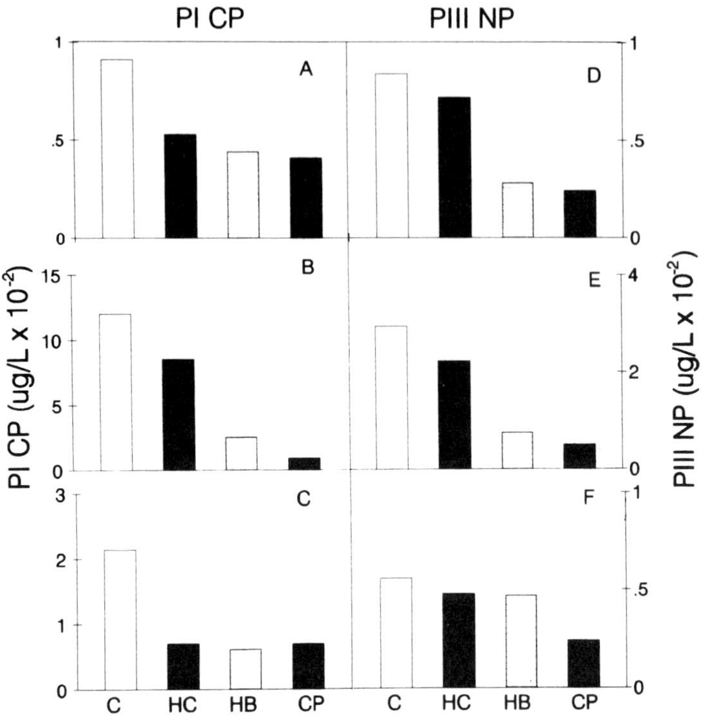

Figure 26.3 Topical glucocorticoids clobetasol-17-propionate (CP), hydrocortisone (HC), and hydrocortisone-17-butyrate (HB) decrease the concentrations of PICP and PIIINP in blister fluids. Clobetasol-17-propionate, hydrocortisone-17-butyrate, hydrocortisone, or vehicle was applied on the abdominal skin of three subjects three times a day for 2 days, and blister fluid samples were collected immediately after blister induction. The PIIINP levels in D–F were determined from the same blister fluid as PICP levels in panel A–C. The values are the means of duplicate assays (modified with permission from the original study, Ref. 5).

Glucocorticoids inhibit various stages of the inflammatory process, such as leukocyte chemotaxis, capillary dilatation, and fibroblast proliferation [6, 7]. In addition, glucocorticoids block the effects of various lymphokines, and decrease the formation of eicosanoids (prostaglandins, leukotrienes). Recent studies have shown that mediators of inflammatory cells modulate connective tissue metabolism. The inhibition of inflammatory processes by glucocorticoids could drastically alter connective tissue synthesis and degradation. For example, glucocorticoids inhibit the synthesis of leukocyte elastase and collagenase. Thus glucocorticoids diminish the tissue destruction by leukocytes in various inflammatory and autoimmune diseases.

From a dermatologic point of view, a very interesting finding has been the induction of plasminogen activator inhibitor by glucocorticoids [8]. Plasminogen–plasmin activator has an important role in tumor metastasis, cell migration, and tissue destruction (i.e., bullous diseases) [9]. Thus the use of glucocorticoids in the treatment of bullous diseases (pemphigus, pemphigoid) has a solid theoretical justification: by inducing plasminogen activator inhibitor, glucocorticoids could prevent the activation of plasminogen to plasmin and thus inhibit the proteolysis of basement membranes and intercellular proteins responsible for cell adhesion.

The knowledge of glucocorticoid action on connective tissue as described above gives a rational basis to the treatment of various fibrotic and degenerative diseases. Glucocorticoids, by inhibiting collagen synthesis, would be effective in early stages of fibrotic processes such as in keloids and localized scleroderma. In contrast, mature fibrotic lesions such as fully developed keloids may not respond to glucocorticoids. One reason for this could be that there is no more active collagen deposition in old keloids and, furthermore glucocorticoids, by inhibiting collagen-degrading enzymes, may in fact prevent the resolution of fibrotic processes.

In certain granulomatous and degenerative diseases glucocorticoids may be very useful. For example, in granuloma annulare there is both degeneration of collagen and active collagen deposition. In lichen sclerosus et atrophicus there is also degeneration process and active collagen synthesis. In these disease models potent glucocorticoids under occlusion could be very effective, since they affect both the synthesis and degradation of connective tissue.

Other Hormones

Considerably less is known about the effects of other hormones. Somatomedin has been shown to increase collagen synthesis. Progesterone was shown to inhibit collagen synthesis, whereas estrogens and androgens had no effect. Sex hormones, however, have definitely marked effects on collagen synthesis and catabolism in the uterus. Thyroxin is able to increase the catabolism of connective tissue, which causes an increase in urinary hydroxyproline. Thyroid hormones modulate markedly glycosaminoglycan synthesis: when thyroid hormone is deficient, more GAGs are synthesized, and the addition of thyroid hormone to cell cultures inhibits GAG synthesis [10].

VITAMINS

Vitamin C (Ascorbic Acid)

A deficient intake of vitamin C leads to scurvy, which is characterized by pathologic changes in the bones and blood vessels. Typical symptoms are the resorption of dentin, bleeding of the gums, and loosening of teeth. Changes in the cells of capillary walls result in hemorrhages in skin, muscles, bones, and gums. On histologic examination the amount of collagen bundles is decreased.

The role of vitamin C in the synthesis of collagen has been extensively studied. Vitamin C is an essential cofactor for prolyl and lysyl hydroxylases, enzymes involved in the biosynthesis of collagen. The synthesis of hydroxyproline from prolyl residues is essential for the functional triplehelical structure of collagen. The role of ascorbate in prolyl hydroxylase reactions has been studied in detail, and it has been suggested that in the absence of ascorbate the enzyme cannot be reactivated for new reactions. Thus in the absence of ascorbate, the collagen synthesized is under-hydroxylated and cannot achieve a stable triple helical conformation, and is rapidly degraded intracellularly.

In addition, ascorbate has been shown to stimulate collagen synthesis at the level of translation in the range of concentration found in serum of healthy young adults [10].

The role of ascorbate in scurvy has recently been doubted since, in some scorbutic animal models, the hydroxylation of proline was not markedly altered, suggesting that some unknown humoral factor other than ascorbate is responsible for scurvy [11].

In general, there is no need for treatment of patients with vitamin C except in those with severe malnutrition or following specific diets. In dermatologic, practice, vitamin C treatment has been suggested to be beneficial in patients with Ehlers-Danlos type VI, in whom there is a deficiency of lysyl hydroxylase.

Retinoids

The analogs of vitamin A have recently gained considerable use in dermatology. 13-*cis*-Retinoic acid is used for treatment of severe acne, and etretinate (acitretin) for hyperproliferative diseases such as psoriasis. All-*trans* retinoic acid (tretinoin) has been used for decades for the treatment of acne, and during recent years for actinic damage.

In 1984 Kligman et al. published a classic work on the effects of tretinoin on sun damage to nude mouse skin [12]. The most important finding was that the newly synthesized connective tissue layer under the epidermis in tretinoin-treated skin was broader that that in vehicle-treated animals, showing that tretinoin somehow stimulated skin regeneration. This finding was later verified in human skin [13]. A double-blind, vehicle-controlled trial showed that the number of fine wrinkles had decreased after 4 months of treatment with 0.1 % tretinoin cream (Retin-A): the skin was smoother and its color was pinkish. On histologic examination the thickness of the epidermis was about three times that of the vehicle-treated skin, while the most consistent finding at the dermal site was hypertrophy of the blood vessels. No apparent changes were observed in the collagen or elastin fibers. In another large series investigators were able to show the formation of new connective tissue beneath the epidermis when the patients were treated with tretinoin for a long time. In addition, fibroblasts seemed to be active in the treated skin, showing a dilated endoplasmic reticulum.

It is not known how retinoids could enhance the regeneration of connective tissue. The action of retinoids on carcinomas and cellular functions has been studied intensively and various hypotheses proposed; for instance, that retinoids may affect the glycosylation of proteins, cellular differentiation, growth factors, or immunosystems and angiogenesis, all of which could participate in skin regeneration.

The mode of retinoic action is not fully understood, although a great step forward was the finding of a family of specific nuclear receptors for retinoic acid that belonged to a superfamily of steroid and thyroid hormone receptors. One especially interesting finding is a close structural relationship between thyroid hormone and retinoic acid receptors. Indeed, it has been shown that thyroid hormone and retinoic acid receptors coregulate various genes such as that for growth hormone, a finding that has given a new insight into the essential role of retinoids in the growth and differentiation of organs and the regulation of morphogenesis. Although epithelial tissues are their main targets, these compounds also affect connective tissue, as shown in retinoic acid-induced skeletal alterations [14]. It is also possible that retinoids may directly stimulate connective tissue formation in the skin, even though it has been shown previously that retinoids in high concentrations have an inhibitory effect on collagen synthesis and mRNA levels under certain in vitro cell culture conditions [15]. Several in vivo findings, however, suggest that retinoids have a stimulatory effect on the expression of many connective tissue components. First, early research showed that vitamin A could reverse the inhibitory effect of glucocorticoids on wound healing. Second, one of the side effects of retinoid treatment is the formation of excessive connective tissue, especially in the bones and skeleton, where extra ossification can be seen. Third, retinoids also affect the healing of dermabrasion in acne patients, leading to hypertrophic scars. Fourth, there are some reports that retinoids have a beneficial effect on skin regeneration in lichen sclerosus et atrophicus, which has been characterized histologically as a form of connective tissue degeneration. Fifth, topical tretinoin has recently been used to prevent glucocorticoid-induced dermal atrophy.

One of the mechanisms by which retinoids may regulate the metabolism of connective tissue is through inhibition of collagenase activity, which could alter the balance between synthesis and degradation of collagen and lead to an excessive accumulation of connective tissue. One recent speculation has been that the increase in the anchoring fibrils that connect the basement membrane to the dermis (type VII collagen) noted after topical tretinoin treatment could be due to collagenase inhibition.

Vitamin D

Calcium and phosphate metabolism are regulated by vitamin D, parathyroid hormone, and thyrocalcitonin. Fat-soluble vitamin D could be regarded as a hormone, since it has several similarities with steroid hormones [16]. The deficiency of vitamin D results in several skeletal alterations known as rickets.These changes are due to the crucial role of vitamin D in the growth and modeling of bone, especially during childhood. Vitamin D also has effects on other tissues such as intestinal mucosa, kidney, and skin. One of the target tissue of vitamin D might be the skin, in which specific receptors of vitamin D have been found. The direct effects of vitamin D on connective tissue components are not known in detail. In fetal rat calvaria, vitamin D analogs and parathyroid hormone reduced collagen synthesis and mRNA levels. In human skin fibroblasts, vitamin D increased fibronectin synthesis [10, 16].

PENICILLAMINE, B-AMINOPROPRIONITRILE, COLCHICINE

The D isomer of penicillamine is an effective chelator of copper and some other metals. D-Penicillamine has been used for the treatment of Wilson's disease, lead and mercury poisoning, and cystinuria. In addition, D-penicillamine has been useful in the treatment of systemic scleroderma and extensive localized scleroderma. In a large clinical study, the treatment of patients with D-penicillamine resulted in a better survival rate and in softening of the skin. The effect was visible only after a relatively long (24 months) period of treatment [17]. D-penicillamine, by chelating copper, prevents the activity of lysyl oxidase, an enzyme involved in cross-link formation of collagen and elastin. In the absence of lysyl oxidase, collagen and elastin are not able to form stable fibrils, and are easily degraded. D-Penicillamine also affects cross-link formation, by reacting with lysine-and hydroxylysine-derived aldehydes (Fig. 26.4). D-Penicillamine could be useful to diminish collagen accumulation, but its use is limited due to toxicity [10, 18].

B-aminoproprionitrile is also an inhibitor of lysyl-oxidase, and has been used in some patients with pulmonary fibrosis, urethral strictures, and tendon adhesions. However, the toxicity of B-aminoproprionitrile and other similar copounds has not been documented in extensive studies [10, 18].

Colchicine, which is used for the treatment of gout, disrupts the microtubules and is able to reduce collagen synthesis and increase collagenase production. Colchicine has been used for the treatment of fibrotic processes. The use of colchicine in treatment of systemic sclerosis or other fibrotic diseases in limited and more studies are needed to show its usefulness in these diseases [10].

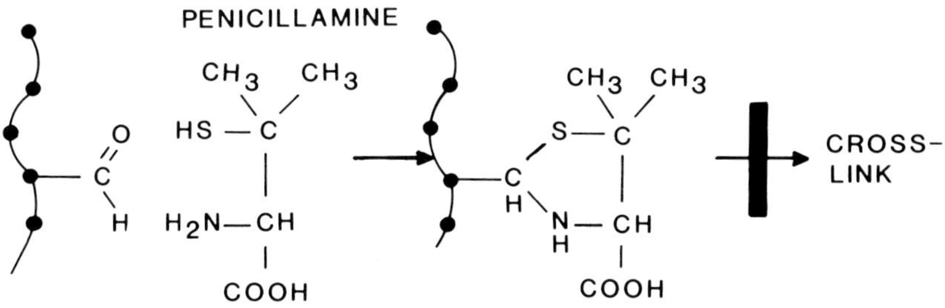

Figure 26.4 Inhibition of collagen cross-linking by penicillamine. Penicillamine inhibits collagen cross-linking by reacting with allysyl residues. The formation of the thiazolidine ring makes the aldehyde unavailable for cross-linking.

PREVENTION OF COLLAGEN ACCUMULATION BY EXPERIMENTAL COMPOUNDS

Inhibition of Prolyl Hydroxylase

Since the 4-hydroxylation of proline residues by prolyl-4-hydroxylase has a central role in the intracellular biosynthesis of collagen, many efforts have been made to develop inhibitors of prolyl 4-hydroxylase. Some divalent cations, of which Zn^{2+} is most effective, have been shown to inhibit prolyl-4-hydroxylase activity and have been used succesfully to prevent liver and lung fibrosis in rats [18].

Other compounds (Fig. 26.5) such as pyridine 2,5-dicarboxylate and analogs inhibit prolyl 4-hydroxylase reaction competetively with respect to 2-oxoglutarate, which is needed in the reaction. Irreversible inhibitors of prolyl-4-hydroxylase have been developed recently, that inhibit the enzyme by a suicide mechanism (Fig. 26.5). For example doxorubicin, which is used for cancer therapy, belongs to this class of inhibitors. Many of these inhibitors have low membrane permeability, and are ineffective in cell cultures and in vivo. However, modulation of this kind of compounds will overcome this drawback in order to allow the development of compounds that pass cell membranes and become activated inside the cell, and that might be useful for the treatment of fibrotic diseases [11, 18].

Inhibition of Triple Helix Formation

Some proline analogs are incorporated into the collagen polypeptide chains. These analogs cannot be hydroxylated, and thus the collagen chains are not able to attain the stable triple helical conformation. As a result, collagen is slowly secreted and easily degraded. These compounds seem to be promising for the

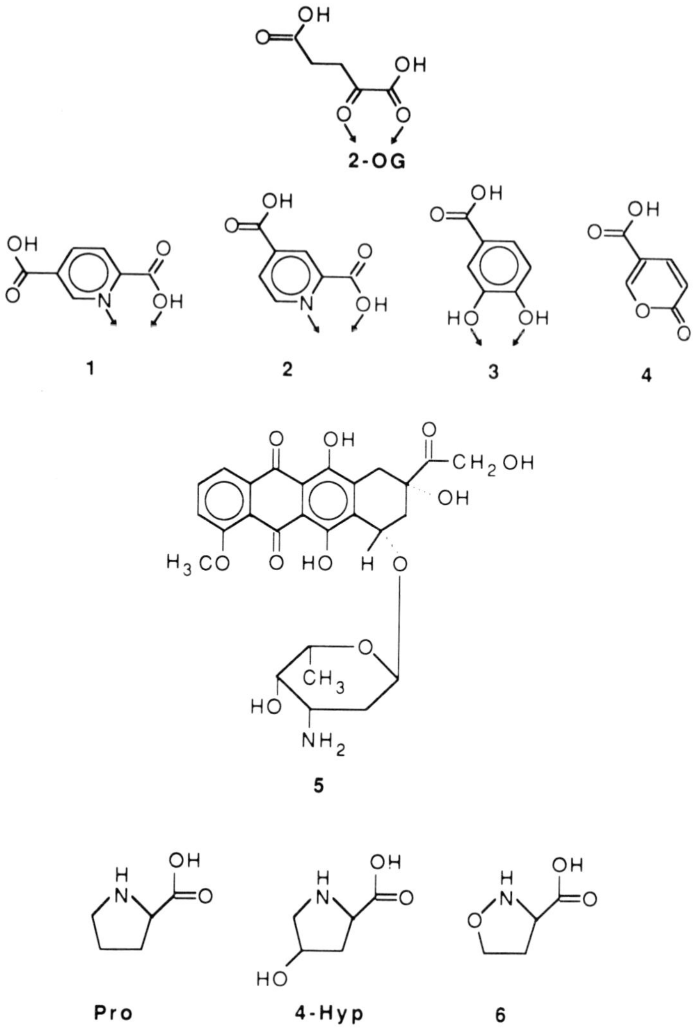

Figure 26.5 Structures of some compounds that inhibit or inactivate prolyl 4-hydroxylase. Pyridine 2,5-dicarboxylate (1), pyridine 2,4-dicarboxylate (2), and 3,4-dihydroxybenzoate (3) inhibit the prolyl 4-hydroxylase reaction competitively with respect to 2-oxoglutarate (2-OG), 3,4-dihydroxybenzoate being also a competitive inhibitor with respect to ascorbate. Coumalic acid (4), doxorubicin (5), and peptides containing 5-oxaproline (6) probably inactivate prolyl 4-hydroxylase by a suicide mechanism (modified from [11] with permission of the publisher).

treatment of fibrotic processes. However, they have not been used in humans [18, 19].

Inhibition of Conversion of Procollagen to Collagen

Conversion of procollagen to collagen in the extracellular space is essential for stable fibril formation. Some divalent cations, polyamines and lysine derivatives, are able to inhibit the conversion process. Further development of analogs of these compounds could provide tools for inhibiting collagen production [19].

Intracellular Degradation

A marked proportion of newly synthesized collagen polypeptides are degraded intracellularly. Some compounds, such as cAMP, increase the intracellular degradation of collagen, resulting in diminished net synthesis of collagen. Compounds such as prostaglandin E_1, E_2, or the B-agonist isoproterenol, which increases cAMP in cells likewise enhance intracellular degradation [10].

DRUGS INDUCING ACCUMULATION OF CONNECTIVE TISSUE

Connective tissue changes are frequently found during phenytoin treatment. Gingival hyperplasia is observed in 50% of patients treated with phenytoin. The basic mechanism of gingival overgrowth is still unknown. Gingival hypertrophy is also found during cyclosporin treatment, in patients receiving renal transplants. Phenytoin- and cyclosporin-induced hyperplasia are similar on both clinical and histopathologic examination [7].

Increased deposition of connective tissue is also found during bleomycin treatment. Lung fibrosis is one of the main side effects of bleomycin therapy.

Another cytostatic drug methotrexate, which is extensively used for treatment of severe psoriasis, can induce liver cirrhosis. Recently, the development of specific and sensitive assays to measure collagen synthesis activity by assaying propeptides of collagen has provided tools to evaluate the development of liver fibrosis in methotrexate-treated patients without using numerous liver biopsies.

IMMUNOMODULATORS: GROWTH FACTORS

Alterations in the immune system may play an important role in many fibrotic skin diseases such as scleroderma. Our knowledge of the mediators involved in connective tissue activation has increased in recent years, and several mediators have now been characterized and cloned and may be of potential use in clinical conditions. For example, interferons have been shown to reduce collagen synthesis by lowering collagen mRNA levels and γ-interferon has been used to treat systemic sclerosis. More extensive clinical trails are needed to establish the role of interferons for treatment of systemic sclerosis. Another interesting mediator, transforming growth factor β (TGFβ), has been shown to increase connective tissue formation by stimulating the synthesis of collagen and fibronectin and by reducing their degradation [20]. Thus, this agent may be a potential method for inducing new connective tissue formation in certain clinical conditions, such as deficient wound healing.

Recently, the activation of collagen gene expression by TGFβ has been shown to be suppressed by tumor necrosis factor α- and γ-interferon, further emphasizing that certain cytokines may be useful for treatment of such fibrotic processes in which TGFβ is an important mediator.

The use of anti-inflammatory and immunosuppressive agents for treating fibrotic diseases has been relatively common, but the survival rate for patients with scleroderma was not improved by treatment with immunosuppressive drugs, and there is no evidence that these could improve the fibrosis involved in this disease [21]. Cyclosporin A has been tried in some patients with systemic scleroderma recently, and results indicate that it may be effective in selected patients. The number of patients with scleroderma treated with this drug is, however, relatively small.

ACKNOWLEDGMENTS

The original research by A. Oikarinen summarized in this overview was supported in part by grants from the Medical Research Council of the Academy of Finland and the Paulo Foundation. The author gratefully acknowledges the helpful comments and suggestions made by Professors Kari I. Kivirikko and Matti Hannuksela. The author thanks Miss Anna Autio for her expert secretarial assistance.

REFERENCES

1. Cutroneo KR, Rokowski R, Counts DF. Glucocorticoids and collagen synthesis: comparison in in vivo and cell culture studies. Collagen Rel Res 1981; 1: 557–68.
2. Oikarinen AI, Uitto J, Oikarinen J. Glucocorticoid action on connective tissue: from molecular mechanisms to clinical practice. Med Biol 1986; 64: 221–30.
3. Oikarinen A, Autio P. New aspects of the mechanism of corticosteroid-induced dermal atrophy. Clin Exp Dermatol 1991; 16: 416–9.
4. Oikarinen A, Autio, P, Vuori J, et al. Systemic glucocorticoid treatment decreases serum concentrations of carboxyterminal propeptide of type I procollagen and aminoterminal propeptide of type III procollagen. Br J Dermatol 1992; 126: 172–8.

5. Oikarinen A, Autio P, Kiistala U, et al. A new method to measure type I and III collagen synthesis in human skin in vivo: demonstration of decreased collagen synthesis after topical glucocorticoid treatment. J Invest Dermatol 1992; 98: 220–5.
6. Parrillo JE, Fauci AJ. Mechanisms of glucocorticoid action on immune processes. Annu Rev Pharmacol Toxicol 1979; 19: 179–201.
7. Seymour RA, Heasman PA. Drugs and periodontium. J Clin Periodontol 1988; 15: 1–16.
8. Andreasen PA, Christensen TH, Huang J-Y, et al. Hormonal regulation of extracellular plasminogen activators and M 54000 plasminogen activator inhibitor in human neoplastic cell lines, studied with monoclonal antibodies. Mol Cell Endocrinol 1986; 45: 137–47.
9. Saksela O. Plasminogen activation and regulation of pericellular proteolysis. Biochim Biophys Acta 1985; 823: 35–65.
10. Pinnell SR, Murad S. Collagen. In: Goldsmith LA, ed. Biochemistry and physiology of the skin. New York: Oxford University Press, 1983: 385–410.
11. Kivirikko KI, Myllylä R, Pihlajaniemi T. Protein hydroxylation: prolyl 4-hydroxylase, an enzyme with four cosubstrates and a multifunctional subunit. FASEB J 1988; 3: 1609–17.
12. Kligman LH, Chen HD, Kligman AM. Topical retinoic acid enhances the repair of ultraviolet damaged dermal connective tissue. Connect Tissue Res 1984; 12: 139–50.
13. Weiss JS, Ellis CN, Headington JT, et al. Topical tretinoin improves photodamaged skin: a double-blind vehicle-controlled study. JAMA 1988; 527–32.
14. Ellis CN, Pennes DR, Madison KC, et al. Skeletal radiographic changes during retinoid therapy. In: Saurat JH, ed. Retinoids: new trends in research and therapy. Karger: Basel, New York, 1984: 440–4.
15. Oikarinen H, Oikarinen AI, Tan EML, et al. Modulation of procollagen expression by retinoids. Inhibition of collagen production by retinoic acid accompanied by reduced type I procollagen messenger ribonucleic acid levels in human skin fibroblast cultures. J Clin Invest 1985; 75: 1545–53.
16. Reichel H, Koeffler HP, Norman AW. The role of vitamin D endocrine system in health and disease. N Engl J Med 1989; 320: 980–91.
17. Steen VD, Medsger TA Jr, Rodnan GP. D-Penicillamine therapy in progressive systemic sclerosis (scleroderma). A retrospective study. Ann Intern Med 1982; 97: 652–9.
18. Kivirikko KI, Savolainen ER. Hepatic collagen metabolism and its modification by drugs. In: Testa B, Perrissound D, eds. Liver drugs: from experimental pharmacology to therapeutic application. Boca Raton, FL: CRC Press, 1988: 193–222.
19. Uitto J, Ryhänen L, Tan EML, et al. Pharmacological inhibition of excessive collagen deposition in fibrotic diseases. Fed Proc 1984; 43: 2815–20.
20. Roberts AB, Sporn MB, Assoian RK, et al. Transforming growth factor type-beta: rapid induction of fibrosis and angiogenesis in vivo and stimulation of collagen formation in vitro. Proc Natl Acad Sci USA 1986; 83: 4167–71.
21. Krieg T, Meurer M. Systemic scleroderma. Clinical and pathophysiological aspects. J Am Acad Dermatol 1988; 18: 457 –81.

Index

About the Editors

CHARLES M. LAPIÈRE is Professor of Dermatology and Venerology, Chairman of the Dermatology Department, and Director of the Experimental Dermatology Laboratory at the University of Liège, Belgium. The author or coauthor of over 300 professional papers and book chapters, Dr. Lapière serves on the editorial boards of numerous journals. He is an international honorary member of the American Dermatological Association, an honorary member of the Society for Investigative Dermatology, a founding member of the European Society for Dermatological Research and of the European Tissue Repair Society, and a member of the American Academy of Dermatology and several European dermatological societies, among others. Dr. Lapière received the M.D. degree (1956) and the Ph.D. degree (1964) in biomedical science from the University of Liège, Belgium.

THOMAS KRIEG is Professor of Dermatology and Venerology and Chairman of the Dermatology Department at the University of Cologne, Germany. The coauthor of more than 200 professional papers, Dr. Krieg is a member of the board of the European Society for Dermatological Research and the European Tissue Repair Society. He is also a member of the Society of Investigative Dermatology, among others. He received the M.D. degree (1975) from the Free University of Berlin, Germany.